ENCYCLOPAEDIA OF
NURSING

ENCYCLOPAEDIA OF NURSING

Dr. Sanjeev Singh

ANMOL PUBLICATIONS PVT. LTD.
NEW DELHI - 110 002 (INDIA)

ANMOL PUBLICATIONS PVT. LTD.
H.O.: 4374/4B, Ansari Road, Darya Ganj,
New Delhi-110 002 (India)
Ph.: 23278000, 23261597

B.O.: No. 1015, Ist Main Road, BSK IIIrd Stage
IIIrd Phase, IIIrd Block
Bangalore - 560 085 (India)
Visit us at: www.anmolpublications.com

Encyclopaedia of Nursing

First Published, 2006

ISBN 81-261-3071-7

PRINTED IN INDIA

Printed at Mehra Offset Press, Delhi.

Preface

Nursing field today is not what it was a few years back. The scope of nursing and nursing education has stretched significantly in recent years. Both practitioners and students now need to understand a variety of issues in depth.

Encyclopaedia of Nursing covers all aspects of Nursing, including general nursing, special nursing care, adult nursing, critical care, oncology, child health, various therapies, information technology, learning disabilities, policy issues, ethics, nutrition, pharmacology, public health, terminology from physiotherapy, speech and language therapy, occupational therapy and radiology.

To better meet the needs of beginning students, care has been taken to clearly explain each and every term in a clear and lucid language and wherever possible, illustrations are given. This volume is ideal for the Nursing professional and student as well as general readers. It provides a comprehensive overview of Nursing with up-to-date entries covering all related disciplines.

It will also be a major source of reference for professionals and students, who require an authoritative and up-to-date guide to assist them in their work. In preparation of this book, the author has freely consulted large number of books and journals so no authenticity is claimed. Author is especially thankful to Anmol Publications Pvt. Ltd., New Delhi for shaping this book in its final form. Suggestions for further improvement of this book are not only welcome but also greatly appreciated.

Author

A

A (Retinol) Vitamin A is a vitamin with antioxidant properties, important for eye protection and bone growth; protein and hormone synthesis (including GH and testosterone); supports tissue maintenance. Helps reduce susceptibility to infection. Essential for healthy skin, good blood, strong bones and teeth, kidneys, bladder, lungs and membranes.

Abbreviated Standard Survey An on-site survey that focuses on specific complaints or specific provider issues related to change of provider ownership, management or Director of Nursing. The abbreviated survey does not cover all the aspects contained in the standard survey, but rather concentrates on a particular area(s) of concern. An abbreviated standard survey may be conducted to substantiate a complaint.

Abdominal and pelvic cavity The lower part of the ventral (abdominopelvic) cavity can be further divided into two portions: abdominal portion and pelvic portion. The abdominal cavity contains most of the gastrointestinal tract as well as the kidneys and adrenal glands. The abdominal cavity is bound cranially by the diaphragm, laterally by the body wall, and caudally by the pelvic cavity. The pelvic cavity contains most of the urogenital system as well as the rectum. The pelvic cavity is bounded cranially by the abdominal cavity, dorsally by the sacrum, and laterally by the pelvis.

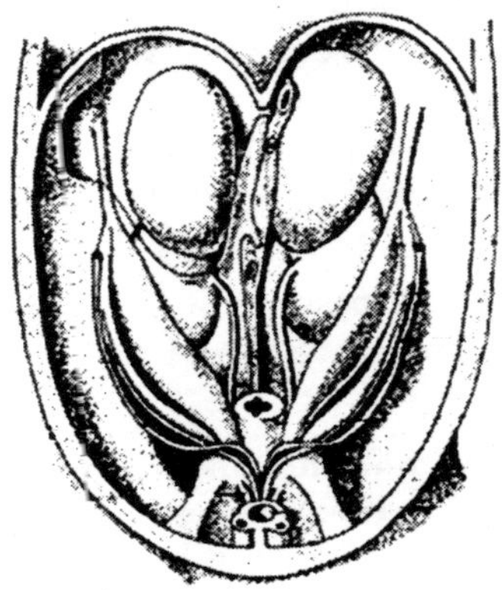

Fig. Abdominal and pelvic cavity

Abdominal aorta The continuation into the abdomen of the thoracic aorta, which divides into the two common iliac arteries.

Abdominal ultrasound A diagnostic imaging technique which creates images from the rebound of high-frequency sound waves in the internal organs.

Abdominal x-ray A simple study that will give the physician an idea of how the internal organs look.

Abduct A movement away from the medial plane. In the orbit, the abducens nerve supplies the lateral rectus muscle that pulls the eye laterally outward. Vocal Cords abducted and adducted (laryngeal tomograms).

Abortion Abortion is a termination or end of pregnancy. Giving birth to an embryo or fetus before it can live outside the womb, usually defined as before 20 weeks of gestation. Abortion may be spontaneous, often called a miscarriage, or induced as in a medical or therapeutic abortion performed to terminate a pregnancy.

Abruptio placenta Abruptio placenta is a premature separation of the placenta from the uterus.

Abscess A localized collection of pus in a cavity formed by the disintegration of tissue.

Absorbent Products Pads and garments, disposable or reusable, worn to absorb leaked urine. Absorbent products include shields, undergarment pads, combination pad-pant systems, diaperlike garments, and bed pads.

Absorption The passage of nutrients in food from the small intestine into the cells in the body.

Abuse Willful intent to cause harm. Abuse may be resident (patient) to resident (patient) or staff to resident (patient) harm.

AC/A ratio Accommodative convergence / accommodative (measured in prism diopters/diopters). The convergence response of an individual (amount the eyes turn inward) in relation to the amount of stimulus of accommodation (eye focusing). The normal ratio is 4:1.

ACAS Aged Care Assessment Services ACAS are an integral part of the aged care system. They provide assessment, information, advice and assistance to older people who are becoming, or have become, frail and wish to remain at home or who are thinking about moving into an aged residential care facility. Younger people with a disability are also eligible for assessment services in some circumstances. ACAS are a linkage point for all aged, health, community and residential services within their ACAS catchment area.

ACAT Aged Care Assessment Team Aged Care Assessment Teams are usually linked to a hospital, geriatric centre or community health centre. An ACAT team in your area is likely to include a doctor, nurse, social worker, occupational therapist and physiotherapist. Upon request you can visit them or they will visit you in your home. Their purpose is to decide what level of care and support services are best for a person and whether this can best be provided in the home, in a hostel or a nursing home.

Accelerated Benefits Benefits which can be drawn out of a life insurance policy prior to death to pay for care needs.

Accessibility Removal of barriers that would hinder a person with a disability from entering, functioning, and working within a building. Modifications that would make a home more accessible include widening doorways, adding a wheelchair ramp, and adding hand rails in a bathroom.

Accessory Apartment Apartments built into the homes of children or other relatives.

Acclimatization The biological process whereby an organism adapts to a new environment. One example is the process of developing microorganisms that degrade toxic wastes in the environment.

Accommodation (eye focusing) The eye's ability to adjust its focus by the action of the ciliary muscle, which increases the lens focusing power. When this accommodation skill is working properly, the eye can focus and refocus quickly and effortlessly, which is similar to an automatic focus feature on a camera. The ciliary muscles must contract to adjust for near vision, which causes the eye's crystalline lens, which is flexible, to be squashed. For distant vision, the ciliary muscle must relax and the eye's crystalline lens is stretched out. The ability of the eye to accommodate does decrease with age due to the crystalline lens becoming less flexible causing a condition called presbyopia.

Accommodation Bond Accommodation payments bonds and charges are a contribution to the cost of accommodation in a residential care facility. If a person's assets exceed a set amount when they enter low level (hostel) care, they may be asked to pay a bond. A person receiving care on an extra service basis may also be asked to pay a bond regardless of whether they need high or low level care. The amount of the bond will be negotiated with the service provider. The provider can only keep a certain amount from the bond annually. The balance of the bond will be repaid to the resident or beneficiaries when they leave.

Accommodation schedule Defines all areas that can influence unit operations required for manufacturing, and relationships and flows between them.

Accommodative esotropia (clinical condition) When an individual is focusing on a near object and his or her eyes are turning inward too much. It is caused by either uncorrected hyperopic refractive error and/or a high accommodative convergence/accommodation (AC/A) ratio. The average age of onset is 2 1/2 years. It is most noticeable when the child is tired or sick. This is treated with plus lenses (glasses or contacts) to help straighten the eyes. In some cases, vision therapy and corrective lenses are prescribed.

Accommodative excess (AE) This clinical condition is also called accommodative spasm. It is an over focusing, over stimulation of the focusing action of the crystalline lens causing an inability to relax the focusing system which may result in blurry vision when focusing at distance objects. Other symptoms include holding near work closer than normal, headaches with near work (such as reading or using a computer), eyestrain associated with near work, and possible double vision. Clinical signs include: patient accepts more minus on accommodative rock but blurs with plus lenses, lower NRA than PRA, dynamic retinoscopy findings indication of over accommodation and/or slow relaxation of accommodation, and reduced or erratic distance visual acuity. Treatment includes a low plus lens and/or vision therapy.

Accommodative fatigue This clinical condition is also called Ill-Sustained Accommodation. It is the inability of the eye to adequately sustain sufficient focusing over an extended time period. The most common sign or symptom is blurred vision after prolonged near work such as reading and using a computer. In addition, such patients often have asthenopia (eyestrain), general fatigue, headaches and nausea, excess tearing, and an unusual sensitivity to light. Clinical signs include: normal amplitude of accommodation, decreased PRA, and the patient generally fails the +/-2.00 D flipper test. Plus lenses (glasses or contacts) and vision therapy are effective in treating this condition.

Accommodative insufficiency (AI) This clinical condition is also called non-presbyopic accommodative insufficiency. It is an under focusing, a lack of focusing ability at a near distance. Symptoms include eyestrain, blurred vision, occasional or constant when doing near work (such as reading or using a computer), occasional unusual sensitivity to light, excess tearing, headaches, and general fatigue. Clinical signs include: patient will have difficulty with a minus lens, low amplitude of accommodation, low PRA and higher NRA. Vision therapy is an effective treatment option.

Accommodative vergence A convergence response (to turn the eyes inward) which occurs as a direct result of accommodation (eye focusing).

Account policy Specifies how passwords must be defined and employed for all user accounts on a system. It specifically addresses the issues of password aging, password uniqueness, and locking a user account because of invalid logon attempts. CFR 21 Part 11 mandates technical controls in these areas specifically.

Accountability Responsibility for the decisions and capability to explain to others or the public all undertaken activities to carry out what was obliged to do; to ensure reaching or making progress towards planned objectives or targets.

Accreditation A process whereby a program of study or an institution is recognized by an external body as meeting certain predetermined standards. Accreditation is often carried out by non-governmental organizations created for the purpose of assuring the public of the quality of the accredited institution or program. Public or private payment programs often require accreditation as a condition of payment for covered services. For long term care facilities, accreditation standards usually include stipulations about the physical plant, governing body, administration, and medical and other staff.

Acesulfame-K An artificial sweetener. Approved in 1988, this sweetener is 200 times sweeter than sugar, yet has a bitter taste. The 'K' in its name stands or potassium. Acesulfame-K is not metabolized by the body. You can cook and bake with it. There are no reported side effects with this sweetener although it may increase insulun secretion, which can cause concern for diabetics.

Acetabulum A large cup-shaped cavity that is the point of articulation between the femur and the os coxae of the pelvis.

Acetyl-L-Carnitine (ALC) The acetyl ester of carnitine, ALC acts as an antioxidant, has protective effects in the brain, and stimulates hormone (including testosterone) release.

Achalasia A condition characterized by severe unremitting spasm of the lower esophagus and lack of peristalsis in the remaining esophagus.

Acid A compound of an electronegative element or radical with hydrogen; it form salts by replacing all or part of the hydrogen with an electropositive element or radical. Or, a hydrogen-containing substance that when dissolved in water dissociates to produce one or more hydrogen ions (H+).

Acid feed Injection of an acid into a liquid stream to make it less alkaline (pH adjustment).

Acrodermatitis Inflammation of the skin of the extremities, particularly of the paws or feet.

e.g. lethal acrodermatitis - an inherited autosomal recessive disease in bull terriers relating to zinc metabolism.

Acromioclavicular joint The articulation between the acromion process and clavicle.

Acromion process The vertical extension of the scapula, above the glenohumeral joint. (from the Greek "acros", literally the "end" or the "top" - like the "acropolis" in Athens, the "top" of the city).

Action point A value set to identify when a parameter has drifted outside the operating range (Acceptance Criteria). A documented response is usually required.

Activated carbon Material used to adsorb organic impurities from water. Derived from wood, lignite, pulp-mill char, blood, etc. The source material is initially charred at high temperature to convert it to carbon. The carbon is then "activated" by oxidation from exposure to high temperature steam. It comes in granular or powdered form.

Active immunity The formation of an antibody that can be stimulated by infection or vaccination.

Active ingredient Any component that is intended to furnish pharmacological activity or other direct effect in the diagnosis, cure, mitigation, treatment, or prevention of disease, or to affect the structure or any function of the body of man or other animals. The term includes those components that may undergo chemical change in the manufacture of the drug product and are present in the drug product in a modified form intended to furnish the specified activity or effect.

Active site The region of a protein molecule that binds the specific substrate and chemically modifies it into the new product (in an enzyme) or interacts with it (in a receptor).

Active transport Energy-requiring transport of a solution across a membrane in the direction of increasing concentration.

Active Treatment An ongoing organized effort to help each resident (patient) maintain their developmental capacity through their regular participation, according to an individualized plan, in a program of activities designed to enable the resident (patient) to attain or maintain the optimal physical, social, intellectual, and vocational levels of functioning.

Activities of Daily Living The core daily personal care activities which are necessary for people to be able to live independently. ADLs are not always defined the same, but generally include Ambulation, Bathing, Continence, Dressing, Eating, Toileting, and Transferring. The level of assistance people need with ADLs is a measure of the type and amount of long term care they need. Problems with ADLs may trigger eligibility to receive benefits from long term care insurance, or may be a requirement for admission to an assisted living facility or nursing home.

Activity Therapist (AT) An allied health professional trained to develop and provide leisure time activities for facility residents (patients).

Actual yield The quantity that is actually produced at any appropriate phase of manufacture, processing, or packaging of a particular drug product.

Acuity Clearness of eyesight. Depends on the sharpness of images and the sensitivity of nerve elements in the retina.

Acupressure Based on the principles of acupuncture, this ancient chinese technique involves the use of finger pressure on specific points along the body to treat ailments such as tension, stress, aches, pains, cramps or arthritis.

Acute Severe; sharp; begins quickly.

Acute Care Care for illness or injury that has developed rapidly, has pronounced symptoms and is finite in length. The goal of acute care is to cure disease and restore the person to an improved level of functioning. In-patient hospital care is acute care, as are doctor's visits, surgery, and X-rays. Acute care services are covered by health insurance policies and by both Medicare, although there are various co-payments, deductibles, and limits to coverage.

Acute Cholecystitis Acute inflammation and infection of the gallbladder caused by obstruction of the cystic duct from stones formed within the gallbladder.

Acute Illness Illness that is usually short-term and that often comes on quickly.

Add Prescription strength of a plus lens which is used for near vision. A plus lens can be added to another lens such as a minus lens for distance vision.

Additus ad antrum The mastoid air spaces connecting the mastoid antrum with the epitympanic recess.

Adduct (adductor magnus) A movement toward the midline. The adductor magnus muscle in the thigh pulls the leg toward the medial plane.

Adenine (A) A purine base, 6-aminopurine, occurring in RNA (ribonucleic acid) and DNA (deoxyribonucleic acid) and as a component of adenosine triphosphate.

Adeno (prefix) Gland. e.g. adenitis - inflammation of a gland.

Adenocarcinoma A malignant tumor of epithelial cells arranged in glandular patterns.

Adenoma A benign epithelial tumor in which the cells form glandular structures or are derived from glandular epithelium.

Adjustment In chiropractic, a small controlled thrust that moves a joint slightly beyond its normal range of motion.

Administer The direct application of a vaccine or a prescribed drug or device, whether by injection, ingestion or any other means, to the body of a resident (patient).

Administration A system whereby public or private enterprises conduct their business. Administration is concerned with planning, programming and evaluation. Along with administration there must be consideration of management, which as a part of administration, is a rational technique enabling administrators to fully develop their human, technical and financial resources. The term administration is often used to denote broad policy and the term "management" to be the execution of such policy and a matter of subordinate concern.

Admission Entrance into a facility or program. Each resident who enters a nursing home for the first time counts as an admission. A resident returning to the facility after an intervening stay elsewhere would be a re-admission.

ADR See: adverse drug reaction.

Adrenal gland The gland located superior to the kidney which is responsible for the production of epinephrine. ("epi" - above + "nephros" - kidney).

Adsorption Adhesion of the molecules of a gas, liquid or dissolved substance to a surface because of chemical or electrical attraction - typically accomplished with granular activated carbon to remove dissolved organics and chlorine. The attachment of charged particles to the chemically active groups on the surface and in the pores of an ion exchanger.

Adult Day Care A daytime community-based program that provides a variety of health, social, and related support services in a protective setting. Programs are designed to meet the needs of functionally and/or cognitively impaired adults who can no longer be left at home alone. Adult day centers offer protected settings which are normally open five days a week during business hours and include a mixture of health, social and support services. Many programs provide meals and transportation services to and from a patients home, and specialized programs for individuals with Alzheimer's disease or related disorders. These programs often provide a respite, or break for family caregivers.

Adult Day Health Care A category of Adult Day Care which provides comprehensive, professional support in a protected environment including on-site nurses, physical therapists, social workers, and/or other professionals for adults who are experiencing a decrease in physical, mental, and social functioning and require tailored medical and/or psychiatric supervision. Such centers normally offer a wide range of therapeutic and rehabilitative activities as well as social activities, meals, and transportation.

Adult Foster Care A live-in arrangement where one adult lives with and is provided care and/or services by an unrelated individual or family. Such arrangements may be certified by the state or managed independently.

Adult Protective Services A state or community-based service that investigates cases of suspected elder abuse, neglect or endangerment.

Advance Directives Include healthcare power of attorney or proxy, living will, Do Not Recessitate (DNR) or other advanced directions to guide healthcare decision-making if a person is unable to make or express decisions on his or her own behalf.

Advanced Clinician At this level the clinician experience allows them to "read" the situation and respond appropriately. The clinician intuitively understands the situation but at this stage still needs to think analytically about what to do.

Adventitious agents Acquired, sporadic, accidental contaminants.

Adverse agents Undesired effects or toxicity due to exposure (often but not limited to a drug or medical device).

Adverse Drug Reaction (ADR) Any unintended response to a drug which is injurious or harmful to health and which occurs at normal doses.

Advisory alarm An alarm indicating a drift of a monitored parameter toward an out-of-spec condition. It is advisory in that no GMP violation has occurred, and is used to advise corrective action before an action alarm can happen.

Aerobe An organism that can live and grow only in the presence of oxygen. 1. Facultative aerobe: one which normally thrives in the absence of oxygen, but which may acquire the faculty of living in the presence of oxygen.

2. Obligate aerobe: one that cannot live without air.

Aerobia The plural of aerobe.

Aerobic Living in air.

Aerobic bacteria Bacteria capable of growing in the presence of Oxygen.

Aerosol A product that is dispensed by a propellant from a metal can up to a maximum size of 33.8 fluid ounces (1000 mL) or a glass or plastic bottle up to a size of 4 fluid ounces (118.3 mL), other than a rim-vented container.

Aerosol photometer Light-scattering mass concentration indicating instrument with a threshold sensitivity of at least 10 to the negative third power microgram per liter for 0.3µm diameter DOP (Dioctyl Phthalate) concentrations over a range of 10 to the fifth power times the threshold sensitivity. Photometers may include hand-held remote meter probes that can scan for airborne contaminants in HEPA filters, in penetrations around frames, seals and plenums, and in hoods and work stations.

AES See: auger electron spectroscopy.

After image The eye's ability to still see an image during eye blinks and even after the viewed object is no longer present. The most common example is seeing light after the flash of a camera.

Afterbirth Afterbirth is the organ inside the uterus that is attached to the baby by the umbilical cord. Essential during pregnancy for growth and development of the embryo and fetus. Also called the placenta.

Agar A complex mixture of polysaccharides obtained from marine red algae, used as an emulsion stabilizer in foods, as a sizing in fabrics, as a gelling agent and as a solid substrate or media for the laboratory culture of microorganisms. Agar melts at 100°C and when cooled below 44°C forms a stiff and transparent gel. Microorganisms are seeded and grown on the surface of the gel.

Agarose A highly purified form of agar.

Agarose gel electrophoresis A method used to separate, identify, and purify molecules of different molecular weight and/or structure. It is specifically applied to the separation of protein or DNA fragments where it is rapid, simple, and accurate, and the separated molecules can be visualized directly by staining with dyes. The electrophoretic migration rate of molecules through agarose gel is dependent on the following parameters:

1. Molecular size: molecules pass through the gel at rates that are inversely proportional to the log of their molecular weight.

2. Agarose concentration: a molecule of a given size migrates at different rates through gels containing different concentrations of agarose.

3. Molecular conformation: a molecule of the same molecular weight but of a different conformation will migrate at different rates. Generally, closed circular or globular forms will migrate faster than linear forms.

4. Electric current: at low voltages the rate of migration is proportional to the voltage, but as the voltage is increased the rate of migration of high molecular weight fragments is increased differentially.

Ageing in Place A concept that allows a resident to choose to remain in his/her living environment regardless of the physical and or mental decline that may occur with the aging process of aging.

Agene Nitrogen Trichloride (NCl_3).

Agenesis Absence, failure of formation or imperfect development of any part.

Agglomerate Suspended solids clustered together to form larger clumps or masses that are easier to remove by filtration or settling.

Agglutination The sticking together of insoluble antigens such as bacteria, viruses or erythrocytes by a particular antibody. Agglutination assays are used to type human blood before a transfusion.

Aging in Place The concept of allowing an older person to remain in the same place as their care needs change, rather than requiring a move to another type of facility. Aging in place is a desired goal of many older people, but current regulations in many states limit the types of services which can be provided in various facilities, necessitating a move. A Continuing Care Retirement Community may promote itself as a place where residents can age in place, but even these facilities will require residents to move to various buildings within the campus as their care needs change.

AHF (antihemophilic factor) In the clotting of blood it is also known as Factor VIII.

Air change rate The number of times the total air volume of a defined space is replaced in a given unit of time. This is computed by dividing the total volume of the subject space (in cubic feet) into the total volume of air exhausted from (or supplied to) the space per unit of time.

Air cleaners Filtration systems that may be freestanding or installed in a ceiling or wall to remove contaminants such as bacteria, viruses, and dust from the air. Air cleaners may incorporate HEPA filters.

Air velocity meters/monitors Meters to measure and indicate the force and speed of airflow. Meters may use a variety of probes for measuring near HEPA filters and at right angles. Monitors check and record air velocity.

Airborne particulate cleanliness classes Statistically allowable number of particles equal to, or larger than 0.5μm in size per cubic foot of air. According to ISO 14644-1, a classification number, N, shall designate airborne particulate cleanliness.

Airflow visualization Using chemical smoke or fog to visualize flow patterns in a cleanroom or clean space.

Air-lift bioreactor A reactor in which the source of agitation is air sparged upwards through a draft tube - most widely used for cell culture applications and monoclonal antibody production.

Airlock A room or space designed to act as a means of segregating areas of different air classification or quality. It may contain a method to remove particulate contamination from clean room garments as personnel pass through, and usually includes HEPA filtered air supply and interlocking doors. Airlocks pressure will "float" between those of the spaces being protected. With all doors closed, the airlock pressure will be somewhere between that of the highest adjoining room and that of the lowest adjoining room as air flows through it from room to room. "Ventilated airlocks" are in neutral ducted air balance (supply CFM = return CFM).

Alanine An amino acid. BCAAs are used as a source of energy for muscle cells. During prolonged exercise, BCAAs are released from skeletal muscles and their carbon backbones are used as fuel, while their nitrogen portion is used to form another amino acid, Alanine. Alanine is then converted to Glucose by the liver. This form of energy production is called the Alanine-Glucose cycle, and it plays a major role in maintaining the body's blood sugar balance.

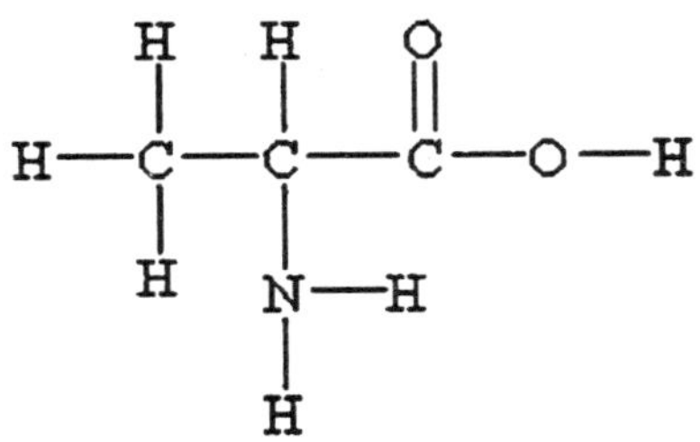

Fig. Alanine

Alarms Audible or visual signals used to warn of unacceptable conditions at monitored sites. They may be buzzers, horns, speakers, bells, or warning lights. They can be Advisory, Alert, or Action alarms. The first two are for operation and maintenance information, to alert of abnormal situations that do not compromise product SISPQ. The Action alarm is for GMP records, indicating that product SISPQ may have been compromised, but Alert alarms are also usually recorded.

Albinism Pigmentation is deficient or absent. May occur in skin, hair, and eyes. Ocular albinism is a pigmentation deficiency occurring mainly in the eyes. Individuals with albinism including ocular albinism commonly have decreased visual acuity (20/70 -20/200), strabismus, photophobia, and nystagmus. There is no known treatment. Individuals may benefit from low-vision aids. Treatment options for strabismus and nystagmus does apply to these individuals.

Albumin Commonly, the white of egg is a simple protein widely distributed throughout the tissues and fluid of plants and animals. Soluble in pure water it is also precipitable from a solution by mineral acids, and coagulable by heat in acid or neutral solution.

Albuminoid Resembling albumin, a simple protein present in horny and cartilaginous tissues, insoluble in neutral solvents. Keratin, elastin, and collagen are albuminoids.

Albuminuria Albuminuria is term used when protein is found in the urine. Protein in the urine can be symptomatic of some prental complications and is probably tested for at your prenatal visits.

Alert point Used in determining when a parameter is drifting toward extremes of the operating range.

Alexander technique F. Matthias alexander created the method after concluding that bad posture was responsible for his own chronic voice loss. Practitioners use gentle hands-on guidance, verbal instruction, teach simple, efficient ways of moving as a means of improving balance, posture, coordination and to relieve tension and pain.

Alignment Proper fusing (uniting) of images to each eye.

Aliquot Of, pertaining to, or designating an exact divisor or factor of a quantity, specially of an integer. To divide out a sample to multiple containers for multiple analytical tests.

Alkalinity An expression of the total amount of basic anions (hydroxyl groups) present in a solution. In water analysis, it also represents the presence of carbonate, bicarbonate, and occasionally borate, silicate, and phosphate salts that react to produce hydroxyl groups. Bicarbonate and carbonate ions are expected to be in most waters. Hydroxide may occur in water that has been softened by the lime soda process or has been in contact with fresh concrete. Alkalinity furnishes a guide in choosing appropriate treatment of either raw water or plant effluents.

Allantoic fluid The clear white portion of an egg. In influenza vaccine manufacturing, the virus is propagated in the embryonic chick and sloughed into the allantoic fluid that is harvested to produce the vaccine.

Allele Alternative form of a genetic locus; a single allele for each locus is inherited separately from each parent (e.g., at a locus for eye color the allele might result in blue or brown eyes).

Allergenic extract An extract in a solvent of a substance that causes an allergic reaction. They are relative crude drugs by contemporary standards and are manufactured by specialty companies and in some cases, by a practiçing allergist. Also, allergenic extracts are generally difficult to filter since they most frequently are extracts of natural substances such as foods, house dust, animal hair, etc.

Allergy A condition in which the body is not able to tolerate eating certain foods, or exposure to certain animals, plants, or other substances.

Allopathy The treatment of disease by creating conditions that are opposite or hostile to the conditions resulting from the disease itself; from greek roots meaning other and disease. Drugs and surgery are allopathic treatments. The term is sometimes used to refer to conventional western medicine to contrast it with alternative therapies, particularly homeopathy, which is based on like curing like.

Alopecia Areata A disease of unknown cause in which hair suddenly falls out, leaving bald patches on the scalp. In half the people affected, the hair grows back within a year. After giving birth, many women experience hairloss.

Alpha fetoprotein screening This blood test measures the levels of a substance called alpha-fetoprotein in the mother's blood. Abnormal levels can indicate a brain or spinal cord defect, the presence of twins, a miscalculated due date, or an increased risk of Down syndrome.

Alpha Lipoic Acid (ALA) A sulfur bearing phytonutrient with antioxidant properties; amplifies effects of other antioxidants. It is an insulin potentiator that may be, in some respects, the very best insulin mimicker. An analogy of what ALA does is that if ALA was an individual, he would be the one which yells at the muscle cells to pick up the key, open the door, and help bring in the creatine.

ALA is a sulfur bearing compound with antioxidant properties. It plays a role in energy metabolism. ALA amplifies the ability of other antioxidants to combat free redicals and enhance recovery. Also may enhance insulin sensitivity, improving the body's ability to add lean mass and reduce fat.

Alphafetoprotein Alphafetoprotein (AFP) is a substance produced by the unborn baby as it grows inside the uterus. Large amounts of AFP are found in the amniotic fluid. Larger-than normal amounts are found in the maternal bloodstream if neural-tube defects are present in the fetus.

Alt A special key on most computer keyboards that allows users to access alternate features and keyboard "hotkeys". Alt is almost always used in conjunction with another key, such as "F4" or "Ctrl".

Alternate Plan of Care Benefit Used by some long term care insurance policies that include home care benefits. A provision for payment for a special arrangement of services specifically designed to allow the person to reside in a setting other than a nursing facility, like services to provide assistance and capital improvements such as ramps, grab bars and/or durable medical equipment. These provisions are designed to delay a move to a nursing home for as long as possible, and might be covered so long as these expenses would cost no more than a the nursing home.

Alum Aluminum sulfate, commonly added during municipal water treatment to cause insoluble colloids to coalesce into larger particles that can be removed by settling.

Alveus A layer of myelinated fibers overlying the ventricular surface of the hippocampus. It arises from cells within the hippocampus and converges medially to form the fimbria, the beginning of the fornix.

Alzheimer Unit Special living units within a Nursing Home or an Assisted Living Facility specifically providing care and services for those with Alzheimers Disease.

Alzheimer's A progressive, neurodegenerative disease characterised by loss of function and death of nerve cells in several areas of the brain, leading to loss of mental functions such as memory and learning. Alzheimer's disease is the most common cause of dementia.

Ambient The normal environment conditions such as temperature, relative humidity, or room pressure of a particular area under consideration.

Amblyopia (clinical condition) Reduced visual acuity (poorer than 20/20) which is not correctable by glasses or contacts and is not caused by structural or pathological anomalies. This condition is often called "lazy eye" because it is typically the result of disuse. It is usually marked by blurred vision in one eye and favoring one eye over the other. About two percent of the population is affected.

Types of functional (reversible) amblyopia:

refractive- anisometropia (the two eyes have different refractive powers), or other amblyopiogenic refractive errors (hyperopia, myopia, or astigmatism)

strabismic- misalignment of the two eyes in which they point in different directions

form deprivation (may also be referred to as amblyopia ex anopsia)- caused by conditions that prevent light from entering the eye. These may include congenital ptosis (droopy eyelid), corneal opacity, or cataract.

Treatment options for functional amblyopia are eye patching, prescription lenses, prisms, and vision therapy.

Ambulation One of the Activities of Daily Living (ADLs). The ability to walk both inside and outside your residence with or without a cane, crutches or brace.

Ambulatory Able to walk with or without difficulty or help.

Ambulatory Care All types of health services which are provided on an outpatient basis, in contrast to services provided in the home or to persons who are inpatients. While many inpatients may be ambulatory, the term ambulatory care usually implies that the patient must travel to a location to receive services which do not require an overnight stay.

Amelanotic In reference to a melanoma, amelanotic refers to a melanoma that contains little or no pigment.

American medical association (AMA) According to its mission statement, this professional association represents the voice of the American medical profession and constitutes the partnership of physicians and their professional associations dedicated to promoting the art and science of medicine and the betterment of public health. The AMA serves physicians and their patients by establishing and promoting ethical, educational, and clinical standards for the medical profession and by advocating the highest principle of all: the integrity of the physician/patient relationship.

Ames test A simple bacterial test for carcinogens.

Ametropia Any optical error such as hyperopia, myopia, or astigmatism. Also called refractive error.

Amine A substance that may be derived from ammonia by the replacement of one or more of the hydrogen atoms by hydrocarbon radicals.

Amino acids Any of a group of twenty hydrocarbon molecules (containing the radical group NH2) linked together in various combinations to form proteins in living things. Synthesized by living cells or obtained as essential components of the diet of human and animals, these twenty amino acids are divided into four (4) groups on the basis of their side-chain properties:

1. Neutral, hydrophobic side chains,
2. Neutral, hydrophilic side chains,
3. Acid, hydrophilic side chains,
4. Basic, hydrophilic side chains.

In addition to the twenty common amino acids there are less common derivatives (e.g. hydroxyproline, found in collagen) formed by the modification of a common amino acid.

Amma therapy System of bodywork therapy that uses traditional oriental medical principles for assessing and evaluating imbalances in the energetic system. It aims to restore, promote and maintain optimum health through the treatment of the physical body, bio-energy and emotions. Used for a wide range of conditions.

Amniocentesis Amniocentesis is the process of removing amniotic fluid from the amniotic sac. Fluid is tested for some genetic defects. If necessary, this test is performed between 15 and 20 weeks of pregnancy and can indicate chromosomal abnormalities such as Down syndrome, or genetic disorders such as Tay Sachs disease, sickle cell disease, cystic fibrosis, and others. It also can detect the baby's sex and risk of spina bifida (a condition in which the brain or spine do not develop properly). There are some risks involved with having an amniocentesis.

Amniocytes Cells shed by the developing fetus and found in the surrounding amniotic fluid.

Amnion nodosum Rounded or oval opaque elevations in the placenta, 1 to 6 mm in diameter, that are seen in the part of the amnion in contact with the chorionic plate and near the insertion of the cord into the placenta. These are usually associated with prolonged oligohydramnios.

Amnion The amnion is the membrane around the fetus. It surrounds the amniotic cavity.

Amniorrhea Escape of the amniotic fluid.

Amniorrhexis Rupture of the amnion .

Amniotic fluid The amniotic fluid is the liquid surrounding the baby inside the amniotic sac.

Amniotic sac The amniotic sac is the sac that surrounds baby inside the uterus. It contains the baby, the placenta and the amniotic fluid.

Ampholyte Amphoteric electrolyte. Electrolyte that can either give up or take on a hydrogen ion and can thus behave as either an acid or a base.

Amphoteric Having two opposite characteristics.

Ampicillin An antibiotic widely used in clinical treatment and rDNA research. It is a derivative of penicillin, which kills bacteria by interfering with the synthesis of the cell wall.

Amplification The production of additional copies of a chromosomal sequence, found as either intrachromosomal or extrachromosomal DNA.

Amplitude of accommodation (AA) A measurement of the eye's ability to focus clearly on objects at near distances. This eye focusing range for a child is usually about

2-3 inches. For a young adult, it is 4-6 inches. The focus range for a 45-year-old adult is about 20 inches. For an 80-year-old adult, it is 60 inches.

Ampoule or ampule A small glass vial sealed after filling and one of the earliest devices developed for safe storage of sterile injectable unit.

Amygdala A complex of nuclei located in the dorsomedial temporal lobe just deep to the uncus. This nuclear complex is in contact with the tail of the caudate nucleus and is a component of the basal ganglia known as the archi striatum. It has olfactory, visceral, endocrine, and behavioral functions and may be involved with emotional changes associated with Alzheimer's disease and in Schizophrenia.

Amyotrophic lateral sclerosis An inherited, fatal degenerative nerve disorder, also known as Lou Gehrig's disease.

Anabolic Metabolic condition in which new molecules are synthesized (growth).

Anabolism The intracellular process involved in the synthesis of more complex compounds than those involved in catabolism (for example, glucose to glycogen) and requires energy.

Anaerobe A microorganism that thrives best, or only, when deprived of oxygen.

1. Facultative anaerobe: one able to grow in the presence or absence of free oxygen.

2. Obligate or obligatory anaerobe: one that will grow only in the absence of free oxygen.

Anaerobic Relating to an anaerobe.

Anaerobic bacteria Bacteria capable of growing in the absence of Oxygen.

Anal fissure A small tear in the anus that can cause bleeding, itching, or pain.

Analog Refers to information processing techniques that send data as a directly representative electronic signal. (e.g. a voice is transmitted across a telephone line as an electrical signal with the same amplitude and frequency as spoken words.)

Analytical data interchange (ANDI) A generic file format. It was common practice to save information from analytical instruments in this file format. The disadvantage now is that the approach does not allow replaying of data on a different system to yield the same result.

Analytical method Small scale process used to characterize and/or separate a mixture, a compound, or an unknown material into its constituent parts or elements.

Anastomosis Connection, natural or surgically created, between two tubular structures.

Ancestor worship Ritualized propitiation and invocation of dead kin, based on the belief that spirits influence the fate of the living. A widespread ancient practice.

Ancillary material Material used in preparing drugs that does not become a component of the drug (e.g. steam, air, N2, DI water).

Ancillary Services Services other than primary care services, which may include physical, occupational, or speech therapy, X-ray, and laboratory services.

Androstenedione An androgen (male hormone). Androgens are produced in two sites in the male body - most originate in the testes, but some potent male hormones are produced by the adrenal glands, located just above the kidneys. Androstenedione is a pivotal adrenal steroid that's actually one step closer to being converted to testosterone than DHEA. It raises your testosterone levels and can provide more strength.

Androstenedione really does raise testosterone above normal levels and could be hazardous. Side effects include acne, male baldness, and a decrease in 'good' cholesterol, which may lead to heart disease. This supplement might be reclassified as a steroid by the FDA, and it is banned in the NFL, Olympics, and other major sports organizations.

Anemia Anemia is marked by a decreased count of red blood cells in the body, which affects the blood's ability to carry oxygen to various organs in the body. Anemia can be a standalone disorder, but it is often a symptom of a concurrent disease. There are several types of anemia, depending on the cause. Anemia can be caused by iron deficiency, malnutrition, blood loss, certain medications, a chronic illness or a genetic disorder.

Anemometer A device that measures air speed.

Anencephaly Anencephaly is the defective development of the brain combined with the absence of the bones normally surrounding the brain. Anencephaly is a rare birth defect resulting in little or no brain and a malformed skull.

Aneuploidy Extra or missing chromosomes; other than the normal number of each per cell.

Aneurysm The dilation of the wall of an artery, vein, or the heart, that forms a sac-like structure.

Angina (angina pectoris) An intense, steady pain or feeling of pressure in the region of the heart caused by a decreased blood flow to the heart muscle.

Angio (suffix) Vessel.

e.g. lymphangitis - inflammation of a lymph vessel.

Angiography An radiologic procedure that produces images of blood vessels (ateries and veins). Angiographic images can be constructed by MR (MRA), CT (CTA), and by conventional X-ray techniques using a cather injection.

Angioma Angioma is a tumor, usually benign, or swelling composed of lymph and blood vessels.

Angle of louis The point of junction between the manubrium and the body of the sternum.

Angstrom (A°+A219) A unit of length equal to one hundred-millionth of a centimeter (one ten-thousandth of a micron) used especially to specify radiation wavelengths.

Animism Belief that a spirit or force resides in every animate and inanimate object, every dream and idea, giving individuality to each. The related polynesian concept of mana holds that the spirit in all things is responsible for good and evil.

Anion A negatively charged particle or ion.

Anion exchange resin An ion exchange material that removes anions from solution by exchanging them with hydroxyl ions.

Anis, aniso (prefix) Unequal; dissimilar.

e.g. anisokaryosis - inequality in the size of the nuclei of cells.

Aniseikonia A difference in the size or shape of two visual images when the images should be the same size and/or shape.

Anisometropia The condition in which the two eyes have different refractive powers.

Ankle joint A "mortise and tenon" joint between the two bones of the lower leg (tibia and fibula) and the talus of the foot.

Ankylosing spondylitis This is a chronic condition caused by inflammation of the joints and ligaments of the back, which affects the spine and may lead to stiffness in the back.

Anneal The process by which the complementary base pairs in DNA strands combine.

Annealing A treatment process for steel in which the metal is heated and held at a suitable temperature and then cooled at a suitable rate for the purpose of reducing hardness, improving machinability, facilitating cold working, producing a desired microstructure, or obtaining desired mechanical, physical, or other properties.

Annual Assessment An annual assessment of a resident's (patient's) physical, mental, emotional, cognitive, and functional status.

Anomalous retinal correspondence (ARC) A type of retinal projection, occurring frequently in strabismus, in which the foveae (center of the retina that produces the sharpest eyesight) of the two eyes do not facilitate a common visual direction; the fovea of one eye has the same functional direction with an extrafoveal (non-fovea) area of the other eye.

Anorectal atresia Absence of a normal opening between the anus and the rectum.

Anosmia Loss of the sense of smell.

Anovulatory Anovulatory is the lack of or cessation of ovulation.

Ansa lenticularis An efferent fiber bundle arising from the internal division of the globus pallidus. It utlimately joins the thalamic fasciculus which projects to the ventral anterior and lateral thalamic nuclei.

Antacids Medicines that neutralize stomach acid.

Ante (prefix) Before in time or space.

e.g. ante mortem - before death.

Antenatal care coverage Percentage of women attended at least once during pregnancy by skilled health personnel because of their pregnancy.

Anterior arch (C1) The curved structure located at the forward part of the atlas (ventral side of body).

Anterior clinoid process The bony process located on the medial end of the posterior border of the lesser wing of the sphenoid bone.

Anterior or ventral Front (example, the kneecap is located on the anterior side of the leg).

Anterior Position When the baby faces the back of the mother's pelvis in utero and/or during labor.

Anterior rib The portion of the rib locted on the ventral side of the body.

Anterior tibial artery Artery originating from the popliteal artery and branching into the posterior and anterior tibial recurrent, and lateral and medial anterior malleolar arteries, and lateral and medial malleolar retes.

Anterior urethra The part of the male urethra that extends from the bulb to the meatus of the glans penis.

Anti (prefix) Against; counteracting.

e.g. antitoxin - an antibody to a toxin.

Antianxiety Medication Psychoactive medications given to reduce anxiety (e.g., Ativan, Valium, Xanax).

Antibiotic An organic substance of microbial origin (usually mold or actinomycete bacteria) that is either toxic or growth inhibiting for other organisms. Also with the advent of synthetic methods of production, a substance produced by a microorganism or a similar substance (produced wholly or partly by chemical synthesis) which, in low concentrations, inhibits the growth of other microorganisms. Penicillin, tetracycline, and erythromycin are examples of antibiotics.

Antibody A modified protein molecule present in the blood serum or plasma (and other body fluids), whose activity is associated chiefly with gamma globulin. Produced by the immune system in response to exposure to a foreign substance, it is the body's protective mechanism against infection and disease. An antibody is characterized by a structure complementary to the foreign substance, the antigen that provokes its formation, and is thus capable of binding specifically to the foreign substance to neutralize it.

Anticholinergic Side Effects Dry eyes, dry mouth, blurred vision, constipation, urinary retention, behavior changes, loss of cognitive function.

Anticholinergics Medicines that help calm spasms in the intestine.

Antidepressant Medication Psychoactive medications given to relieve depression (e.g., Celexa, Paxil, Prozac, Zoloft)

Antidiarrheals Medicines that help control diarrhea.

Antiemetics Medicines that help prevent and control nausea and vomiting.

Antigen Any of various foreign substances such as bacteria, viruses, endotoxins, exotoxins, foreign proteins, pollen, and vaccines, whose entry into an organism induces an immune response (antibody production, lymphokine production, or both) directed specifically against that molecule. Response may be demonstrated as an increased reaction, such as hypersensitivity (usually protein or a complex of protein and polysaccharide, or occasionally a polysaccharide of high molecular weight), a circulating antibody that reacts with the antigen, or some degree of immunity to infectious disease if the antigen was a microorganism or its products.

Anti-inflammatory medications Anti-inflammatory medications are drugs to relieve pain or inflammation.

Anti-interferon An antibody to an interferon. Used for the purification of interferons.

Antioxidants Any substances that prevent or impede cell oxidation (destruction) by free radicals, etc.

Antipsychotic Medication Psychoactive medications given to reduce or control psychotic (withdrawal from reality) symptoms (e.g., Haldol, Prolixin, Risperdal, Zyprexa, and Seroquel).

Antiresorptive Drugs A class of drugs used to prevent thinning of the bones

Antiseptic Acting against sepsis. An antiseptic agent is one that has been formulated for use on living tissue such as mucous membranes or skin to prevent or inhibit growth or action of organisms. Antiseptics should not be used to decontaminate inanimate objects.

Antiserum The blood serum obtained from an animal after has been immunized with a particular antigen. It contains antibodies specific for that antigen as well as antibodies specific for any other antigens with which the animal has previously been immunized.

Antispasmodics Medicines that help reduce or stop muscle spasms in the intestines.

Antistatic Reducing static electric charges by retaining enough moisture to provide electrical conduction.

Antistatic cleaners Liquid cleaners that enhance surface conductivity of cleanroom tabletops, workstations, and other surfaces.

Antitachycardia pacing A method of treating ventricular tachycardia (too-fast heartbeat) by stimulating the heart with a preset rapid series of small electrical pulses.

Antitoxin An antibody that is capable of neutralizing the specific toxin that stimulated its production in the body. Antitoxins are produced in animals for medical purposes by injection of a toxin or toxoid, with the resulting serum being used to counteract the toxin in other individuals.

Antrum The portion of the stomach where food collects prior to passage into the small intestine, also contains the acid secreting cells.

Antrum of stomach The dilated portion of the pyloric region of the stomach, near the junction with the duodenum.

Anus The opening at the end of the digestive tract where bowel movements leave the body.

Anxiety A debilitating condition of fear, which interferes with normal life functions.

Aorta The main trunk of the arterial system which originates from the left ventricle of the heart and extends to the level of the fourth lumbar vertebra.

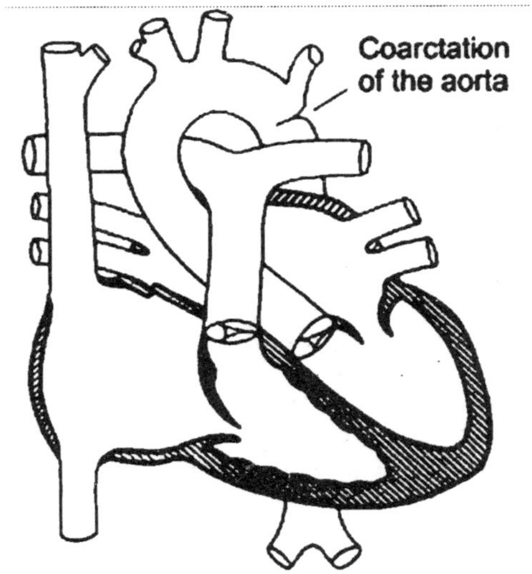

Fig. Aorta

Aortic arch The portion of the aorta which bends over inorder to extend into the thorax.

Aortic bifurcation The point where the abdominal aorta divides into the two common iliac arteries.

Aortic sinus Dilations of the aortic wall superior to each valve.

Ap view A front to back view of the body.

Aperture rule A stick-like instrument used in vision therapy to develop convergence and divergence (eye teaming) skills.

Apex The pointed part of the heart's left lower chamber (ventricle).

Apex of heart The bottom most portion of the heart, formed by the left ventricle.

Apgar Score The first test most babies are given (at one and five minutes after birth). Assesses five basic indicators of health: respiration, pulse, activity level, response to stimulation, and appearance.

Aphasia Loss of the ability to use or understand language.

API (active pharmaceutical ingredient) Also called Drug Substance. Any substance or mixture of substances intended to be used in the manufacture of a drug (medicinal) product and that when used in the production of a drug becomes an active ingredient of the drug product. Such substances are intended to furnish pharmacological activity or other direct effect in the diagnosis, cure, mitigation, treatment, or prevention of disease or to affect the structure and function of the body.

API starting material A material used in the production of an API which is itself or is incorporated as a significant structural fragment into the structure of the API. A starting material may be an article of commerce, a material purchased from one or more suppliers under contract or commercial agreement, or it may be produced in-house. Starting materials are normally of defined chemical properties and structure.

Aplasia Defective development or congenital absence of an organ or tissue.

Apoenzyme The protein moiety of an enzyme - determines the specifity of the enzyme reaction.

Appendectomy An operation to remove the appendix.

Appendicitis Irritation, inflammation, and pain in the appendix, caused by infection, scarring, or obstruction (blockage).

Appendix (Veriform appendix) Appendage of the cecum.

Application Software Software that is designed and written for a specific personal, organizational, or processing task, such as graphics software.

Applied kinesiology A diagnostic technique and therapy developed in the 1960s by a chiropractor (george goodheart). Applied kinesiology posits that organ or gland dysfunctions show up as weaknesses in certain muscles. Using gentle pressure, applied kinesiologists test muscle strength to identify health problems and nutritional deficiencies. After diagnosis, treatment may involve exercises to strengthen a muscle, hands-on manipulation of the muscles and bones, and vitamin or mineral supplements.

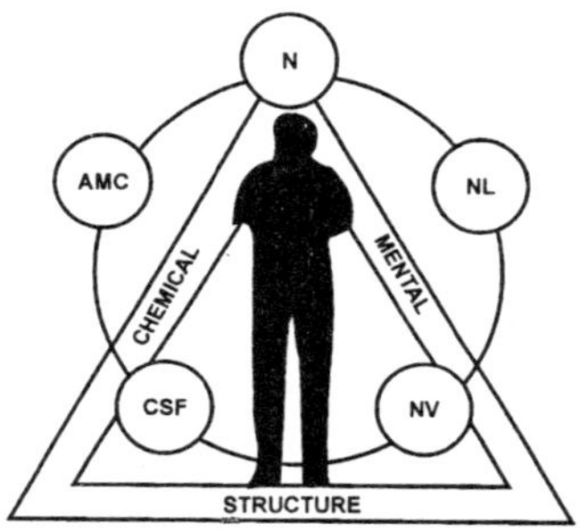

Fig. Applied kinesiology

Appropriated login or impersonation Someone using the authorization code, usually user ID and password of another person to secure access to network resources for which he or she does not have privileges or authorization. Can be intentional or not. CFR 21 Part 11 mandates technical controls that prevent this.

Aquifer An underground layer of permeable rock, sand, or gravel that contains water for wells or springs.

Arachnoid Mater The middle of the three meninges enclosing the brain and spinal cord. It is a thin, translucent membrane closely adherent to the dura mater. Trabeculae extend from its inner surface across the subarachnoid spa ce to the pia. Also forms the outer membrane of the leptomeninges.

Arachnoid villi (granulations) Microscopic tufts of pia-arachnoid mater that pierce the dura and open into venous sinuses, lacunae or extradural veins. They permit unidirectional flow of cerebrospinal fluid from the subarachnoid space to the venous system.

Archicerebellum The phylogenetically oldest part of the cerebellum represented by the nodulus and paired flocculi (flocculonodular lobe). Closely related to the vestibular system.

Archistriatum The phylogenetically oldest component of the basal ganglia; the amygdaloid nuclear complex.

Area of Rescue Assistance (ARA) A room or stairwell landing used for safe refuge in a fire or other emergency by residents (patients) who are unable to negotiate stairs.

Areola The areola is the pigmented or colored ring surrounding the nipple of the breast. During pregnancy, the areola often beomes darker in color.

Arginine A conditionally essential amino acid with anabolic and immune system supportive effects. It is required for growth, immune function, wound healing and many aspects of protein metabolism. Arginine is necessary for the production of growth hormone. It is also a precursor for nitric oxide, a critical substance that helps regulate the function of cardiovascular, nervous and immune systems and which is essential for muscle growth.Arginine is essential for sperm formation, so it plays a vital role in male fertility.

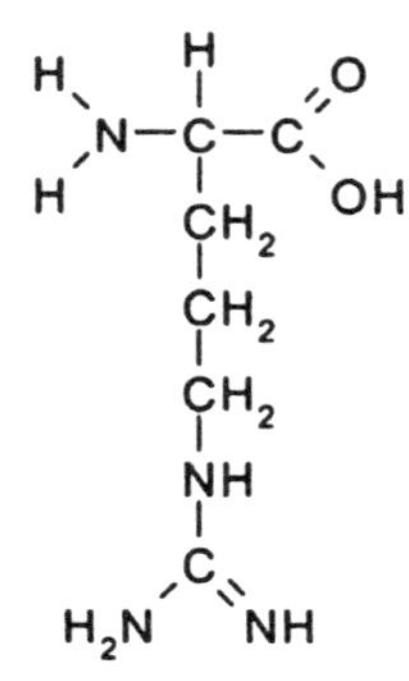

Fig. Arginine

Arithmetic average roughness (Ra) The arithmetic average height of roughness component irregularities from the mean line measured within the sample length (L).

Aromatherapy Uses essential oils from flowers, trees, roots, herbs, berries and fruits, to treat emotional disorders such as stress and anxiety as well as a wide range of other ailments and to promote physical, mental and emotional wellness. Oils are either massaged into the skin in diluted form, inhaled, placed in baths, or applied on and around the body. Aromatherapy is often used in conjunction with massage therapy, acupuncture, reflexology, herbology, chiropractic and other wholistic healing.

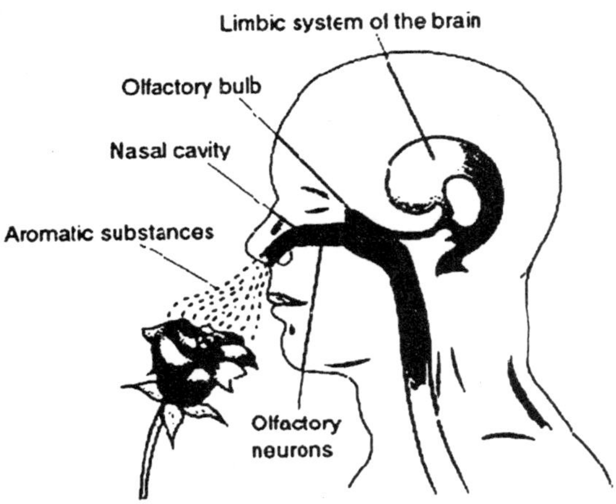

Fig. Aromatherapy

Array A lead consisting of three electronically common elements joined at a yoke. The SQ array is used as part of an AICD system.

Arrest The stopping of a function. Cardiac arrest is the stopping of the heartbeat and the heart's function.

Arrhythmia Arrhythmia is an irregular or missed heartbeat.

Arrow Keys A set of 4 keys at the right of the computer keyboard that can be used to control the movement of the cursor on the screen up, down, left, and right.

Arteriogram A radiograph of arteries after they have been injected with a contrast material.

Artery A blood vessel that carries blood away from the heart

Arthr(o) (prefix) Joint; articulation.

e.g. arthrolith - a calculous deposit within a joint.

Arthritis Arthritis is chronic condition marked by inflammation, pain and stiffness in the joints. More than 100 diseases fall under the arthritis category, each with its own subset of symptoms, causes and complications.

Arthrogram A roentgenographic record of a joint after the introduction of contrast material.

ArthrographyA radiographic examination of a joint after the injection of a dye-like contrast material and/or air to outline the soft tissue and joint structures on the images

Articular cartilage Usually hyaline, located on the articular surfaces of bones within a synovial joint.

Articular fossa A hollow of depressed area within a joint.

Articular surface The surfaces of bone or cartilage which form a joint.

Artificial Insemination (AI) More recently known as intrauterine insemination, or IUI. Using a catheter, doctors put sperm directly into a woman's uterus near a Fallopian tube.

Artificial rupture of the membranes (AROM) This when your caregiver breaks your bag of waters for you. They use a plastic tool called an amniotome that looks a little like a very long crochet hook. It doesn't hurt because there are no nerve endings in the amniotic membranes.

Artificial sphincter Sometimes complicated cases of incontinence require implantation of a device known as an artificial urinary sphincter. People who might benefit from this treatment include those who are incontinent after surgery for prostate cancer or stress incontinence, trauma victims and people with congenital defects in the urinary system. The artificial sphincter has three components, including a pump, balloon reservoir, and a cuff that encircles the urethra and prevents urine from leaking out. The cuff is connected to the pump, which is surgically implanted in the scrotum (in men) or labia (in women). The pump can be activated (usually by squeezing or pressing a button) to deflate the cuff and permit the bladder to empty. After a brief interval, the cuff refills itself and the urethra is again closed. Because the artificial sphincter is an implant, it is subject to the risks common to implants, such as infection, erosion (breaking down of tissue) and mechanical malfunction. Yet with appropriate pre-surgical evaluation, operative techniques and postoperative follow-up, many problems can be avoided and incontinent patients can experience an improved quality of life with this device.

Arytenoid cartilage Paired cartilage of the larynx which articulates with the lamina of the cricoid cartilage.

Ascending aorta The portion of the aorta that originates from the left ventricle and gives rise to the right and left coronary arteries.

Ascending colon The portion of the large intestine that is on the right side of the abdomen.

Ascites Fluid that fills the abdomen when the liver is not functioning properly.

Ascomycetes A family of fungi marked by long spore-containing cells. Form sexual spores called ascospores, which are contained within a sac (a capsule structure). Ergot, truffles, some molds of the genera Neurospora and Aspergillus, and yeasts belong to this category.

Ascorbic Acid Also known as Vitamin C. A water soluble vitamin, and an antioxidant. Your body cannot store Vitamin C, so you must supplement it regularly. It is not resistant to heat, so cooking will destroy it. Vitamin C functions primarily in the formation of collagen, the chief protein substance of your body's framework. It also helps in the production of vital body chemicals. Vitamin C also is a detoxifier (helping cleanse your body of toxins).

Asepsis A condition in which living pathogenic (causing or capable of causing disease) organisms are absent.

Aseptic Marked by or relating to asepsis.

Aseptic processing Processing conditions designed to achieve a sterile product.

Aseptic processing area Area in which sterile product is formulated, filled into containers, and sealed.

Aseptic transfer (in Isolators) The key issue in all contained aseptic environments. Aseptic transfer is essential for change parts, components, and even product to enter and exit an isolator system without sterility challenges. There are an increasing number of ways to make an aseptic transfer. The following is a brief list of some of the key techniques:

1. Alpha Beta Systems Double Door Systems: also called RTPs (Rapid Transfer Ports) and HCT (High Containment Transfer). When mated, the two ports act as one door, protecting the internal and external environments.

2. Alpha Beta Dry Heat Sterilized: similar to Alpha Beta port with the additional safeguard of a heat sterilized seal.

3. UV and Pulsed Light: light sterilization/ sanitization. Sterilizing the system by making use of a wide spectrum of light within the transfer chamber.

4. One Shot Systems: basically, two halves coming together. Similar to an Alpha Beta port but simpler, cheaper, and capable of only a single connection.

5. Heat Welded Bag Systems: passed in or passed out using a continuous polyethylene

liner which is heat sealed and cut to maintain the integrity of the internal and external environments.

6. Steam Sterilized: the liquid component or powder path is clean steam sterilized after connection and prior to transfer.

7. Autoclave/Depyrogenation/Dryheat: pass through for batch. Use of conventional autoclave to sterilize a canister provided with an Alpha Beta port and filters to allow the passage of steam and safe aspiration on cooling. Depyrogenation/Dryheat uses dry heat to sterilize and at sufficient temperature depyrogenate components, typically glassware, in a batch oven

8. Depyrogenation Tunnel: standard volume glassware entry. Depyrogenation/Dry heat uses dry heat to sterilize and at sufficient temperature to depyrogenate components, typically glassware, in a tunnel allowing continuous input.

Aspartame An artificial sweetener. Known by the trade name NutraSweet, it is an artificial sweetener. Certain people should avoid products that contain Aspartame. They are people who cannot metabolize the amino acid Phenylalanine, which is an ingredient in aspartame; and people who are suspectable to headaches.

It is nearly 200 times sweeter than sugar. Aspartame is produced from the amino acids L-asartic acid and L=phenylalannine. It has been approved for use in certain goods since 1981. Heat causes aspartame to lose its sweetness, therefore, you can't bake with it. Unlike some sweetners, it has no aftertaste.

Aspiration Aspiration is swallowing or sucking a foreign body or fluid, such as vomit, into an airway.

Aspirin Can reduce soreness after a hard workout, or lower your risk of heart disease. Can also reduce your risk for throat or stomach cancer.

Assay A technique (test) for measuring a biological response or for determining characteristics such as composition, purity, activity, and weight.

Assessment A system of evaluation of professional accomplishments using defined criteria and usually including an attempt at measurement either by grading on a rough scale or by assigning numerical value. The purpose of assessment in an educational context is to make a judgment about the level of skills or knowledge, to measure improvement over time, to evaluate strengths and weaknesses, to rank students for selection or exclusion, or to motivate. Assessment should be as objective and reproducible as possible. A reliable test should produce the same or similar scores on two or more occasions or if given by two or more assessors. The validity of a test is determined by the extent to which it measures whatever it sets out to measure. One can distinguish three types of assessment:

Formative assessment is testing that is part of the developmental or ongoing teaching/learning process. It should include delivery of feedback to the student.

Summative assessment is testing which often occurs at the end of a term or course, used primarily to provide information about how much the student has learned and how well the course was taught.

Criterion-referenced assessment refers to testing against an absolute standard such as an individual's performance against a benchmark.

Assimilation The formation of cellular material utilizing small food molecules and energy.

Assistant Director of Nursing (ADON) A registered nurse who acts as the assistant to the Director of a facility's nursing services.

Assistant Midwife A midwife who works as an assistant to the primary midwife. In a country, province or state where midwifery is not recognized by law, a midwife who works under the supervision of another health care professional.

Assisted Living A facility which provides care to residents who cannot live independently, but who do not require around-the-clock nursing care or extensive medical supervision. Defined broadly, assisted living is any group residential program not licensed as a nursing home that can respond to unscheduled needs for assistance. ALFs are usually more residential than nursing homes, and emphasize privacy and autonomy while providing supervision and oversight. Generally, residents of an ALF need assistance with Activities of Daily Living (ADLs), but are otherwise able to care for themselves. ALFs do not provide a level of care sufficient to be certified as Medicare providers. Terminology varies from state to state, and a facility which is called an Assisted Living Facility in one state might be called other things in other states, i.e. a Residential Care Facility (RCF), a Board and Care Home, a Domiciliary Care Facility, an Adult Care Home, or a Community-Based Care Facility.

Assisted Reproductive Technologies (ART) The new forms of fertility treatment incorporate many methods of sperm retrieval and preparation. Once the sperm have been processed to ensure optimal fertilizing potential, they are used in a variety of procedures that aid the process of conception. These procedures include artificial insemination (AI), in vitro fertilization (IVF), and sperm microinjection techniques.

Assisted Resident An assisted resident is a person who can only afford to pay a small accommodation bond or charge because, among other things, the value of their assets is less than four times the basic age pension. Providers receive an additional supplement for assisted residents.

Assistive Devices Tools designed to substitute for missing or impaired body functions. Examples include special telephones for people with hearing impairments, walking aids, elevated toilet seats, communication devices, and reachers which allow people in wheelchairs to reach objects in high places.

Associate of the college of optometrists in vision development Individual who is licensed optometrist for at least two years and provides developmental and behavioral vision care services including vision therapy. Associate members must obtain at least 10 hours of continuing education annually in functional / developmental/ behavioral / rehabilitation vision care. The optometrist has not sat for his/her certification exams, therefore is not Board Certified in Vision Development and Therapy.

Association Linking a document with the program that created it so that both can be opened with a single command. For example, double-clicking a DOC file opens Word for Windows and loads the selected document.

Asthenopia Eyestrain, symptoms include excessive tearing, itching, burning, visual fatigue, and headache. It can be caused from an uncorrected refractive error, accommodation (eye focusing) disorder, binocularity (eye teaming) disorder, or by extended, intense use of the eyes.

Asthma Asthma is a disease marked by recurrent attacks of shortness of breath and difficulty breathing. Often caused by an allergic reaction.

Astigmatism Light rays entering the eye do not all meet at the same point (similar to a frayed string), which results in blurred or distorted vision. An abnormally shaped cornea typically causes this condition. Occasionally astigmatism exists in the lens of the eye. This condition is corrected by a cylindrical (toric) eyeglass or contact lens.

Astrocyte Largest and most numerous type of neuroglial cell within the central nervous system. These cells of ectodermal origin are of two types; fibrous and protoplasmic astrocytes

Asynchrony A condition in which the heart fails to maintain a normal time sequence between atrial and ventricular contractions.

At rest HVAC room condition when unmanned, and without machinery operating. Previously called "static condition".

Atherectomy A minimally invasive CAD intervention procedure which involves the excision and removal of blockages by catheters with miniature cutting systems. not found in EuroDicautom

Atherosclerosis Narrowing or blockage of arteries caused by a buildup of fat (cholesterol) within the artery wall. The build-up is sometimes referred to as "plaque."

Atlas and axis C1 (the atlas) sits atop C2 (the axis) and can rotate about the dens - a vertical post from C2.

FX C2 Axis.

Atmospheric tank (fire code) A storage tank designed to operate at pressures from atmospheric through 0.5 pounds per square inch (psig) (3.4 kPa).

Atomic absorption spectrophotometry A highly sensitive instrumental technique for identifying and measuring metals in water.

Atonic colon Lack of normal muscle strength in the large intestine; caused by overuse of laxatives or by a disease called Hirschsprung's disease.

Atonic uterus An atonic uterus is flaccid; relaxed; lack of tone.

ATP (Adenosine Triphosphate) The body's energy currency, released when fuel molecules are broken down.

Atresia Lack of a normal opening, from the esophagus, the intestines, or the anus.

Atria The upper chambers of the heart, specifically the right atrium and left atrium. The 2 atria collect blood as it comes into the heart and fill the ventricles (lower chambers) with blood.

Atrial appendage The ear-shaped appendage of either atrium of the heart.

Atrio ventricular (AV) node A cluster of muscle cells located in the wall between the right and left atrium, just above the ventricles. This part of the heart's electrical pathway helps carry signals from the atria to the ventricles.

Atrio ventricular synchrony AV synchrony - The normal physiologic sequencing of atrial contraction followed, after a fraction of a second, by a ventricular contraction.

Atrium One of two upper chambers of the heart (plural: atria). The atria collect blood as it comes into the heart and fill the lower chambers (ventricles) with blood.

Atrophy A wasting of tissues, organs or the entire body; caused by death and resorption of cells, diminished cellular proliferation, pressure, ischemia, malnutrition, decreased function or hormonal changes.

Au Pair A foreign national who lives with an American family for up to a year, and in exchange for room, board, and a small stipend, helps with childcare and housework. She may or may not have any previous experience caring for children, unlike nannies, who usually do.

Audit comment A feature of the audit trail that aids both originator and reviewer in understanding why the originator performed a specific action. CFR 21 Part 11 does not require entering the reason for a record change, but some predicate rules (such as GLPs) do expect an explanation. It is important that the user interface for entering audit comments prevents users from changing the audit trail itself.

Audit trail A computer-generated and time-stamped record of who did what, when. CFR 21 Part 11 requires audit trails to be generated independently of operators. An audit trail must capture all activities related to creating, modifying, and destroying records on a system.

Auger electron spectroscopy (AES) An alternative surface analysis that can detect all elements with an atomic number greater than that of helium with the additional ability to analyze sub micron-diameter features. It is not as quantitative as ESCA and cannot determine the chemical state of an element. The primary advantage of Auger is that when combined with etching, a chemical depth profile can be measured rapidly and can image the distribution on the surface of spatial limitation resolution of 100 to 1,000 angstroms (depending on the equipment capability).

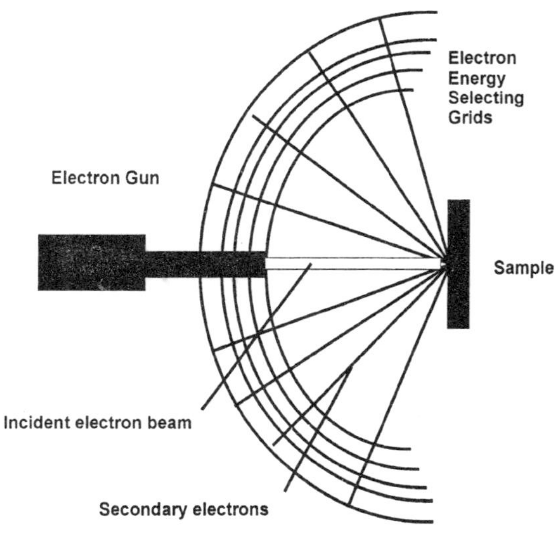

Fig. Auger electron spectroscopy

Austenite A face-centered cubic crystal with high solubility for carbon (about 2%); an allotropic form of iron resulting from steel being heated above the transformation temperature.

Autegoneous weld A weld made by fusion of the base material without the addition of filler.

Authentication The process of identifying a person, system, or company sufficiently to allow access to a system or part of a system.

Authentication mechanisms Also known as authority checks, or authorized signers are mechanisms distinct from authorization that grants or denies access to a network resource, authentication programs are used by system administrators to establish and verify as conclusively as possible that a person logging in to the network is who he or she claims to be. FDA says that "authority checks" are to "ensure that only authorized individuals can use the system, electronically sign a record, access the operation or computer system, input or output device, alter a record, or perform operations".

Autoclave An apparatus into which moist heat (steam) under pressure is introduced to sterilize or decontaminate materials placed within (e.g. filter assemblies, glassware, etc.). Steam pressure is maintained for pre-specified times and then allowed to exhaust. There are two types of autoclaves:

1. Gravity displacement autoclave: this type of autoclave operates at 121°C. Steam enters at the top of the loaded inner chamber, displacing the air below through a discharge outlet.

2. Vacuum autoclave: this type of autoclave can operate with a reduced sterilization cycle time. The air is pumped out of the loaded chamber before it is filled with steam.

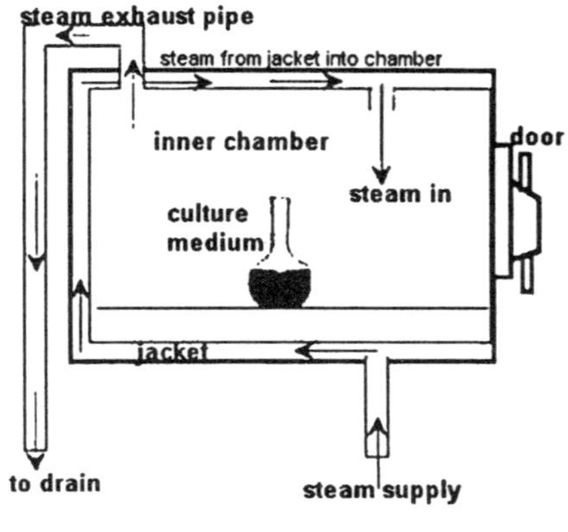

Fig. Autoclave

Autoexec.bat In DOS and Windows based PCs, the file that contains a list of commands that are automatically executed on system start up.

Autoimmune diseases A host of diseases caused by the immune system mistakenly attacking the body's own cells, tissues and organs. Auto-immune diseases are marked by inflammation, but symptoms and complications vary greatly. Some of the most common auto-immune diseases are rheumatoid arthritis, lupus, scleroderma, multiple sclerosis and diabetes mellitus.

Autologous Derived from the same individual.

Automated refractor Also called auto refractor. This method determines the eye's refractive error and the best corrective lenses to be prescribed by using a computerized device that varies its optical power mechanically and prints out the results.

Automated system Any facility system or piece of equipment that is controlled with limited or no manual intervention.

Automatic implantable cardioverter defibrillator (AICD) A surgically implanted device that monitors the heartbeat and delivers electrical impulses to correct an abnormal rhythm and restore a regular heartbeat. The AICD system usually consists of an implanted pulse generator and one or more leads. The system is adjusted using an external programming device.

Automatic welding Welding with equipment that performs the welding operation without adjustment of the controls by a welding operator. The equipment may or may not perform the loading and unloading of the work.

Autoradiography A technique that uses X-ray film to visualize radioactively labeled molecules or fragments of molecules; used in analyzing length and number of DNA fragments after they are separated by gel electrophoresis.

Autosome A chromosome not involved in sex determination. The diploid human genome consists of 46 chromosomes, 22 pairs of autosomes, and 1 pair of sex chromosomes.

Autotrophs One of two categories in which microorganisms are classified on the basis of their carbon source. Autotrophs use carbon dioxide as a carbon source.

Av groove A groove on the surface of the heart which separates the atria from the ventricles.

Avatar In multiuser internet environments and games, an avatar is a user's own graphical representation.

Avoidable Decline Reduction or loss of a resident's (patient's) physical, mental, emotional, cognitive, or functional well being attributable to actions or lack of actions by a facility.

Axial Plane (Transverse Plane) A horizontal plane; divides the body or any of its parts into upper and lower parts.

Axial view The axial imaging plane is a "cross-section" - perpendicular to the long axis of a cylinder.

Note For vertebrate anatomy, this is parallel to the floor for humans (bipedal) and perpendicular to the floor for quadruped.

Axilla The region of the body commonly referred to as the armpit.

Axillary Relating to the axilla.

Axillary vein The continuation of the basilic vein which ends at the lateral border of the first rib, becoming the subclavian vein.

Axis The alignment of the len's cylindrical part; used for correcting astigmatism. This measurement is given in degrees. The values are typically from 90 degrees to 180 degrees.

Axon The process of a neuron that conducts impulses away from the cell body. Typically a single process, extending for variable distances, enveloped in a myelin sheath and establishing specialized junctional contacts.

Ayurvedic medicine practiced in India for over 5,000 years. Ayurvedic tradition holds that illness is a state of imbalance among the body's systems and can be detected through such diagnostic procedures as reading the pulse and observing the tongue. Nutritional counseling, massage, natural medications, meditation and other modalities are used to address a spectrum of ailments, from allergies to AIDS.

Azoospermia The complete absence of sperm. It can result from obstruction of the vas deferens (the duct that takes the sperm from the testicles to the urethra) or from failure of the testicles to produce sperm.

Azygoesophageal recess An area of lucency on the frontal chest image, representing a portion of the Right lower lobe that crosses the midline anterior to the spine, and ends at the azygous vein and or the esophagus.

Azygous arch The point where the azygous vein arches over the root of the right lung to empty into the superior vena cava.

Azygous lobe A normal variant produced by an indentation in the R. upper lobe of the lung by four layers of pleura (two layers of visceral pleura and two layers of parietal pleura). It is produced by invagination of the azygous vein. This is not a true lobe, since it does not have a separate bronchus. Azygous Lobe.

Azygous vein A vertical paraspinal vein that connects the superior venae cava with abdominal veins.

B

B-1 (Thiamin) A vitamin which maintains energy levels, supports brain function (memory). Aids in digestion. Necessary for metabolism of sugar and starch to provide energy. Maintains a healthy nervous system. Alcohol can cause deficiencies of this vitamin and all the B-complex vitamins.

B-12 (Cobalamin) Necessary for carbohydrate, protein and fat metabolism. Important to amino acid and fatty acid synthesis; essential for hemoglobin and nerve cell growth and maintenance. The anti-stress vitamin, sometimes prescribed for stress reduction.

B-2 (Riboflavin) A vitamin which helps with energy production and amino acid production. Helps body obtain energy from protein, carbohydrates, and fats. Helps maintain good vision and healthy skin.

B-3 (Niacin) A vitamin Important in carbohydrate metabolism, formation of testosterone and other hormones, formation of red blood cells and maintaining the integrity of all cells. Helps body utilize protein, fats, and carbohydrates. Necessary for a healthy nervous system and digestive system. It also lowers elevated blood cholesterol levels when taken in large amounts of more than 1,000 milligrams a day.

B-5 (Pantothenic Acid) A vitamin which supports carbohydrate, protein and fat metabolism; hemoglobin synthesis. Helps release energy from protein, carbohydrates, and fat. Needed to support a variety of body functions, including the maintenance of a healthy digestive system.

B-6 (Pyridoxine) A vitamin which supports glycogen and nitrogen metabolism; production and transport of amino acids; production and maintenance of red blood cells (hemoglobin) Essential for the body's utilization of protein. Needed for the production of red blood cells, nerve tissues, and antibodies. Women taking oral contraceptives have lower levels of B-6.

Baby Blues Mild depression that may last a couple of weeks following childbirth, usually the result of dramatic hormonal swings and the letdown after the excitement of labor and birth.

BAC (bacterial artificial chromosome) A vector used to clone DNA fragments (100-kb to 300-kb insert size; average, 150-kb) in E. Coli cells. Based on naturally occurring F-factor plasmid found in the bacterium E. coli.

Back labor Back labor is when the pain of labor is felt in the lower back.

Back up copy A magnetic copy of data, software, user-developed application, or operating parameters associated with an automated system and not considered the original.

Background contamination Contamination introduced accidentally in reagents, dilution water, solvents, rinse water, etc., which can be confused with constituents in samples being analyzed.

Background environment The environment that surrounds a critical area.

Background Operation A job performed by a program when another program is in the active window. For example, printing, or creating a backup, can be done by Windows 98 as a background operation.

Backup To create a copy of a disk's contents on another location for safe keeping. Since hard drives are not infallible, it is recommended that you backup its contents regularly.

Backward compatibility A new version of a computer program that can use files and data created with an older version of the same program. A computer is said to be backward compatible if it can run the same software as the previous model. Backward compatibility is important because it eliminates the need to start over when you upgrade to a newer product, but is sometimes sacrificed in favor of a new technology.

Backwash The countercurrent flow of water through equipment, usually to clean or to recover performance, such as in a resin bed (flow-in at the bottom of the exchanger unit and out at the top) to clean and reclassify the bed after exhaustion. This process of reversing flow may also be applied to filters in order to force contaminants out of plugged pores and passages.

Bacteria The plural of Bacterium.

Bactericide An agent that kills vegetative bacteria but not mycobacteria or spores.

Bacteriophage A virus that exclusively infects bacteria. A protein coat surrounds the genome (DNA or RNA). One of the bacteriophages most extensively studied is the lambda phage, which is also one of the most important viral vectors used in rDNA work. Lambda promoters have been used to express eukaryotic proteins in E.coli.

Bacteriostatic Inhibiting growth of bacterial organisms without necessarily killing them or their spores.

Bacteriostatic water For Injection, water that serves the same purposes as Sterile Water for Injection, it meets the same standards, with the exception that it may be packaged in either single-dose or multiple-dose containers of not larger than 30-mL size.

Bacterium Any of a large group of microscopic organisms having round, rod-shaped, spiral, or filamentous unicellular or noncellular bodies that are often aggregated into colonies, are enclosed by a cell wall or membrane (prokaryotes), and lack fully differentiated nuclei. Bacteria range in size from 0.4μm to 2.0μm and may exist as free-living organisms in soil, water, organic matter, or as parasites in the live bodies of plants. Some are disease producing, but most perform necessary functions such as digestion, fermentation, and nitrification. Most of the forms are variously grouped under generic names such as: Alcaligenes, Dialister, Escherichia, Klebsiella, Kurthia, Pasteurella, Salmonella, and Shigella.

Barometer Instrument used to measure atmospheric pressure.

Bag of waters The bag of waters is the sac that surrounds baby inside the uterus. It contains the baby, the placenta and the amniotic fluid.

Bandwidth Maximum rage of signal frequencies, amount of data, or number of users a data carrier can handle.

Bariatric referring to surgery for the purpose of inducing weight loss.

Barium A liquid used to coat the inside of organs so they will show up on an x-ray.

Barium enema A procedure done to evaluate the large intestine for abnormalities. A fluid called barium that shows up well on x-rays is given into the rectum as an enema. An x-ray of the abdomen shows strictures (narrowed areas), obstructions (blockages), and other problems.

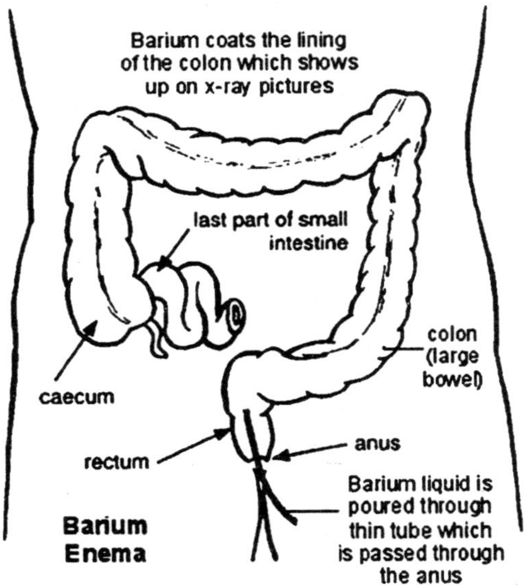

Fig. Barium enema

Barrett's esophagus A condition in which normal cells that line the esophagus, called squamous cells, turn into abnormal cells, called specialized columnar cells. Damage to the lining of the esophagus causes the cells to change; often occurs with long-term acid reflux.

Barrier isolator A containment device that utilizes barrier technology for the enclosure of a controlled workspace. There are two main types of isolator: 1. Type 1 Isolator: An isolator designed to protect the product from process-generated and external factors that would compromise its quality.

2. Type 2 Isolator: An isolator designed to protect the product from process-generated and external factors that would compromise its quality and to protect the operator from hazards associated with the product.

Barrier technology The technology of using separating environments, whether protecting the world from a product or the product from the world. Containment, barrier isolation and isolation all refer to the same technology, which is enclosing an environment. There are, however, some redefining terms that are gaining favor: 1. Containment - protect the world from the product (as in the case of highly potent compounds or a toxic).

2. Isolation - protect the product from the world (as in the case of a sterile product).

Basal Body Temperature (BBT) The temperature of your body upon first waking up in the morning. The basal body temperature rises by about 1/2 to 1 1/2 degrees around ovulation, which is how many women determine when they're fertile.

Basal ganglia Subcortical masses of grey matter (nuclei) located within the medullary center of each cerebral hemisphere. Usually includes the caudate nucleus, putamen, globus pallidus, amygdala and claustrum. The ter m is now used to refer to the corpus striatum, subthalamic nucleus and substantia nigra.

Base An electropositive element or radical that unites with an acid to form a salt. Or, a substance that when dissolved in water, dissociates to produce one or more hydroxyl ions (OH-).

Base down (BD) prism A wedge-shaped lens which is thicker on one edge than the other. The thicker edge (base) is turned down. Prisms bend light (opposite direction from its thicker end) so the base-down prism turns the light upward thus causing the eye to also move up. This prism is used to measure an eye misalignment and/or treat a binocular dysfunction (eye teaming problem). Prisms are sometimes added to glasses to help improve eyesight due to a misalignment or visual field loss.

Base In (BI) prism A wedge-shaped lens which is thicker on one edge than the other. The thicker edge (base) is turned inward, closest to the nose. Prisms bend light (opposite direction from its thicker end) so the base-in prism turns the light outward (toward the ear) thus causing the eye to also move outward. This prism is used to measure an eye misalignment and/or treat a binocular dysfunction (eye teaming problem). Prisms are sometimes added to glasses to help improve eyesight due to a misalignment or visual field loss.

Base out (BO) prism A wedge-shaped lens which is thicker on one edge than the other. The thicker edge (base) is turned outward, closest to the ear. Prisms bend light (opposite direction from its thicker end) so the base-out prism turns the light inward (toward the nose) thus causing the eye to also move inward. This prism is used to measure an eye misalignment and/or treat a binocular dysfunction (eye teaming problem). Prisms are sometimes added to glasses to help improve eyesight due to a misalignment or visual field loss.

Base pair (BP) Two nucleotides that are in different nucleic acid chains and whose bases pair by hydrogen bonding. In DNA, the nucleotide bases are adenine (A) that always pairs with thymine (T) and guanine (G) which pairs with cytosine (C). In RNA molecules, adenine (A) joins the uracil (U). Two strands of DNA are held together in the shape of a double helix by the bonds between these pairs.

Base sequence Analysis A method, sometimes automated, for determining the base sequence.

Base up (BU) prism A wedge-shaped lens which is thicker on one edge than the other. The thicker edge (base) is turned up. Prisms bend light (opposite direction from its thicker end (base)) so the base-up prism turns the light downward thus causing the eye to also move down. This prism is used to measure an eye misalignment and/or treat a binocular dysfunction (eye teaming problem). Prisms are sometimes added to glasses to help improve eyesight due to a misalignment or visual field loss.

Baseline In some analytical procedures a sample is dissolved in water or combined with other reagents for analysis. A "blank" or standard consisting of the same reagents may be analyzed without sample present. This provides a comparative reference point, or baseline, so that the test results can be attributed solely to the sample itself.

Baseline pharmaceutical engineering guides (ISPE) A series of industry publications developed in partnership with the US food and drug administration (FDA). Each volume in the series is a collaborative effort of industry leaders representing a broad cross-section of manufacturers and other industry experts. The Guides document current industry practice for facilities and systems used for production of pharmaceutical products and medical devices. They are intended to:

Establish a baseline approach to new and renovated facility design, construction, commissioning, and qualification that is based upon clear understanding of the type of product and its manufacturing process.

Prioritize facility design features based upon the impact on product and process.

Avoid unnecessary spending on facility features that do not contribute to consistent production of quality products.

The Guides include five product manufacturing operation based guides (vertical guides), and three support system/ function based guides (horizontal guides):

1. Volume I - Bulk Pharmaceutical Chemicals (1996)

2. Volume II - Oral Solid Dosage Forms (1998)

3. Volume III - Sterile Manufacturing Facilities (1999)

4. Volume VI - Biotech (in progress)

5. Volume -Oral Liquids and Aerosols

6. Volume IV - Water and Steam Systems (in progress)

7. Volume V - Commissioning and Qualification Guide (in progress)

8. Volume VII - Packaging and Warehousing

Basic Care Fee Residents of residential aged care homes will be asked to pay a daily fee for the care they receive. This includes a basic daily care fee for residents and a daily income-tested fee for some residents, depending on their income.

Basic science years A term that usually refers to the initial two years of a medical school's program. However, in some schools, this may entail more or less than two years. With the introduction of new learning methodologies such as Problem-Based Learning (PBL) and early exposure to patients, basic science learning has become more integrated with clinical instruction and the division between basic science years and clinical years has eroded.

Basidiomycetes Reproduce by basidiospores, which are extended from the stalks of specialized cells called the basidia. The class comprises Photobasidiomycetes (smuts and rusts) and the Hymenomycetes (mushrooms and puffballs).

Basilar artery The artery that originates from the junction of the two (L & R) vertebral arteries (VA) and runs along the dorsal clivus (base of the skull), anterior to the brainstem, before dividing in a terminal bifurcation into the two posterior cerebral arteries (PCA).

Basis of design A design document that describes what the purpose of a given system is and how the system will accomplish its required task. This document is created and approved before the issuance of bid specifications and is often used to develop them. Until the system is developed this is a conceptual document.

Basis pedunculi Ventral most part of the midbrain cerebral peduncle consisting of corticospinal, corticobulbar, and corticopontine fiber tracts. Also known as the crus cerebri.

Batch A specific quantity of material produced in a process or series of processes so that is expected to be homogeneous within specified limits. In the case of continuous production a batch may correspond to a defined fraction of the production, characterized by its intended homogeneity. The batch size may be defined either by fixed quantity or the amount produced in a fixed time interval.

Batch fermentation The process in which a fixed volume of sterile medium in a vessel is inoculated with a desired organism. The broth is fermented for a defined period to completion, without further additions of media. After discharging the batch, the fermenter is cleaned and rebatched with medium for another cycle. Two other types of fermentation cycles are fed batch and continuous.

Batchwise Control The use of validated in-process sampling and testing methods such that results prove the process has done what it purports to do for the specific batch concerned, assuming control parameters have been appropriately maintained.

Batch number A unique combination of numbers and/or letters which specifically identify a batch or lot and from which the production and distribution history can be determined.

Bathing One of the Activities of Daily Living (ADLs). The ability to wash oneself completely in a tub, a shower or by sponge bath, with or without the aid of equipment.

These activities include getting a basin of water, managing faucets, getting in and out of a tub or shower, and reaching head and body parts for soaping, rinsing and drying.

Baud Rate The speed at which telecommunicated data is transmitted, measured in bytes-per-second (BPS).

BBS Bulletin Board Systems. Users dial into the BBS or access it on the world wide web, and exchange information between users such as news, opinions, and information. Users can "talk" to other users who are on the BBS at the same time.

BCAA's (Branch Chain Amino Acids) Leucine, Valine, and Isoleucine are called "branch chain" aminos due to their molecular structure, and are important essential amino acids well known for their anticatabolic (muscle-saving) benefits. They are called BCAA's because they structurally branch off another chain of atoms instead of forming a line. Studies have shown that BCAA's postively affect skeletal muscle growth, enhance fat loss, help to stimulate protein synthesis and inhibit its breakdown, so BCAA's have powerful anabolic and anticatabolic effects on the body. They may also potentiate the release of some anabolic hormones, such as growth hormone. Regular ingestion of BCAA's help to keep the body in a state of postive nitrogen balance. In this state, your body much more readily builds muscle and burns fat. Studies have shown that athletes taking extra BCAA's have shown a loss of more bodyfat than those not taking BCAA's.

BCAAs are used as a source of energy for muscle cells. During prolonged exercise, BCAAs are released from skeletal muscles and their carbon backbones are used as fuel, while their nitrogen portion is used to form another amino acid, Alanine. Alanine is then converted to Glucose by the liver. This form of energy production is called the Alanine-Glucose cycle, and it plays a major role in maintaining the body's blood sugar balance.

B-Complex Vitamins A group of eleven known vitamins that work together in your body. All play vital roles in the conversion of food into energy. Essential for the normal functioning of the nervous system, and the maintenance of good digestion. Helps promote healthy skin, hair, and eyes. These are water soluble vitamins, which means they cannot be stored by your body and must be replaced every day.

Bed Column of carbon, sand, chromatography, or ion exchange resins through which a liquid passes during operation.

Bed depth The height of the exchange or capture material in a column after proper backwashing for effective operation.

Bed expansion The effect produced during backwashing; resin particles separate and rise in the column. Regulating backwash flow may control bed expansion caused by the increase in space between resin particles.

Bed Hold Reservation of a bed in a nursing facility, often during a therapeutic leave or other temporary absence from the facility. Some facilities also offer bed holds to prospective residents not yet ready to be admitted who want to be sure to have a bed available. Facilities often charge private-paying residents for bed holds at a lower rate than the standard bed rate.

Bed Reservation Benefit Long term care insurance terminology. Pays the cost of reserving a place in a care facility, a Bed Hold, if the person needs to be hospitalized during a covered stay.

Bedside teaching A part of clinical rounds where both student and instructor attends the patient's bedside to discuss the case and/or demonstrate a clinical procedure. This is the student's opportunity to see how the attending physician relates to the patient and to get hands-on instruction in interviewing a patient, physical examination, and counseling skills.

Behavior therapy/modification Aims at modifying behavior by reinforcing acceptable behavior and suppressing undesirable behavior. The therapist employs any of various techniques of reward and punishment including aversion therapy, desensitization, or guided imagery. The learning theory of the psychologist B.F. Skinner and others is the basis for most behavior therapies. In Skinner's principle of extinction, a behavior pattern that is not reinforced, or rewarded, will be extinguished or rendered inoperative. For example, if smoking is made unpleasant for the smoker, then the smoking habit may be curbed or given up. Behavior therapy is used in private and institutional therapy, in group and individual settings, to treat such disorders as drug addiction, alcoholism, and phobias.

Behavioral Intervention Non-drug interventions used to change the resident's (patient's) behavior or environment to lessen or accommodate the resident's (patient's) behavioral symptoms.

Behavioral optometrist also called functional optometrist or developmental optometrist An optometrist who specializes in all aspects of vision as it is related to an individual's development and to the role of vision in relation to reading, computer monitor use, and sports. The optometrist may use prescription lenses and/or vision therapy to improve an individual's visual function and performance. Behavioral optometry had its origins in orthoptics, which is a non-surgical treatment for strabismus, and in case analysis systems which were developed to resolve eyestrain symptoms that include excessive tearing, itching, burning, visual fatigue, and headache in nonstrabismic individuals. Behavioral optometry's emphasize of visual care is in prevention, remediation, rehabilitation, and enhancement.

Behavioral Techniques Different methods to help "retrain" the bladder and get rid of the urgency to urinate.

Beneficiary The individual or organization who is entitled to the benefits or proceeds of a will, trust or insurance policy.

Benefit Period The number of days or years of coverage included in an insurance policy. Many Long Term Care Insurance policies will offer between three and five years and some will offer lifetime benefits.

Medicare has a different definition of the term. In Medicare, a Benefit Period is a spell or period of illness. Medicare benefits, deductibles and co-insurance are based on a benefit period which begins when a coverable event happens, like a hospitalization, and ends when the person has gone 60 days without the need for coverable services.

Benefit Triggers Term used by insurance companies to describe when they will begin to pay benefits. In a Long Term Care Insurance policy, the triggers are generally tied to deficits in two or more Activities of Daily Living, or to Cognitive Impairment.

Benign Prostatic Hyperplasia A condition in which the prostate becomes enlarged as part of the aging process.

Benign Senescent Forgetfulness Age-related memory loss, which results from the slowing of neural processes with age.

Benign Tumor A tumor that is not cancerous.

Best evidence based assessment (BEBA) An evaluation performed by properly selected measurement methods under methodological rigor with which the instruments are constructed and administered; assessment must be congruent with evaluation questions and designed to demonstrate acquired competencies. Proper choice of measurement methods and construction of measurement instruments is a crucial step in the evaluation process because it determines the quality of data that will be collected securing robust and valid results. The methodological rigor is necessary for reliability and validity of the evaluation.

The best evidence-based assessment approach reflects a present focus on the quality of evaluation process and has been initiated by recent developments of so-called quantified tests, standardized patient examinations and computer case simulations and the use of relevant research data and information to validate the preferred assessment procedures.

Best evidence medical education (BEME) Methods and approaches used by teachers of medical education based on the best available evidence as opposed to opinion-based education. BEME should take into account these factors: how reliable the evidence is as well as its utility, extent, strength, validity and relevance. It calls for critical appraisal of available literature and existing databases and identifying any existing gaps.

Beta adrenergics Beta-adrenergics are substances that interfere with transmission of stimuli. They affect the autonomic nervous system.

Beta carotene A phytonutrient carotenoid with antioxidant and provitamin A activity. In addition to providing the body with a safe source of Vitamin A, beta carotene works with other natural protectors to defend your cells from harmful free radical damage. This is an important micrinutrient in helping the body with metabolic functions, such as recovery from exercise. Beta-Carotene is the plant derived form of Vitamin A, which is important for several bodily functiosn, including eyesight, immune function and even bone growth. Beta-Carotene is nontoxic. Good sources of Beta Carotene include Carrots, Sweet Potatoes, Pumpkins, Cantaloupes, Acricots, Spinach and Broccoli.

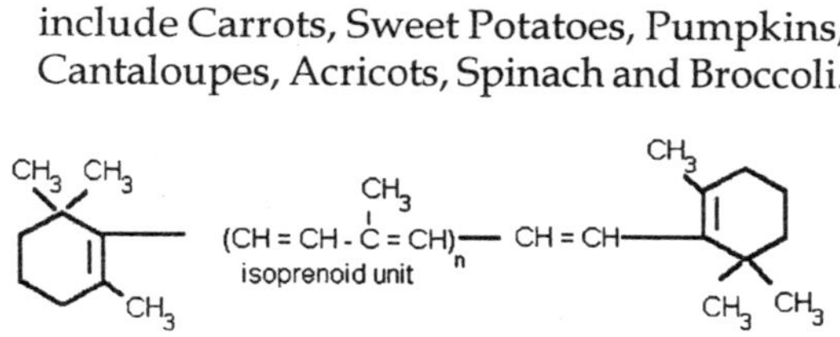

beta carotene

Fig. Beta carotene

Beta Hydroxy Beta-Methylbutyrate (HMB) It is a compound mande in the body and a metabolite of the essential amino acid Leucine. Studies have found that HMB has a decrease in stress-induced muscle protein breakdown. Studies also found that HMB may enhance increases in both muscle size and strength when combined with resistance training.

There are a number of theories why you may need HMB. The first, is that under stressful conditions, the body may not make enough HMB to satisfy the increased needs of tissues. It could also be that stress may alter enzymes or concentration of certain biochemicals that decrease normal HMB production. Another theory is that HMB may regulated enzymes sresponsible for muscle tissue breakdown.

Bi lateral integration/ gross motor coordination Visual guidance of body movements and the coordination between both sides of the body.

Bi ocularity Using both eyes, but not together as a team.

Bicornuate Uterus A uterus shape where the two ducts that form the uterus do not fuse and form a single open area, but remain two distinct uterine cavities that may be fused only at the bottom, or even half way. This condition significantly increases the chance for miscarriage and infertility. Depending on the severity of the shape, surgery may be an option to correct the uterus or improve the uterus' ability to carry a pregnancy to term.

Bifocal glasses Used to correct vision at two distances, composed of two ophthalmic lenses such as a plus lens for near vision and a minus lens for distance vision.

Bifurcation The point where a structure divides into two branches (e.g. the abdominal aorta bifurcates into the common iliac aa. and the trachea bifurcates into the L and R mainstem bronchi).

Bilateral A term describing a condition that affects both sides of the body or two paired organs, such as kidneys.

Bile A digestive fluid made by the liver and stored in the gallbladder which helps digest fats.

Bile ducts Tubes that take bile from the liver to the gallbladder and small intestine to aid in digestion.

Biliary atresia Bile ducts do not have normal openings, preventing bile from leaving the liver. This causes jaundice (a yellow skin color) and liver damage known as cirrhosis. Biliary atresia is a birth defect.

Biliary Colic syndrome of right upper quadrant abdominal pain seen after eating, associated with nausea; caused by gallstones.

Bilirubin Bilirubin is a breakdown product of pigment formed in the liver from hemoglobin during the destruction of red blood cells. Related terms: —Bilirubin count —Bilirubin lights —Jaundice

Binary Refers to the 'language' computers speak. Binary code (or machine language) consists only of zeroes and ones (i.e. a choice is either on or off), called bits. Letters and other information have a specific binary representation, made up of up to 8 bits (one byte).

Binary explosive An explosive material composed of separate components, each of which is safe for storage and transportation and would not in itself be considered as an explosive.

Binocular fusion dysfunction A clinical condition in which the eyes are not working as a team. Vision therapy is an effective treatment option.

Binocular vision The simultaneous use of the two eyes.

Binocularity The ability to use both eyes as a team and to be able to fuse (unite) two visual images into one, three-dimensional image .

Bioactivity A protein's ability to function correctly after it has been delivered to the active site of the body (in vivo).

Bioassay The determination of the biological activity of a substance (e.g. a drug) by observing its effect on an organism (or organ) compared to a standard preparation.

Bioaugmentation A strategy involved in bioremediation that increases the activity of an organism to break down or metabolize a pollutant. This involves reseeding a waste site with bacteria as they die.

Bioburden The level and type of microorganisms which may be present in raw materials, API (Active Pharmaceutical Ingredient) starting materials, intermediates, or APIs which have defined limits and should not affect the quality of the API. Bioburden should not be considered contamination unless the levels have been exceeded or defined objectionable organisms have been detected.

Biochemistry The study of chemical processes in living things. Despite the dramatic differences in the appearance of living things, the basic chemistry of all organisms is strikingly similar. Even tiny, one-celled creatures carry out essentially the same reactions that each cell of a complex organism, such as man, carries out.

Biocide An agent that can kill all pathogenic and non-pathogenic living organisms, including spores. More general than bacteriocide, biocide includes insecticides and any compound toxic to any living thing.

Biodegradable Material that can be broken down by biological action.

Bioenergetics Holds that repressed emotions and desires affect the body and psyche by creating chronic muscular tension and diminished vitality and energy. Through physical exercises, breathing techniques, verbal psychotherapy, or other forms of emotional-release work, the therapist attempts to loosen this character armor and restore natural well-being.

Bioequivalency A scientific basis on which generic and brand name drugs are compared with one another. Drugs are bioequivalent if they enter circulation at the same rate when given in similar doses under similar conditions.

Biofeedback Technique used especially for stress-related conditions such as asthma, migraines, insomnia and high blood pressure. Biofeedback is a way of monitoring minute metabolic changes in ones body with the aid of sensitive machines.

Biofield An energy field that suffuses living bodies and extends several inches beyond the body. This concept is employed in therapies such as healing touch, medical qigong, therapeutic touch, and reiki. In these therapies, the biofield from a practitioners hands is joined to the recipients biofield in order to treat an illness or to promote health. There is no consensus on what biofield is; some say it is spiritual energy, others say it is an electromagnetic field.

Biogenerator A contained system, such as a fermentor, into which biological agents are introduced along with other materials so as to effect their multiplication or their production of other substances by reaction with the other materials. Biogenerators are generally fitted with devices for regulation, control, connection, material addition, and material withdrawal.

Biohazard An infectious agent(s), or part thereof, presenting a real or potential risk to human, other animals, or plants, directly through infection or indirectly through disruption of the environment.

Bioinformatics The use of computers in the life sciences, electronic databases of genomes and protein sequences, and computer modeling of biomolecules and biologic systems.

Biologic A therapeutic agent derived from living things.

Biological barrier An impediment (naturally occurring or introduced) to the infectivity and/or survival of a microbiological agent or eukaryotic cell once it has been released into the environment.

Biological Impurities Impurities resulting from living matter (bacteria, virus, algae, protozoa, microfungi) and their by-products, including pyrogens (endotoxins).

Biological indicators Resistant microorganisms placed into or on various materials to confirm that a sterilization process is effective. They may for instance be placed within a filter in order to determine if a proposed autoclave cycle is effective. After autoclave, they are removed and culture tests are performed to see if the microorganisms were killed.

Biological Value (BV) An attempt to measure how efficiently protein us used in the body. Biological Value is derived from providing a measure intake of protein, then noting the nitrogen uptake versus nitrogen excretion. The actually process is much more complicated though. In theory, a BV value of 100 is maximal. Some studies claim they have a higher BV than 100, but they refer to a chemical score, not the biological value of whey.

Biologics "Any virus, therapeutic serum, toxin, antitoxin, vaccine, blood, blood component or derivative, allergenic product, or analogous product... applicable to the prevention, treatment, or cure of diseases or injuries of man...".

Biomass The entire assemblage of living organisms (both plant and animal), of a particular region, considered collectively.

Biometabolism Physical and chemical processes that occur within a cell or an organism, for example, the conversion of nutrients into energy.

Biometrics A method of verifying an individual's identity based on measurement of his/her physical feature(s) or repeatable action(s) where those features and/or actions are both measurable and unique to that individual. The main types of biometrics are: face recognition, finger scanning, hand geometry, finger geometry, iris recognition, palm, retina, signature, and voice recognition.

Bionics An interscience discipline for constructing artificial systems, which resemble or have the characteristics of living systems.

Biopharmaceuticals Ethical pharmaceutical drugs derived through bioprocessing.

Biophysical profile Biophysical profile is a method of evaluating a fetus before birth.

Bioprocess engineering Process that uses complete living cells or their components (e.g., enzymes, chloroplast) to effect desired physical or chemical changes.

Bioprocessing The creation of a product utilizing a living organism.

Biopsy The gross and microscopic examination of tissues or cells removed from a living patient, for the purpose of diagnosis or prognosis of disease, or for the confirmation of normal conditions.

Biopure water Water that is sterile, pyrogen free and has a total solids content of less than 1 ppm.

Bioreactor A closed system used for bioprocessing (flask, roller bottle, tank, vessel, or other container), which supports the growth of cells, mammalian or bacterial, in a culture medium. A bacterial reaction usually is said to take place in a fermenter, and cell culture in a bioreactor.

BIOS (Basic Input Output System)+A539. Provides a way for software to access computer hardware. This contains important information about the computer, i.e. the type and location of drives, amount of memory, etc.

Biosphere All the living matter on or in the earth, the oceans and seas, and the atmosphere.

Biosynthesis The production, by biological synthesis or degradation, of compounds by a living organism (e.g. amino acid synthesis, nucleotide synthesis).

Biotechnology An industry that creates, develops, and markets a variety of techniques that use living organisms, or substances from those organisms, to make or modify a product by microbial and biochemical processes. A common misconception is that biotechnology refers only to recombinant DNA or gene splicing work. Recombinant DNA is only one of the many techniques used to derive products for organisms, plants, and parts of both for the biotechnology industry. A list of areas covered by the term biotechnology would more properly include: plant tissue culture, cell fusion techniques (especially for the production of monoclonal antibodies), enzyme systems, plant breeding, meristem culture, fermentation, and others.

Biotin A vitamin that helps with energy metabolism, fatty acid and nucleic acid synthesis.

Biowaste Inactivation The inactivation or "killing" of biological organisms using heat or chemicals. This step is done at the end of the processing to ensure that there are no living organisms remaining in the effluent that is sent to the sanitary sewer system. Heat is usually applied at 130°C (266°F) for mammalian cells. Chemicals used include caustic or acid.

Birth Canal The passageway made up of the cervix, vagina, and vulva the baby travels through during birth.

Birth weight The first weight of the fetus or newborn obtained after birth. This weight is best measured within the first hour of life before significant postnatal weight loss occurs.

Birthing center A birthing center is a facility in which a woman labors, delivers and recovers in the same room. It may be part of a hospital or a freestanding unit. Also called birth centers.

Birthing room A place designed and equipped for women giving birth. Some are in hospitals, others are totally separate facilities.

Bit The smallest unit of information recognized by a computer and its related equipment.

Bitmap A data presentation format in which every pixel of an image is stored as bits in a file, each "mapped" to a specific area of the total image.

BLA (biologics license application) The required application for marketing a biologic product in the United States. Most biopharmaceuticals are biologics.

Bladder The musculomembraneous sac used for urine collection from the kidneys (via the ureters) and discharge through the urethra.

Bladder Training A behavioral technique that teaches the patient to resist or inhibit the urge to urinate, and to urinate according to a schedule rather than urinating at the urge.

Blank A preliminary analysis omitting only the sample to provide an unbiased reference point or baseline for comparison. It is important to minimize extraneous contamination that could be confused with constituents in the sample itself.

Blastomere Blastomere is what one of the cells egg divides into after it has been fertilized.

Blighted Ovum A condition where the egg creates a sac and the pregnancy seems to progress normally, but an ultrasound reveals that the baby never formed.

Blind weld A "blind weld" is defined as a pipe or tube joint welded automatically in which there is no physical way to inspect the weld either visually or with a borescope.

Blinding Clinical trial technique in which, to eliminate bias in a research study, subjects and/or clinical investigators remain unaware of which investigational product is provided.

Blood borne pathogens Infectious microorganisms that are carried in the blood of infected humans or animals and that can be transmitted through contact with infected blood, body fluids, tissues, or organs. Blood-borne pathogens are implicated in diseases such as malaria, syphilis, brucellosis, tuberculosis, hepatitis B, and AIDS (Acquired Immunodeficiency Syndrome). Workplace transmission of a blood-borne pathogen can occur via accidental inoculation with a contaminated "sharp" exposure through open cuts, skin abrasions, and mucous membranes of eyes and mouth indirect transmission (e.g., touching mouth, eyes, nose or open cuts with contaminated hands).

Blood corpuscle A cell that circulates in the blood.

Blood plasma Blood from which all blood corpuscles, with the exception of platelet cells, have been removed (e.g. by centrifugation) resulting in a clear, straw-colored fluid, which clots as easily as whole blood.

Blood platelets Small, disc-shaped, metabolically active cells circulating in the blood. They are essential in the blood clotting process since they aggregate to form a plug on the injured surface of the blood vessel.

Blood serum The liquid expressed from clotted blood or clotted blood plasma.

Bloody show Bloody show is a small amount of vaginal bleeding late in pregnancy; it often precedes labor.

Blowdown The bleeding-off of fixed quantities of accumulated feed water to reduce concentrated impurities. If these impurities are permitted to accumulate, they may pass through the distillation process and contaminate the distillate or foul the distillation system.

Blurred vision Lack of visual clarity or acuity.

BME (basic medium eagles) One of the most common tissue culture media composed of isotonic salts, carbohydrates and vitamins.

When combined with animal serum. BME is a good medium for cell proliferation.

Board and Care Home Residence, sometimes a single family home, which offers housing and personal care services for a small number of residents. Services like meals, supervision, and transportation are generally provided. In some states, this type of home is classified as an Assisted Living Facility.

BOD (biochemical oxygen demand) The amount of oxygen required to oxidize the dissolved organic matter in a water sample by aerobic (bacterial) decay. A measure of the oxygen depletion that would result from discharging organic impurities into a waterway.

Body mind centering Amovement-reeducation approach that explores how the body's systems contribute to movement and self-awareness. The approach also emphasizes movement patterns that develop during infancy and childhood. Incorporates guided movement, exercise, imagery and hands-on work.

Body of pancreas The mid portion of the pancreas. The pancreas has both endocrine ("internal") and exocrine ("external") glands, including the islets of Langerhans - cell clusters that produce insulin and the pancreatic acini that secrete pancreatic digestive juices for the small intestine.

Body of sternum The portion of the sternum between the angle of Louis and the xiphoid process.

Body oriented psychotherapy Seeks to enhance the psychotherapeutic process by incorporating a range of massage, bodywork and movement techniques. Acknowledging the mind-body link, practitioners may use light touch, soft or deep-tissue manipulation, breathing techniques, movement, exercise or body awareness techniques to help address emotional issues.

Bone Density Bone density is measured by the amount of mineral in bones. Loss of mineral matter in the bone is one of several factors that can make the bones more brittle, which can lead to osteoporosis. Bone density is measured by a test called dual energy X-ray absorptiometry (DXA).

Boot To start a computer. A "cold boot" refers to the process of turning a computer on at the power source (switching it on). A "warm boot" (or "re-boot") refers to, basically, restarting the operating system.

Boot Disk The disk on which the operating system is stored.

Boron It is a trace mineral. Studies show that Boron helps the body retain minerals, such as Calcium and Magnesium. Large amounts of Boron, over 10 milligrams a day, can be toxic, particularly to the organs that manufacture testosterone. You can find traces of Boron in all the food groups, even in wine, with the greatest concentration in prunes, raisins, parsley flakes, and almonds. A 1987 study showed that Boron could dramatically increase testosterone levels, however, the study was for postmenopausal women who had testosterone deficiencies. Once their boron-rich diets brought their testosterone levels back up to normal, those levels stabilized, and they didn't get any higher no matter how many more prunes or parsley flakes that they ate. Thus, it is somewhat unproven that boron can help build muscle mass by increasing your testosterone levels. However, a lack of boron in your diet may have a 'negative' impact on energy utilization.

Botryoid Shaped like a bunch of grapes.

Botulinum toxin type a (oculinum, botox) An injection of this poison has been used as an alternative to conventional surgery in selected strabismic patients. It causes a temporary paralysis of an extraocular muscle that leads to a change in eye position. This change has been reported to result in long-lasting and permanent alteration in eye alignment. Although one injection is often sufficient to produce positive results, one-third to one-half of patients may require additional injections. This technique has been most successful when used in adults with small-angle misalignments. It is not commonly used in children. This treatment is also used in patients who have blepharospam (an uncontrollable eye lid spasm).

Bougie Along tapered tube of soft plastic used in esophageal surgery to dilate strictures.

Bovine cartilage A source of mucopolysaccharides which have anti-inflamatory and joint protective properties.

Bovine Colostrum Usually from cows, a dairy product that has similar properties to human colostrum. Normally, adults cannot absorb colotrum's antobodies and growth factors the way a newborn can. But it still has superior nutritional values which may make it a useful supplement.

Bowel Small and large intestine.

Bowel movement Passage of stool (body wastes) from the large intestine through the rectum and anus.

BPC (bulk pharmaceutical chemical) A pharmaceutical product derived by chemical synthesis, in bulk form, for later dispensing, formulation or compounding, and filling in a pharmaceutical finishing facility.

Breakthrough Passage of a substance through a bed, filter, or process designed to eliminate it. For ion exchange processes, the first signs are leakage of ions (in mixed beds, usually Silica) and the resultant increase in conductivity. For organic removal beds, usually small, volatile compounds (Trihalomethanes (THMs) are common in activated carbon).

Brachiocephalic trunk (innominate) The first branch of the arch of the aorta which further divides into the right common carotid and right subclavian arteries. ("innominate" - literally "nameless").

Brachiocephalic vein Two veins formed at the root of the neck from the union of the ipsilateral internal jugular vein (IJV) and the subclavian veins. The two brachiocepalic veins later combine to form the superior vena cava (SVC).

Brachytherapy Involves the placement of tiny radioactive pellets into the Prostate gland. By utilizing ultrasound to place the seed pellets, damage to surrounding tissues is minimized. Approximately 13,500-16,000 rads of radiation energy is delivered directly to the Prostate. This procedure is performed on an outpatient basis. It is a one time procedure with very effective results. The 10-year follow-up outcome data parallels that of Radical Prostatectomy.

Brady pacing A method of treating a slow or irregular heartbeat by periodically stimulating the heart with small electrical pulses.

Bradycardia A slow heartbeat, typically less than 60 beats per minute. It may be caused by the sinoatrial node not working properly, or by a condition called heart block.

Brainstem Term that denotes the medulla, pons and midbrain exclusive of the cerebellum.

Brawny Edema The skin changes that occur in post-phlebitic extremities due to increased venous pressure and deposit of breakdown product of blood.

Braxton Hicks contractions Braxton-Hicks contractions are irregular, painless tightening of uterus during pregnancy.

Braze welding A welding process using nonferrous filler metal that has a melting point below that of the base metals, but above 427°C (800°F). The filler metal is not distributed in the joint by capillary attraction. This type of welding has been also called Bronze welding, a misnomer.

Brazing A metal joining process wherein coalescence is produced by use of a nonferrous filler metal having a melting point above 427°C (800°F), but lower than that of the base metals being joined. The filler metal is distributed between the closely fitted surfaces of the joint by capillary action.

Break point The point at which a person can no longer fuse (unite) two images into one. A blur point will occur before the this point.

Breakthrough The first appearance in the effluent of an ion-exchange unit of unadsorbed components similar to those that deplete the activity of the resin bed. Breakthrough indicates that the resin is exhausted and needs to be regenerated.

Breast A "modified sebaceous gland" in the superficial tissues of the anterior chest wall. Consists of a variable mixture of milk-producing glandular tissue, fat, and supporting connective tissue (Cooper's ligaments). Several major medical groups recommend routine mammograms for early detection of breast cancer. There is continued discussion about the benefits of screening mammograms.

Breast Pump A device to extract milk from a mother's breasts so she can feed her infant later with a bottle. Pumps range from inexpensive manual models to powerful industrial-strength machines that can pump both breasts at the same time within a few minutes.

Breath control shields Typically made of acrylic or plastic materials, shields protect product, equipment, or the work from particulate contamination expelled by people.

Breathwork General term for a variety of techniques that use patterned breathing to promote physical, mental and/or spiritual well-being. Some techniques use the breath in a calm, peaceful way to induce relaxation or manage pain, while others use stronger breathing to stimulate emotions and emotional release.

Breech Position When the baby's bottom or feet rather than the head face the mother's cervix as labor nears. Three to four percent of full-term babies are positioned this way.

Breech presentation Breech presentation is an abnormal position of the fetus where the buttocks or legs come into the birth canal ahead of the head.

Bregma Craniometric term denoting the point on surface of skull where the sagittal and coronal sutures meet.

Brewster stereoscope An instrument used in orthoptics/vision therapy to improve eye teaming skills and near focusing skills. It consists of two parallel viewing tubes with a +5.00 D lens. The distance from the target can be adjusted as well as the pupillary distance. The Bernell-O-Scope and Keystone Ophthalmic Telebinocular are designed essentially the same.

Broad spectrum Over a wide range. A broad-spectrum disinfectant is effective against a wide range of microorganisms including bacterial spores, mycobacteria, non-lipid and lipid viruses, fungi, and vegetative bacteria.

Bronchus intermedius On the right, the segment of bronchus between the origin of the upper lobe bronchus (of the lung) and the bifurcation into the middle and lower lobe bronchi.

Broth The liquid culture medium in which fermentation or cell culture takes place.

Brown Adipose Tissue (BAT) A type of specialized fat that is known to convert fat calories into heat, thereby disspating excess calories.

Browse To search through or examine a directory tree of files, directories, disks, workstations, workgroups, or domains. Often done via a "Browse" button in a dialog box.

Browser A software program that allows users to view content on the Internet and World Wide Web.

BSE (bovine spongiform encephalopathy) Sometimes called "Mad Cow Disease". A disease of cattle presumably caused by a virus or other unidentified entity that affects the brain and causes the cow to behave erratically. Prevalent in parts of Europe but not in the United States. BSE is a contaminant that is undesirable in bovine sera. It is not known whether the causative agent can be filtered out since the causative agent itself is not known. In humans, it is believed to cause Creutzfeld-Jacob, a disease affecting the nervous system.

Bubble point test A filter leakage test in which the filter is wetted and air pressure is applied and slowly increased until water is expelled from the largest pores and bubbles appear from a submerged tube in a downstream collection vessel. Vigorous bubbling, as opposed to a diffusional airflow or occasional bubbles, is indicative of reaching the bubble point. This visual test can be fairly accurate for low area filters, such as discs. When used to evaluate high area filters, it is subject to limitations in observation, test time, collection conditions, and pressurization rates. The bubble point test is not recommended for integrity testing of filter cartridges.

Buckwheat A plan native to Asia that has fragrant white flowers and small triangular seeds. The edible seeds are often ground into flour. According to animal studies, buckwheat is better than casein (a milk protein) for promoting muscle growth and body growth and decreasing blood lipds. For persons allergic to wheat gluten, it provides a gluten-free food with uses similar to gains. Roasted buckwheat is known as Kasha. Buckwheat is usually available as flour.

Buffer A storage device, or area on a storage device, which holds data temporarily, until needed for processing or printing. A buffer can also be used to aid communication between two devices with very different processing speeds (such as two modems, or the CPU and the printer).

Buffer prep Area Section of most biotech facilities devoted to the preparation of controlled bioburden buffer solutions for use in the chromatographic separation area of those facilities.

Bug An error in a computer program or system, or a malfunction in a computer hardware component. One of the final steps in writing a computer program is to debug it, or search and repair any obvious or common errors.

Bulk handling The transferring of flammable or combustible liquids from tanks or drums into smaller containers for distribution.

Bulk oxygen system An assembly of equipment, such as storage containers, pressure regulators, safety devices, vaporizers, manifolds, and interconnecting piping that has a storage capacity of more than 12,000 cubic feet (340 m^3) of oxygen at normal temperature and pressure, connected in service or ready for service, or more than 25,000 cubic feet (708 m^3) of oxygen, including unconnected reserve on hand at the site.

BVD (bovine viral diarrhea) Viral contaminant found in bovine sera. Able to be filtered out using 0.1 μm nylon filters.

Bovine Of, relating to, or from a cow: such as Bovine Blood: blood from a cow.

Byte An abbreviation for binary term. A storage unit capable of holding eight bits or the space required for a single letter or number, a single character.

C

C section A C-section is another term for a cesarean section (delivery), or a delivery of a baby through an abdominal incision rather than through the vagina.

Cache A special type of computer memory that operates at very high speed. It is similar to RAM but is much faster. It is usually used by the CPU as a storage place for processing instructions. When the computer is shut down any information held in the cache memory is lost. An area set aside in RAM or on a disk to save frequently or recently used data.

CACPs Community Aged Care Packages CACP's are coordinated packages of community care services to help people with complex care needs continue living in their own home. Each CACP is designed for an individual person and is based on their particular needs.

Caffeine Alkaloid that stimulates alertness and boosts energy. A herbal compound that enhances alertness and fights fatigue. Caffeine increases endurance during prolonged submaximal activity by increasing blood epinephrine (adrenaline) levels, thereby allowing fat cells to break down more readily during aerobic activity. Caffeine also makes a muscle contraction more forceful.

Calamus scriptorius The tapered caudal part of the fourth ventricle in the region of the vagal and hypoglossal trigones. Likened to the nib of a pen in shape.

Calcaneus The "heel bone" of the foot, located at the back of the tarsus.

Calcar avis Projection or eminence located along the medial wall of the occipital horn of the lateral ventricle caused by the deep calcarine fissure.

Calcitonin A hormone secreted by specialized cells in the thyroid gland, which results in lowering of the serum calcium level.

Calcium A metallic dyad element of a lustrous yellow color, symbol Ca, atomic number 20, atomic weight 40.09, melting point 810°, often found in water usually as dissolved calcium carbonate, chalk (CaCO3). Soluble in water, it causes hardness and subsequent scaling.

Calibration (ICH API defintion) The demonstration that a particular instrument or device produces results within specified limits by comparison with those produced by a reference or traceable standard over an appropriate range of measurements.

Call System A system to allow residents (patients) to communicate with a nurses' station from their rooms and from toilet and bathing facilities.

Calorie Any of several approximately equal units of heat, each measured as the quantity of heat required to raise the temperature of one (1) gram of water by °C from a standard initial temperature, specially from 3.98°C, 14.5°C, or 19.5°C, at a constant pressure of one (1) atmosphere. Also called "gram calorie", "small calorie".

The unit of heat equal to 1/100 the quantity of heat required to raise the temperature of one (1) gram of water from 0°C to 100°C at one (10 atmosphere pressure. Also called "mean calorie".

The unit required to raise the temperature of one (1) Kilogram of water by 1°C at one (1) atmosphere pressure. Also called "kilogram calorie", "large calorie".

Calorimetry Analytical method that measures heat loss or gain resulting from physical or chemical changes in a sample. Differential scanning calorimetry compares the results of heating a sample to those for heating a reference material. For example, a method to measure the temperature at which the sample crystallizes, changes phases, or decomposes.

Cancer A group of neoplastic diseases in which there is a transformation of normal cells into malignant cells. The cells proliferate in an abnormal way resulting in a malignant, cellular tumor.

Candida Yeast that causes irritation and infection, especially of the mucous membranes of the body such as the mouth, vagina, and anus.

Capacity (Facility) The maximum number of residents (patients) and other persons who may reside in the facility at any time under the terms of the facility license.

Capitation A program which reimburses providers and plans based on the number of persons under care, generally on a per member, per month (PMPM) basis. Payments are made at the same level, whether or not the member receives services during the month. Contrast capitation to fee-for-service, where payments are based on the actual units of service provided.

Caps Lock A key that toggles the keyboard between upper-case and lower-case modes. When caps lock is off, striking a key will produce a lower case letter, and holding down the 'shift' key while striking a key will produce a capital letter.

Capsid The external protein shell or coat of a virus particle.

Carbohydrate There are two basic forms of carbohydrates: Simple & Complex. Simple carbs are usually devoid of fiber and include such foods as refined sugars, fruit juices, and apple sauce. The problem with simple carbs is that they promote a large insulin surge, which can lead to hypoglycemia. Complex carbs are absorbed more slowly, so they don't cause as great an insulin surge as the simple type. Primary macronutrient source of energy in the body; burned as glucose and stored in muscle as glycogen (excess stored as fat) and includes all sugars (1 gram yields 4 calories).

Carbon filter A vessel loaded with activated carbon and used to remove organics, chlorine, tastes, and odors from liquids, operating on the principle of adsorption.

Carbon thickness A measurement of surface organic material. Carbon thickness values typically range from 5 to 20 angstroms (Å). Significantly contaminated surfaces can show surface carbon thickness of 20 angstroms (Å) or more.

Carbonate hardness That hardness in water caused by bicarbonates and carbonates of calcium and magnesium. If alkalinity exceeds total hardness, all hardness is carbonate hardness; if hardness exceeds alkalinity, the carbonate hardness equals the alkalinity.

Carcinogen A substance that causes the development of cancerous growths in living tissue. A chemical is considered to be a carcinogen if it has been evaluated by the International Agency for Cancer Research (IARC) and found to be a carcinogen or potential carcinogen, or if it is listed in the Annual Report on Carcinogens published by the National Toxicology Program, or if it is regulated by OSHA as a carcinogen.

Carcinogenic Cancer-causing. Many agents that are carcinogenic are mutagens.

Cardia Relating to that portion of the stomach closest to the heart, where the esophagus enters.

Cardiac arrest The heart stops completely, so that no blood is being pumped out to the body.

Cardiac arrhythmia An abnormal heartbeat. Types of arrhythmias include tachycardias (accelerated heartbeats) and bradycardias (slow heartbeats).

Cardiac catheterization (Angiography) A diagnostic procedure in which catheters are passed through the arteries of the heart. Pressures are measured and blood samples are taken from within the heart and its major blood vessels.

Cardiac rhythm management (CRM) The field of cardiovascular disease which relates to the detection and treatment of abnormally fast tachycardia (Tachy) and abnormally slow bradycardia (Brady) heart rhythms.

Cardiology Medical Specialty dealing with diseases of the heart.

Cardiophrenic angle The angle formed by the heart ("cardio") and the diaphragm ("phrenic") - usually refers to pleural space or a region on the frontal chest film.

Cardioversion The stopping of a fast heart rate by an electrical impulse that is delivered at the same time as the heartbeat. It uses low to moderate energy to restore the heart's normal rhythm.

Care Management Assessment and coordination of the overall care needs of a person, including both medical and social needs. A service in which a professional, typically a nurse or social worker, assists in planning, arranging, monitoring, or coordinating long term care services. Services may include making an assessment, creating a care plan, and arranging for services in multiple locations from numerous people and organizations. A Care Manager or Care Coordinator is a person who provides Care Management. This person can be a doctor, nurse, social worker or other similarly trained and, licensed professional.

Care Plan A comprehensive plan for the care of a resident, developed by a multi-disciplinary team including family members, nurses, dieticians, physicians, therapists, and activities or social services professionals. The plan spells out the type of care to be provided, with stipulated timeframes for completion and assignment of responsibilities to specific staff. Nursing homes are mandated to create and maintain care plans for their residents, and surveyors review the plans for adequacy and follow-through. In some states, Assisted Living Facilities are also mandated to create and maintain care plans.

Caregiver Individuals, often family members or friends, who provide assistance to see that the physical, psychological, and/or social needs of another person are met. Those who do so without pay are often called Informal Caregivers, to distinguish them from people who are paid to provide this assistance. The Primary Caregiver is the person who provides most of the care, and Secondary Caregivers are others who provide assistance on a part-time basis.

Carer A Carer is someone who provides care and support for a parent, partner, child, relative or friend who has a disability, is frail aged, or who has a chronic mental or physical illness. Most people will either give or receive care at some time in their life.. Carers range in age from as young as nine to people well into their nineties but the majority (80%) are aged under 65. Two thirds of Carers are women and most Carers provide care for a parent, partner or child

Carina (trachea) A ridge at the tracheal bifurcation, formed by the last tracheal cartilage that runs anteroposteriorly between the orifices of the two main bronchi. (from "carina" - the "v" shape of the bottom of a boat).

Carnitine (L-Carnitine) Non-structural amino acid that transports fatty acids into muscle cells for use as energy fuel. Carnitine is water-soluble and can be made in the body from the amino acids lysine and methionine with the assistance of vitamins C, B6 and Niacin, which act as coenzymes in the process.

Carnitine as discovered in meat in 1905, and was once called Vitamin T, because they thought it was a vitamin at first. 98% of te body's carntine exists in the heart and skelatal muscles. Carnitine is synthesized in the liver from Lysiine and Methionine, but half of the body's daily requirement for Carnitine comes from foods sources, including meat, poultry, fish and some diary products. Without supplemental carnitine, some people cannot use fat as energy.

Carotid bifurcation The point of division of the common carotid arteries into the internal and external carotid arteries.

Carrier A person who has a recessive mutated gene, together with its normal allele. Carriers do not usually develop disease but can pass the mutated gene on to their children.

Cartilage A hard but slippery coating on the end of each bone. In certain diseases, such as osteoarthritis, cartilage breaks down and wears away.

Cascade To arrange all the windows so that they are neatly stacked; only the title bars show behind the active window.

Cascading Menu A submenu that appears (usually to the left or right of the main menu item) when a menu selection is made.

Case A person in the population or study group identified as having a specific health problem or disease of interest.

Case-Mix Provider reimbursement calculated based on an assessment of the medical needs of the residents under care. A method by which a health care provider measures the service needs of the patient population, which may be based on age, medical diagnosis, severity of illness, or length of stay. Reimbursement is set at a standard amount for each type of care required, rather than the billed charges or the actual cost of providing that care.

Case Study An analysis of a clinical situation where the focus is on the clinician's decision-making regarding a diagnosis and/or set of symptoms.

Casein Primary protein found in milk, along with whey protein. Casein is the insoluble protein fraction of milk. It is absorbed more slowly than whey and provides the body with amino acids over an extended period in comparison to whey protein, the soluble protein fraction in milk.

Caseous Having a consistency like that of cottage cheese.

Cat's Claw An herb used in South American folk medicine for its anti-inflamatory and immune system protective properties.

Catabolic Metabolic condition in which muscle is broken down and energy is released.

CatabolismProtein breakdown in muscles.

Catabolism The intracellular phase of metabolism involved in the energy-yielding degradation of nutrient molecules (for example, glucose to CO_2 and H_2O). Waste products are called catabolites.

Catalase An enzyme that catalyzes the decomposition of hydrogen peroxide and molecular oxygen and water.

Catalyst A compound that increases the rate of a chemical reaction without being consumed or changed. In the biosciences, the term enzyme is used. Enzymes catalyze biological reactions.

Cataract A condition of the crystalline lens, in which the normally clear lens becomes clouded or yellowed, causing blurred or foggy vision. Cataracts may be caused by aging, eye injuries, disease, heredity, or birth defects. Surgery is a treatment option. The affected lens is removed and is replaced with a substitute (implant) lens or with a special type of contact lens. Generally the success rate of cataract surgery is over 90%, if the eye is otherwise healthy.

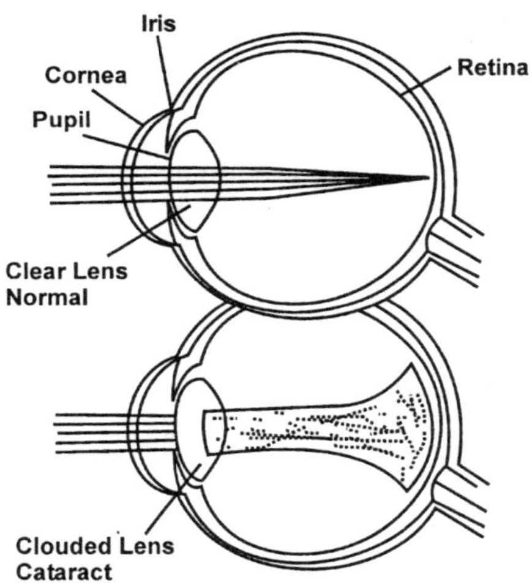

Fig. Cataract

Cataract, congenital A congenital cataract is marked by cloudiness of the eye lens present at birth.

Catarrh Inflammation of a mucous membrane with free discharge.

Catastrophic Illness Illness resulting in a massive and sudden change in a person's health and/or lifestyle, often accompanied by enormous medical bills.

Category Nursing is one profession with two categories of care providers - Registered Nurses (RNs) and Registered Practical Nurses (RPNs). Although all nursing students learn from the same body of nursing knowledge, RNs study it in greater depth and breadth over a longer period of time, and accordingly are able to provide care in more complex situations.

Catheter A tube passed through the body for draining fluids or injecting them into body cavities. It may be made of elastic, elastic web, rubber, glass, metal, or plastic.

Catheterization A test in which a catheter is inserted through the veins or arteries and into the heart to measure pressure, take blood samples and test for abnormalities in the heart.

Cation A positively charged particle or ion.

Cation exchange The displacement of one positively charged particle by another on a cation-exchange material.

Cation exchange resin An Ion exchange resin, which removes positively charged ions (cations) by exchanging them for hydrogen ions.

Cauda equina The lumbar and sacral nerve roots within the lumbar cistern as they descend to emerge from their respective intervertebral and sacral foramina.

Caudate nucleus One of the nuclei belonging to the basal ganglia located lateral to the thalamus. The nucleus consists of an enlarged head that bulges into the lateral wall of the frontal horn of the lateral ventricle, a body adjioning the dorsolateral thalamus and an attenuated tail that extends into the temporal horn of the lateral ventricle within its roof.

Cause specific death rate The number of deaths attributable to a specific disease in a given population in a given time period (usually expressed per 100,000 persons per year)

Cautery a device employing electric current for cutting tissue and controlling bleeding during surgery.

Cavitation A condition of liquid flow where, after partial vaporization of the liquid, the subsequent collapse of vapor bubbles can produce surface damage.

Cavum septum pellucidum Space enclosed within the laminae of the septum pelludicum, the membranous partition that seperates the frontal horns of the ventricle.

Cecum The first portion of the large intestine. Like a "blind pouch", it extends below the "ileocecal valve" - where the small intestine (ileum) joins the colon.

Cele (suffix) Tumor; herniation.

e.g. meningocoele - hernial protrusion of meninges.

Celiac artery The artery which originates from the abdominal aorta and divides into the left gastric, splenic, and common hepatic arteries.

Cell The fundamental unit of life. The living tissue of almost every organism is composed of these fundamental living units. Unicellular organisms, such as yeast or a bacterium, perform all life functions within the one cell. In a higher organism, a multicellular organism, entire populations of cells may be designated a particular task. The cells of muscle tissue, for example, are specialized for movement.

Cell bank Master Cell Bank: The bank of cells, which contain the original unused mutated cells from which, the Manufacturing Working Cell Bank is taken. This is usually kept under lock with very limited access.

Manufacturing Working Cell Bank: The bank of cells derived from the Master Cell Bank, which are used to seed the fermentation manufacturing process.

Cell culture The in vitro propagation of cells removed from organisms in a laboratory environment that has strict sterility, temperature, and nutrient requirement; also used to refer to any particular individual sample. Usually, cell culture takes place in a bioreactor.

Cell differentiation The process whereby descendants of a common parental cell achieve and maintain specialization of structure and function. Muscle cells become muscle cells and bone cells develop. In humans all the different types of cells differentiate from the simple sperm and egg.

Cell fusion The fusing together of two or more cells to become a single cell. This technique has had important consequences in immunology, developmental biology, and genetics. For example, monoclonal antibodies are produced by fusing a spleen cell (producing an antibody specific for the antigen of interest) with a mouse myeloma cell to produce a hybridoma which has an indefinitely long life because of the myeloma component and which secretes a specific antibody. When a human cell is fused with a mouse cell, the human chromosomes are progressively lost from the resultant hybrid and by correlating the presence of proteins in the hybrid with the presence of particular human chromosomes, genes can be assigned to individual chromosomes.

Cell lines When cells from the first culture (taken from the organism) are used to make subsequent cultures, a cell line is established. "Immortal" cell lines can replicate indefinitely.

Cellulitis A diffuse inflammatory process within solid tissues characterized by edema, redness, pain and interference with function. Cellulitis often occurs in the loose tissues beneath the skin, but may also occur in mucous membranes and in muscle bundles surounding organs.

Cellulose A polymer of six-carbon sugars found in all plant matter, the most abundant biological compound on earth.

Census A count of the number of residents in the facility at midnight. Medicare programs require providers to document a midnight census. Since residents may be in more than one facility during a given day, the facility entitled to payment for the day is determined by identifying where the resident is staying at midnight.

Centesis (suffix) Puncture.e.g. thoracentesis - puncture of the pleural cavity.

Centimorgan (cM) A unit of measure of recombination frequency. One centimorgan is equal to a 1% chance that a marker at one genetic locus will be separated from a marker at a second locus due to crossing over in a single generation. In human beings, one centimorgan is equivalent, on average, to one million base pairs.

Central canal (of spinal cord) Narrow ependymal lined channel that extends from the fourth ventricle through the length of the spinal cord within the midline of the transverse gray commissure (lamina X of Rexed). It is usually not patent beyon d the 20th year of life.

Centrifugation Mechanical means of separation based on differences in sedimentation rates due to differences in density between the suspended particles in the liquid.

Centrifuge A centrifuge operates on the principle of centrifugal force, the inertial reaction by which a body tends to move away from a center about which it revolves. This technique is commonly used to separate solids from liquids or liquids of different densities. Centrifugal equipment is divided into two major types, sedimenters and filters.

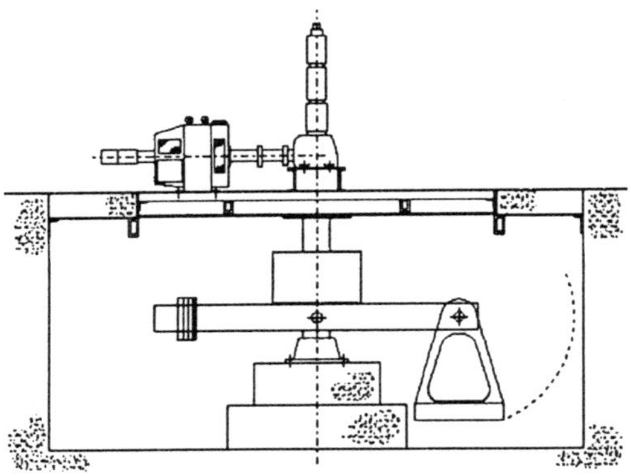

Fig. Centrifuge

Centromere The constricted region usually near the center of a chromosome (at the joining point of chromosome arms) consisting of highly repeated DNA sequences.

Centrum semi(ovale) The semioval area of white matter within either cerebral hemisphere as seen when the brain is cut horizontally just above the level of the corpus callosum or the oval area seen when the two hemispheres are taken together.

Cephalic vein Originates from the dorsal venous arch in the hand and joins the axillary vein.

Cerebellar tonsil A paramedian portion of the cerebellum that is continuous with the uvula of vermis that forms part of the caudal lobe of the cerebellar hemisphere.

Cerebellum Sub-division of the rhombencephalon located in the posterior cranial fossa. It straddles the pons and medulla to which it is connected along with the midbrain by 3 peduncles. It functions in the motor sphere; coordination of muscle activity in movement, maintenance of equilibrium, and muscle tone.

Cerebral aqueduct (of sylvius) The narrow cerebrospinal fluid filled channel of the midbrain that joins the third and fourth ventricles of the brain.

Cerebral hemisphere Pair of rounded structures on either side of the midline of the brain that are partially separated by the longitudinal (interhemispheric) cerebral fissure.

Cerebral peduncle The ventral part of the midbrain consisting of the tegmentum and basis pedunculi (or crus cerebri).

Cerebrospinal fluid A watery, clear, colourless liquid produced largely by the choroid plexuses and contained within the cerebral ventricles, central canal of the spinal cord and the subarachnoid spaces surrounding the central nervous system.

Certificate of Need Issued by the state organization responsible for healthcare facility licensure, a CON program limits the number of healthcare facilities which can be located in a market area, by requiring new providers to demonstrate and document that there is a need for their services. In some states there is a partial or total moratorium on CONs for nursing homes, where the State has determined that there are already too many facilities available for the population of that state.

Certification The process by which governmental, non-governmental or professional organizations or other statutory bodies grant recognition to an individual who has met certain predetermined specified qualifications. In most cases such recognition is on a voluntary basis.

Certified Home Health Aide A home health aide who has completed required State training and competency testing in the skills needed to work as a nurse aide.

Certified Medication Assistant (CMA) Non-licensed personnel who are authorized to administer medications, under the supervision of licensed personnel (e.g., an RN), based on completion and testing in a State approved medication administration course.

Certified Nurse Aide (CNA) A nurse aide who has completed required State training and competency testing in the skills needed to work as a nurse aide.

Certified vendor drawings Drawings prepared by vendors for the fabrication of equipment, specialty components and skid mounted systems. These are certified as fabricated by the vendor and become the official document for the equipment involved.

Cervical Incompetence A condition where a woman's cervix, or opening between the uterus and vaginal tract, is not strong enough to remain closed during pregnancy. During a critical time period of growth, most often from about 16 to 22 weeks, the cervix may open and labor will begin prematurely. A cervical stitch can be used to help hold the cervix closed.

Cervical spine Vertebral column of the neck.

Cervical Stitch A stitch placed around the cervix, or opening between the uterus and vaginal tract, to keep it closed during pregnancy. This is only needed in cases where a woman has a diagnosis of cervical incompetence. This procedure will work for most women, and although early labor may still occur, it will often be past the viability age for the baby.

Cervix The lower end portion of the uterus connecting the isthmus and the ostium uteri with the vaginal canal.

Cesarean delivery Cesarean delivery is to deliver a baby via a cesarean section.

Cesarean section When a woman cannot deliver a baby vaginally, or if a baby is in distress during labor, a cesarean section is performed. An incision is made in a woman's abdomen and her uterus to deliver the baby.

CFU (colony forming unit) A measure of the number of bacteria present in the environment or on the surfaces of an aseptic processing room, measured as part of qualification and ongoing monitoring. Also applied to the testing of purified water samples.

CGMPS (current good manufacturing practices) Current accepted standards of design, operation, practice, and sanitization. The FDA is empowered to inspect drug-manufacturing plants in which drugs are processed, manufactured, packaged, and stored for compliance with these standards.

Chadwick's sign Chadwick's sign is the dark-blue or purple discoloration of the mucosa of the vagina and cervix during pregnancy. It is a normal sign of pregnancy.

Chakras The seven vital energy centers of the body. The chakras extend from the base of spine to the crown of head. Located in the rectal area, near the genitals, behind the navel, at the heart, at the neck, between the eyebrows, and on the crown of the head. Each chakra corresponds to certain colors, emotions, organs, nerve networks, and energies.

Chancre A hard, syphilitic primary ulcer, the first sign of syphilis, appearing approx. 2 to 3 weeks after infection. The ulcer begins as a painless lesion or papule that ulcerates. Occurs generally singly, but sometimes may be multiple.

Change control A formal system by which qualified representatives of appropriate disciplines review proposed or actual changes that might affect a validated process's status. The intent is to determine the need for action that would ensure that the system is maintained in a validated state.

Change over The program by which a processing area is cleared of supplies and components used in the manufacture of a previous product and then readied for production of a new product. This often includes parts change over and/or special cleaning to eliminate cross-contamination.

Channeling Cleavage, cracking, and furrowing of a resin bed due to resin age, a change in one of the feed solutions, or faulty operational procedures. The solution being treated follows the path of least resistance, runs through these furrows, and fails to contact active resin material in other parts of the bed.

Characterization Precisely deciphering and describing all the characteristics of a drug substance that affect its efficacy and its purity. Or the chemical, physical, and sometimes biological properties that are attributes of a specific drug substance.

Charge Nurse The nurse in charge or supervising a particular part of a facility for a given time shift.

Chart stimulated recall oral examination (CSR) A measurement tool for assessing clinical decision-making and the application of medical knowledge using actual patients and a standardized oral examination. A trained and experienced physician/ examiner questions the examinee about the provided care, probing for the reasons behind the work-up diagnoses, interpretation of clinical findings and treatment plans. The examiners rate the examinee using an established protocol and scoring procedure. In an efficiently designed CSR, each patient case (test item) takes 5 to 10 minutes. A typical CSR exam involves one or two physicians as examiners per separate 30 to 60-minute sessions. The examinee's performance is measured by combining scores from all the cases tested for a pass/ fail decision overall, or by scoring for each session. Exam score reliabilities have been reported between 0.65 and 0.88. In assessing recall ability or medical knowledge, multiple-choice questions (MCQ) are more effective than CSR exams.

Chat A feature of the internet that allows users to "talk" to one another in virtual real time. Users communicate by typing messages which are sent instantly to another person or group within the chat room program.

Check Box A square dialog box item that takes an off or on value. Clicking in a check box adds or removes an X in the box, indicating whether the setting is on (checked) or off (unchecked).

Checksum A record of the number of bits transmitted and included with the transmission so that the receiving program can check to see whether the same number of bits arrived. If the counts match, it is assumed that the complete transmission was received.

Cheiroscope An instrument used in orthoptics/vision therapy to train binocular skills and accommodation skills. The Keystone Correct-Eye Scope is an example of a Cheiroscope.

Chelating agents Organic compounds that can withdraw ions from solution, forming insoluble complexes.

Chelation therapy Typically administered in an osteopathic or medical doctor's office, chelation therapy is a series of intravenous injections of the synthetic amino acid EDTA, designed to detoxify the body. Often used to treat arteriosclerosis, angina, Alzheimer's disease. EDTA stands for ethylenediamine-tetruacetic acid (an amino acid). FDA approved for removing lead and other heavy metals from the bloodstream. One theory holds that chelation removes the calcium in arterial plaque; another suggests that EDTA works as an antioxidant. Proponents say that chelation also reverses gangrene, relieves the pain associated with lupus and arthritis, and reverses memory loss.

Chemical Pregnancy Usually a general term to apply to many early miscarriages where a baby never develops. The "chemicals" or hormones of the pregnancy were produced, but a baby did not form. Often the pregnancy itself could not be diagnosed, as the loss happened too early.

Chemical Restraint A psychoactive drug used by a facility for discipline or convenience and not for medical treatment.

Chemoautotrophs Facultative autotrophs that obtain their energy from the oxidation of inorganic compounds.

Chemolysis Certain types of kidney stones can be dissolved with the application chemicals. Uric acid stones, for example, can be dissolved with a solution of sodium bicarbonate in saline. Cystine stones may be treated successfully with a combination of acetylcysteine and sodium bicarbonate in saline. Struvite and carbon apatite stones can be treated with an acidic solution of hemiacidrin. The procedure involves infusing the chemical solution into the affected area by means of a ureteral catheter in a series of treatments over time until the stone is dissolved. The patient's urine must be cultured regularly throughout the course of treatment to guard against urinary infection and prevent the buildup of excessive chemical levels, particularly magnesium, which can cause other health problems.

Chemostat A growth chamber that keeps a bacterial culture at a specific volume and rate of growth by limiting nutrient medium and removing spent culture.

Chemotherapy Treatment of disease by means of chemical substances or drugs.

Chick Embroyo Extract This type of extract contains short amino acid chains called oligopeptides, plus additional essential amino acids and trace elements (iron, copper, cobalt, selenium, and zinc). The peptides in the extract possess both cell stimulating and protective properties. The peptides indicated that they were activating growth factor receptors in them. The extract works as a general tonic and stimulates the adrenal gland, normalizing its function. It also acts as a mild stimulant and an antidepressant; and it improves libido, erectile function, sparmatogenesis and other aspects of sexual function in men and women. It also improves sleep and promotes weight loss.

Chimeric An organism, especially a plant, containing tissues from at least two genetically distinct parents. Type of antibody, partially human and partially mouse.

Chiropractic The chiropractic system is based on the premise that the spine is literally the backbone of human health. Misalignments of the vertebrae caused by poor posture or trauma result in pressure on the spinal nerve roots, which may lead to diminished function and illness. The chiropractor seeks to analyze and correct these misalignments through spinal manipulation or adjustments.

Chitosan Chitosan is a natural product extracted from Chitin (by products of

Crustacean shell extracts). Chitosan and chitin are waste products of the crab and shrimp industry. It can be used to inhibit fat digestion and as a drug delivery transport agent. It also has been used as a cholesterol lowering substance. Chitosan is marketed as a 'fat blocker'. It appears that it can impede fat absorption by 'gelling' with fat in the small intestine. Side effect of Chitosan is that since it is made from sea food, some people have allergic responses to it. Also, you need a high concentration of Chitosan for it to 'gel' with fat.

Chloasma Chloasma are extensive brown patches of irregular shape and size on the face or other parts of the body.

Chloramine A chlorine compound formed by reaction with organic amines or ammonia.

Chlorinated vinyls Thermoplastic chlorinated vinyls include PVC, CPVC, and VDC. PVC and CPVC are very similar materials, the primary difference being the addition of more chlorine to the PVC molecule to synthesize CPVC. This results in a higher glass transition temperature that equates to a higher use temperature for CPVC. The polymerization with chlorine also makes these materials inherently flame resistant. In addition to being resistant to higher temperatures, CPVC is more resistant to process chemicals.

Chlorination Adding chlorine or chlorine compounds to water for disinfection.

Chlorine An element used to kill micro-organisms in water. At room temperature and atmospheric pressure a greenish yellow gas.

Chlorine demand Amount of chlorine used up by reacting with oxidizable substances in water before chlorine residual can be measured.

Chlorine residual Portion of free or combined chlorine that remains active after specified contact period.

Chloroplasts Relatively large, chlorophyll containing, green organelles responsible for photosynthesis in photosynthetic eukaryotes, such as algae and plant cells. Every chloroplast contains an outer membrane and a large number of inner membranes called thylakoids.

Cholangiogram An X-ray study of the bile ducts performed with contrast injected into the ducts.

Cholangiography X-rays of the bile ducts.

Cholangitis Infection with in the bile ducts usually caused by stones.

Cholecystectomy An operation to remove the gallbladder.

Cholecystokinin A hormone secreted by the duodenal mucosa in the presence of fats which causes the gallbladder to contract.

Choledocholithiasis Stones within the bile duct system.

Choledochoscope Highly specialized fiber optic endoscope for looking within the common bile duct.

Cholesterol A substance normally made by the body, but also found in foods from animal sources, like beef, eggs, and butter. Too much cholesterol in the body can lead to narrowing and blockage of the arteries, especially those that feed the heart and keep it healthy. High cholesterol can also cause the formation of gallstones. Ideally, blood cholesterol levels should be less than 200mg/dL.

Choline A B-fatty acid involved in the production of neurotransmitters in the brain that regulate mood, appetite, behavior, memory, etc. Most effective in phosphatidyl choline form. It is beleived to help concentration and alertness. Studies indicate that it improves cognitive performance. Blood levels of choline decrease during prolonged exercise.

Chondroitin Chondroitin is extracted from bovine tracheas or shark cartilage. It is a major component of connective tissue, especially cartilage. Chondroitin can stimulate repair of cartilage cells and also black enzymes that damage joints.

Chorioamnionitis Inflammation of the amnion, usually secondary to bacterial infection. This condition is an obstetric emergency that may cause conditions such as pneumonia, meningitis, or sepsis in the neonate, and bacteremia or sepsis in the mother.

Choriocarcinoma Choriocarcinoma -Highly malignant cancer that grows in the uterus during pregnancy or at the site of an ectopic pregnancy.

Chorion Chorion—Outermost fetal membrane found around the amnion.

Chorionic villus sampling Chorionic villus sampling—Diagnostic test done early in pregnancy. A biopsy of tissue is taken from inside the uterus through the cervical opening to determine abnormalities of pregnancy.

Choroid plexus A vascularized epithelium projecting into the ventricles of the brain that produces the cerebrospinal fluid.

Choroid The vascular membrane between the sclera and the retina of the eye, that extends from the ora serrata to the optic nerve.

Chromatids Copies of a chromosome produced by replication.

Chromatin The complex of DNA and protein in the nucleus of the interphase cell, originally recognized by its reaction with stains specific for DNA.

Chromatography Procedure by which solutes (e.g., proteins and other chemical products) are selectively separated by a dynamic differential migration process in a system consisting of two or more phases, one of which moves continuously in a given direction and in which the individual substances exhibit different mobilities by reason of differences in adsorption, partition, solubility, vapor pressure, molecular size, or ionic charge density. The individual substances thus obtained can be identified or determined by analytical methods. There are several types of chromatography in use with different operating principles:

1. Adsorption - separates products by their different affinities for the surface of a solid medium, either an inorganic carrier such as silica gel, alumina, or hydroxyapatite, or an organic polymer.

2. Ion Exchange - uses ion exchange resin to which ionized functional groups have been attached. At an appropriate pH, target proteins acquire a net surface charge that allows them to selectively bind to an ion exchange resin. Other impurities are eluted through the column.

3. Gel Filtration - employs a neutral cross-linked carrier with a defined pore size for molecular fractionation. Molecules larger than the largest pores cannot enter the matrix and pass directly through the column; smaller molecules enter the carrier and are retarded. Gel filtration thus separates on the basis of molecular size, eluting larger molecules first, followed by progressively smaller species.

4. Affinity - relies on the propensity of each biomolecule to have an affinity for another highly specific biomolecule, such as an antibody-antigen relationship. Once bound together, the drug molecules can be detached by altering various chemical attributes in the column.

5. Hydrophobic - separates by molecule polarity and reverse interaction with water.

6. High Pressure Liquid Chromatography (HPLC)-

Chromium / Chrimium Picolinate Chromium increases the efficiency of the hormone insulin, which the pancreas releases after you eat carbohydrates or protein. Chromium acts to make the receptor of muscle cells more sensitive to insulin (which allows you to store more carbohydrates in the muscle cells as glycogen rather than in fat cells as lipids). Insulin also helps muscles use amino acids for building protein rather than breaking them down. Chromium can promote modest muscular gains and decreases in bodyfat (thus helps build lean mass). Exercise increases the excretion rate of chromium.

Chromium enrichment layer thickness In stainless steel, the same as its maximum depth of enrichment, unless a surface iron layer is present in which case the chromium enrichment layer is calculated as the maximum depth of enrichment minus the thickness of the surface iron oxide layer.

Chromosomal Abnormality Chromosomal Abnormality Chromosomes are the packages of genetic information in every cell of the body. Normally, there are 46 chromosomes in every cell. Down syndrome is the most common chromosome abnormality. Down syndrome occurs when there is an extra copy of chromosome 21. People with Down syndrome have varying degrees of mental retardation and can have other health problems. Babies can have other chromosome problems, some of them more serious than Down syndrome and some of them less serios.

Chromosomal Anomalies Any problem in a person's genetic code, or DNA. Very minor anomalies may not even be noticeable. More serious ones cause problems such as Down's Syndrome and other known genetic disorders. The most dramatic ones will cause the death of the baby, usually during the first trimester, and most often before the mother knew she was pregnant. The chromosomal problem may have started with a poor quality egg, poor quality sperm, during fertilization, or in the early cell divisions.

Chromosome The self-replicating genetic structure of cells containing the cellular DNA that bears in its nucleotide sequence the linear array of genes. In prokaryotes, chromosomal DNA is circular, and the entire genome is carried on one chromosome. Eukaryotic genomes consist of a number of chromosomes whose DNA is associated with different kind of proteins.

Chronic Referring to a disease or disorder that usually develops slowly and lasts for a long period of time.

Chronic Care Continuing care provided over long periods of time without any expectation that the patient's level of functioning will necessarily improve, as opposed to the focus of Acute Care on curing disease and rehabilitation of the patient to a previous functional status. Chronic conditions often begin inconspicuously and symptoms are less pronounced than acute conditions. Chronic care services are provided by both

Chronic Condition A general term that includes both chronic illnesses and impairments, including arthritis, cancer, heart disease, depression, hearing impairments, and vision problems. A disease or condition that lasts over a long period of time and typically cannot be cured. Chronic conditions often result in some type of disability.

Chronically Ill Terminology used in Tax-Qualified Long Term Care Insurance policies. To qualify for coverage in a Tax-Qualified policy, the policyholder be certified as chronically ill by a licensed health care practitioner because they are not able to perform at least two Activities of Daily Living without substantial assistance for a period of at least 90 days, or because they require Substantial Supervision to protect themselves from threats to health and safety due to Severe Cognitive Impairment. Policies that are Tax-Qualified may pay benefits from the beginning of services, providing the services are expected to be needed for at least 90 days.

Chrysin An anti-aromatase, which means it stops a lot of excess testosterone from converting to estrogen. Also, a compound with significant antiviral activity - especially in relation to the HIV. A an effect on the benzodiazapene receptors (which have a calming, antistress effect). It is possible that Chrysin taken in the correct dosage could reduce cortisol secretion due to the body's sensing less stress. Chrysin may act as an antiestrogen by inhibiting aromatase activity, limiting the conversion of testosterone to estrogen.

CHSRA Standard Report Set This is a set of reports similar to what was previously sent out quarterly in the mail from CHSRA. The standard Report Set is available to all users of the ePIP system. While it provides a convenient way to request a group of reports like CHSRA previously mailed, it likely contains more than you would prefer to review if you request reports frequently. Look into Report Sets as a way to customize a series of reports for your facilities needs.

Ciliary body A structure directly behind the iris of the eye and contains the ciliary muscle.

Ciliary muscle A band of muscle and fibers that are attached to the lens that controls the shape of the lens and allows the lens to accommodate (change focus).

Cingulum An association bundle of the cerebrum located within the cingulate gyrus which almost encircles the corpus callosum having connections along its course with adjacent frontal, parietal and temporal lobe cortex.

CIP (clean in place) Internally cleaning a piece of equipment without relocation or disassembly. The equipment is cleaned but not necessarily sterilized. The cleaning is normally done by acid, caustic, or a combination of both, with WFI rinse. The design of a CIP system should considered the operating volume design for the water consumption, chemical and biowaste effluent, and energy required to clean a given circuit or piece of equipment.

Circle of willis The polygonal (hexagon/ pentagon) anastomosis that is made up of the internal carotid, anterior and posterior cerebral arteries, the anterior communicating artery, and the posterior communicating arteries - all in the region of the suprasellar cistern.

Circumduction Movement of a limb or extremity so that the distal end describes a circle while the proximal end remains fixed.

Circumflex artery Any of several paired curving arteries.

Cirrhosis A chronic problem makes it hard for the liver to remove toxins (poisonous substances) from the body. Alcohol, medications, and other substances may build up in the bloodstream and cause problems. Cirrhosis is a result of scarring and damage from other diseases, like biliary atresia and alcoholism.

Cisterna chyli The dilated protion of the thoracic duct (a lymphatic channel) in the lumbar region that recieves fluid from the intestinal, lumbar, and descending intercostal lymph vessels.

Civil Money Penalty (CMP) A fine imposed on facilities for noncompliance.

Classical pharmaceuticals Small-molecule, nonbiotech drugs produced by chemical synthesis.

Classification The level (or the process of specifying or determining the level) of airborne particulate cleanliness applicable to a cleanroom or clean zone, expressed in terms of an ISO Class N, which represents maximum allowable concentrations (in particles per cubic meter of air) for considered sizes of particles.

Classified space A space in which the number of airborne particles is limited. This is accomplished by the strict use of HVAC systems. Areas are classified as Class 10, Class 100, Class 1,000, Class 10,000, and Class 100,000. In pharmaceutical production, only classes 100, 10,000, and 100,000 are used.

Claustrum A thin vertical sheet of gray matter that underlies the cortex of the insula. It is located between the extreme capsule laterally and the external capsule medially. Considered a component of the basal ganglia bu t with no functional relationship.

Clava The protuberance on the dorsal surface of the medulla overlying the gracile nucleus. Also known as the Gracile tubercle.

Clavicle The "collar bone". A curved bone which articulates medially with the sternum and laterally with the scapula, forming the anterior portion of the shoulder girdle.

Clean air device Stand-alone equipment for treating and distributing clean air to achieve defined environmental conditions.

Clean air projector Fan and filter unit used to locally clean room air and deliver it to a desired location. Often called a fan/filter unit.

Clean area An area where particulate and microbial levels are specified (e.g., Filling Room - Class 10,000 "In Operation").

Clean space A room or volume controlled to meet a certain airborne particulate limit (Class or Grade). In pharmaceutical facilities, clean spaces are usually classified and controlled only for aseptic processing facilities, but may also be defined for certain biotech processes. Final non-sterile bulk facilities, oral product, most topical product manufacturing facilities, and warehouses are normally not classified as clean spaces.

Clean steam Steam free from boiler additives that may be purified, filtered, or separated. When condensed, clean steam meets the specification for WFI. Usually utilized to sterilize process equipment.

Clean zone ISO 14644-1 defines it as "a dedicated space in which the concentration of airborne particles is controlled, and which is constructed and used in a manner to minimize the introduction, generation, and retention of particles inside the zone and in which other relevant parameters, e.g. temperature, humidity, and pressure, are controlled as necessary". Additionally, ISO 14644-1 states, "this zone may be open or enclosed and may or may not be located within a cleanroom".

Cleanroom A specially constructed space environmentally controlled with respect to airborne particles (size and count), temperature, humidity, air pressure, airflow patterns, air motion, and lighting. ISO 14644-1 defines it as "a room in which the concentration of airborne particles is controlled, and which is constructed and used in a manner to minimize the introduction, generation, and retention of particles inside the room, and in which other relevant parameters, e.g. temperature, humidity, and pressure, are controlled as necessary."

Cleanroom classification The maximum number of particles greater than or equal to 0.5μm in diameter that may be present in a cubic foot of room air.

Cleavage The splitting up of a complex molecule into two or more simpler molecules. The series of cell divisions occurring in the ovum immediately following its fertilization.

Cleft palate Cleft palate—Defect in the palate, the part of the upper jaw or mouth.

Clenbuterol This drug is classified as a Beta-2 agonist, and is used for treating asthma. It is not an anabolic steroid, or a growth hormone. Currently, it is not approved for sale in the United States, but it is sold in Europe, under various names, such as Spiropent, Monores, and Ventipulmin. Researchers in 1987 noted an unusual effect in animals when using this drug. Their muscles grew, while they lost body fat. The main side effects associated with this drug include tremors, heart rhythm disturbances, headaches, nervousness, excessive sweating and insomnia.

Bodybuilders use it because it mimics the actions of Epinephrine. It simulates a process called Thermogenesis, which turns fat calories into heat and which results in a loss of body fat. The side effects start when you use more than 80 micrograms or more. The dosage that's used to treat asthma is around 20 to 40 micrograms twice a day. The muscle building dose would be over 80 micrograms in humans, but scientists consider it to be dangerous and unethical. Another problem is that any effects you get from it wears off rapidly. Bodybuilders who have used this drug shows that it is better for promoting fat burning than for muscle building.

Clerkships A rotation around the clinical settings of the medical school. Some clerkships are obligatory (e.g., internal medicine, pediatrics, surgery), while others are elective or selective. In the United States, medical students do clerkships in their third and fourth year while in Europe, this typically occurs in the fourth through sixth year of medical school.

Click To depress and release a mouse button quickly. (In Windows, the term "click" usually refers to the left mouse button).

Client The person or persons with whom the nurse is engaged in a professional therapeutic relationship. In most cases, the client is an individual. The client may also be a family, a group (as in psychotherapy) or a community (as in the public health field). In research, the client is a subject or participant, and in education, the client may include students.

Clinical competence The mastery of relevant knowledge and the acquisition of a range of relevant skills at a satisfactory level including interpersonal, clinical and technical components at a certain point of education, such as at graduation. In the case of clinical training, which is primarily based on an apprenticeship model, teachers define what the student is expected to do and then test their ability to do it. However, in actuality, most clinical actions are concerned with problems for which there are no clear answers and no single solution. In such situations, an experienced doctor searches his or her mind and sifts through a wide range of options and in some cases the solution will be something he or she has never arrived at before. Therefore, competence itself is only of value as a prerequisite for performance in a real clinical setting and does not always correlate highly with performance in practice.

Clinical Contraindication to a Psychoactive Dose Reduction The resident (patient) has a specific condition and a history of recurrent psychotic symptoms which have been stabilized with a drug; or there have been two gradual dose reductions attempted in one year that resulted in the return of symptoms; or the resident's (patient's) physician provides in the clinical record a diagnosis, a risk/benefit analysis, and a conclusion why this treatment is necessary.

Clinical endpoint An indicator (such as blood pressure) measured in a human subject to asses the safety, efficacy, or other objective of a clinical trial.

Clinical hold The temporary cessation of a clinical trial by FDA if the agency is concerned about a drug or study protocol. The trial may resume when the problem is solved.

Clinical Links For CHSRA QIs, a mapping of quality indicators that are clinically related to each other and should be considered when investigating care problems within a particular domain of care.

Clinical Narrative A detailed description of a clinical situation including intentions and interpretations of events, chronology of action and outcomes.

Clinical oral examination (COE) Unstructured clinical and oral examination which is the traditional form of clinical examination and continues to be popular in many parts of the world. With face-to-face contact, examiners explore both the breadth and depth of a student's understanding in real-life clinical situations. Aspects of competence which can be tested include the ability to respond to new information, a variety of interpersonal skills, and those aspects of competence that cannot be easily measured by more objective methods, such as an OSCE. Case variability can be reduced by recruiting a small group of patients with the same condition and similar symptoms or by the use of simulated patients. The use of videotapes of students undertaking a long-case examination with subsequent scoring of the performance by the examiner, who then discusses the results with the examinee, enhances the value of this form of examination. Proper briefing and training of examiners and a very structured approach to scoring contribute to the quality of this exam.

Clinical Scholar At this level the clinician's practice is fluid. The clinician intuitively understands the situation and the action to take. The manner and degree of engagement and involvement with patients and families is finely tuned. They skillfully work with and through others.

Clinician Level At this level clinician's have a broad range of experience in caring for patients, develop therapeutic relationships with patients and families and works effectively with all members of the team. When the clinician has consistently demonstrated Clinician Level behavior the manager/director will recognize them as practicing at the Clinician Level. This level must be achieved within two years of hire.

Clip Art A collection of images you can use in various documents. Clip art is often distributed on CD-ROM in large collections (thousands of clip art pieces) organized into categories, or available on the World Wide Web.

Clipboard A temporary storage area in all versions of Windows used for storing various types of data (for example, text, graphics, sound, and video). The clipboard can hold one piece of information at a time for use in a program or to cut/copy and paste information between programs.

Clivus The inclined anterior bony wall of the posterior cranial fossa formed by the occipital and sphenoid bones. The brainstem rest on the clivus.

Clivus A triangular bone, that slopes upward from the foramen magnum to the dorsum sellae, in the posterior cranial fossa. (clivus = "wedge" or "slide").

Clomid Also clomiphene, a drug used to stimulate ovulation in women who may not be ovulating or may have a luteal phase defect . (May be mispelled Chlomid.)

Clone A group of individuals produced from one individual through asexual processes that do not involve the interchange or combination of genetic material. As a result, members of a clone have identical genetic compositions. Protozoa and bacteria, for example, frequently reproduce asexually by a process called binary fission. In binary fission, a single-celled organism undergoes cell division and the result is two cells with identical genetic composition. Next, these two identical cells undergo division and the result is four cells with identical genetic composition. These identical offspring are all members of a clone.

Clone A population of genetically identical cells derived from the multiplication of a single cell. It is the basis of rDNA and monoclonal antibody production.

Cloning vector DNA molecule originating from a virus, a plasmid, or the cell of a higher organism into which another DNA fragment of appropriate size can be integrated without loss of the vectors capacity for self-replication; vectors introduce foreign DNA into host cells, where it can be reproduced in large quantities. Examples are plasmids, cosmids, and yeast artificial chromosomes; vectors are often recombinant molecules containing DNA sequences from several sources.

Closed Record The complete record of a resident (patient) that has died or been discharged by a provider.

Closed system System sterilized-in-place or sterilized while closed prior to use, is pressure or vacuum tight to some predefined leak rate, can be utilized for its intended purpose without breach to the integrity of the system, can be adapted for fluid transfers in or out while maintaining asepsis, and is connectable to other closed systems while maintaining integrity of all closed systems. (From PDA TR-28 for sterile product manufacture).

Clostridium A genus of bacteria, most are obligate anaerobes and form endospores.

Clostridium difficile (Also known as C. diff or C. difficile.) Bacteria normally found in the large intestine, which can cause a serious intestinal infection and diarrhea in some people who are taking antibiotics.

CMC (chemistry, manufacturing, and controls) The section on a BLA (Biologics License Application) or IND (Investigational New Drug) describing the composition, manufacture, and specifications of a drug product and its ingredients.

CMV Cytomegalovirus (CMV) infection- Group of viruses from the herpesvirus family.

Coagulation Adding insoluble compounds to water to neutralize the electrical charge on colloids, causing them to coalesce to form larger particles that can be removed by settling.

Coaguligand A VTA (Vascular Targeting Agent) that utilizes a human coagulation protein to induce tumor blood vessel clotting.

Coccus A bacterium of round, spheroidal, or ovoid form, including micrococcus, staphylococcus, streptococcus, and pneumococcus.

Coccyx The "tail bone" - a caudal extremity of the vertebral column formed by the fussion of four rudimentary vertebrae.

Cochlea A spiral bone tube of the inner ear, which lies against the lateral end of the internal acoustic meatus. The cochlea ("snail") contains the auditory sensory structure.

COD (chemical oxygen demand) The amount of oxygen needed to completely oxidize all oxidizable organic and inorganic substances in water.

Coding sequence The region of a gene (DNA) that encodes the amino acid sequence of a protein.

Coenzyme A non-polypeptide molecule required for the action of certain enzymes; often contains a vitamin as a component.

Coenzyme Q10 This antioxidant is shown to have heart protective and energy productive properties. COQ10 is involved in cellular energy production. Several studies have reported improved endurance after taking CoQ10. It is considered one of the best antioxidants. It may be an ergogenic aid because it plays a pivital role in a cellular process that leads to ATP synthesis and is known as the electron transport system.

Cofactor Small molecular weight, heat stable inorganic or organic substance required for the action of an enzyme.

Cognitive Impairment A loss or deterioration of mental capacity. A deficiency in a person's short or long term memory, orientation as to person, place and time, deductive or abstract reasoning, or judgment. Typically related to an illness or injury, like Alzheimers Disease, stroke, or traumatic brain injury.

Co-Housing Intergenerational communities where all members own their own private homes, but some meals and other community services are provided in shared facilities.

Colic A condition in an otherwise healthy baby characterized by excessive crying.

Coliform bacteria A group of bacteria found in mammalian intestines and soil, used as a measure of fecal pollution in water. They are easy to identify and count in the laboratory because of their ability to ferment lactose.

Colitis Irritation of the colon (large intestine).

Collagen Collagen is a fibrous protein that functions as a building block of the skin, the tendons, the bones, as well as other connective tissues.

Collateral eminence An elevation along the floor of the posterior part of the temporal horn of the lateral ventricle, lateral to the hippocampus caused by the deep collateral sulcus.

Collateral targeting The therapeutic strategy of targeting structures and cell types other than cancer cells common to all solid tumors as a means to attack a solid tumor.

Collateral trigone That part of the lateral ventricle where the occipital horn, temporal horn, and posterior part of the body become confluent.

Colleague A colleague "from outside of your discipline" should be someone who knows your practice and can speak to your work in any or all of the themes of practice. Therefore, a colleague for this purpose is defined as someone with formal clinical training who is "a member of the care team" or a "direct care provider". Examples are pharmacists, chaplains, clinical dieticians, physicians, child-life specialists or any of the six disciplines involved in this program. They are nursing, occupational therapists, physical therapists, respiratory therapists, social workers and speech-language pathologists.

Colliculus C. Superior Bilateral rounded eminences projecting from the surface of the rostral midbrain tectum associated with the visual system.

C. Inferior: Bilateral rounded eminences extending from the surface of the caudal midbrain tectum associated with the auditory system.

C. Facial: Small elevation on the floor of the fourth ventricle medial to the sulcus limitans, produced by the underlying abducent nerve nucleus and the internal genu of the facial nerve.

Colloid A translucent, yellowish material of the consistency of glue, less fluid than mucoid or mucinoid, found in the cells and tissues in a state of colloid degeneration or colloid carcinoma.

A substance, such as gelatin or cytoplasm that because of the size of its molecules, is slowly diffusible rather than soluble in water and is incapable of passing through an animal membrane.

Colon The part of the large intestine that extends from the cecum to the rectum.

Colon hydrotherapy Involves the cleansing of the large intestine with warm purified water. A single colonic treatment is said to be equivalent to several enemas in removing toxic debris from the colon.

Colonoscopy A test using a long, flexible tube with a light and camera lens at the end, which examines the large intestine.

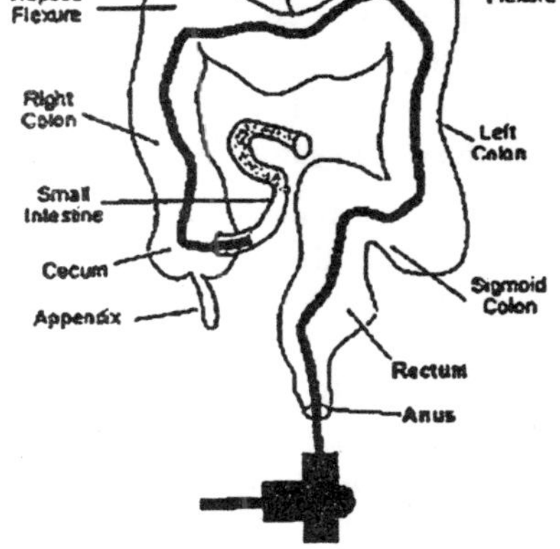

Fig. Colonoscopy

Colony A growth of microorganisms on a solid medium. The growth is visible without magnification.

Color perception test A test that measures the ability to identify and distinguish colors.

Color vision deficiency Also known as colorblindness. It is the absence of or defect in the perception of colors. Color vision is based on perception of red, green, and blue. If there is a defect in the perception of one of these colors, a color will be perceived as if it were composed only of the other two colors. Based on the color or colors for which there is defective perception, a person may suffer from red, green, or blue blindness. Color blindness in which all colors are perceived as gray is termed monochromasia. For people with the common, inherited, types of color deficiency there is no cure.

Colostomy A procedure done when there is an abnormality in the large intestine or rectum that allows stool to leave the body by a different route. Through an operation, an opening is made in the abdomen and the colon (large intestine) is connected to it. Stool passes through the opening to a collection bag on the abdomen. A colostomy may be temporary or permanent, depending on the health of the colon.

Colostrum Colostrum is a fluid produced by the mammary glands of female mammals prior to milk production. It has a high concentration of immunoglobins, antimicrobial agents and hormone. factors. Colostrum provides major immune and gastrointestinal system benefits.

Bovine Colostrum usually comes from cows, a dairy product that has similar properties to human colostrum. Normally, adults cannot absorb colotrum's antobodies and growth factors the way a newborn can. But it still has superior nutritional values which may make it a useful supplement.

Combustible dust Any finely divided solid material that is 420μ or 0.017 inches or less in diameter, or any material capable of passing through an US No. 40 standard sieve that when dispersed in air in the proper proportions, could be ignited by a flame, spark or other source of ignition.

Combustible liquid A liquid having a closed cup flash point at or above 100°F (37.8°C). Combustible liquids do not include compressed gases or cryogenic fluids. Combustible liquids are subdivided as follows:

1. Class II - Liquids having a closed cup flash point at or above 100°F (37.8°C) and below 140°F (60°C)

2. Class III-A - liquids having a closed cup flash point at or above 140°F (60°C) and below 200°F (93.3°C) Class III-B - liquids having a closed cup flash point at or above 200°F (93.3°C).

Comitant strabismus A condition in which the magnitude of deviation remains essentially the same in all positions of gaze and with either eye fixating.

Commissioning The documented process, verifying that equipment and systems are installed according to specifications, placing the equipment and systems into active service and verifying its proper operation. Commissioning is done for good business, but can include many Qualification activities.

Commissure Compact bundles of nerve fibers that cross the midline and interconnect corresponding regions in opposite cerebral hemispheres. The principal commissures are the corpus callosum, anterior and posterior c ommissures.

Common bile duct A tube that moves bile from the liver to the small intestine.

Common carotid artery The major artery for the head and neck, that divides into the internal and external carotid arteries. On the right, it begins at the bifurcation of the brachiocephalic trunk, and on the left - it is a direct branch from the aorta.

Communicating veins Veins found in the thigh, lower leg, and foot that connect superficial and deep veins.

Communication The process by which information and feelings are shared by people through an exchange of verbal and non-verbal messages. In the context of medical education, its primary function is to establish understanding between patient and doctor. In an atmosphere of effective communication, patients improve faster, cope better with post-operative pain, require less psychotropic drugs, and experience numerous other health benefits.

Communication skills Proficiency in the interchange of information. These are essential skills for clinical practitioners because of the large and varied number of people they must communicate with every day. The idea that doctors automatically learn communication through experience or that doctors are inherently either good or bad communicators is being largely abandoned. It is now widely believed that such skills can be taught to both students and doctors by a variety of professionals including doctors and specialists in communication skills as an important part of undergraduate as well as postgraduate and continuing medical education.

Community A group of individuals living together in some form of social organization with cohesion in planning and operation and/or manifesting some unifying trait or common interest. In health care organization, it refers to the most local level of the health system. The form of services provided to a locality will vary according to each country's political, economic, social, cultural and epidemiological patterns.

Community diagnosis Appraisal of the health status of a community in general or limited to specific health conditions, determinants or subgroups.

Community medicine The specialty that deals with the health and disease of a population or of a specified community. The goal is to identify health problems and needs, to identify means by which these needs may be met, and to evaluate the extent to which health services do so. Community medicine is concerned with specified populations rather than individuals.

Community based LTC Community-based LTC refers to community-based programs such as Meals-on-Wheels, home health services, adult foster care centers, adult day care centers, hospice and other.

Comorbidity The presence of two or more conditions or diseases in the same person.

Companionship Services People who provide companionship to elderly and shut-in people, providing conversation, reading, and possibly light errands.

Comparison Group A group of facilities used to calculate comparison group percentages. By default, this is set to all facilities in the project that submit MDS data to CHSRA. Facilities that are part of our Oryx initiative also have the ability to select a Oryx facilities comparison group for its reports. Facilities located in Wisconsin also have the ability to select Wisconsin facilities participating in ePIP as their comparison group.

Competence Possession of a satisfactory level of relevant knowledge and acquisition of a range of relevant skills that include interpersonal and technical components at a certain point in the educational process. Such knowledge and skills are necessary to perform the tasks that reflect the scope of professional practices. Competence may differ from "performance", which denotes actions taken in a real life situation. Competence is therefore not the same as "knowing" on the contrary, it may well be about recognizing one's own limits. The more experienced the professional being tested, the more difficult it is to create a tool to assess their actual understandings and the complex skills of the tasks they undertake. A holistic integration of understandings, abilities and professional judgments i.e. a "generic" model, is one where competence is not necessarily directly observable, but rather can be inferred from performance.

Complaint Investigation An on-site investigation of specific allegations of noncompliance of a provider with State requirements.

Complementary DNA (cDNA) DNA that is synthesized from a messenger RNA template; the single-stranded form is often used as a probe in physical mapping.

Complementary sequence Nucleic acid base sequence that can form a doublestranded structure by matching base pairs with another sequence; the complementary sequence to GTAC is CATG.

Complete Abortion A miscarriage where all tissue has been passed out of the uterus

Compounding The bringing together of excipient and solvent components into a homogeneous mix of active ingredients.

Compressed gas A material, or mixture of materials that are either liquefied, nonliquefied, or in solution having a boiling point of 68°F (20°C) or less at 14.7 psia (101.3 kPa) of pressure. The exceptions to this rule are those gases that have no health or physical hazard properties. These gases are not considered compressed until the pressure in their packaging exceeds 41 psia (282.5 kPa) at 68°F (20°C).

Computed tomography (CT) A computerized imaging technique that take multiple X-ray measurements and then constructs a 2D or 3D image of the body.

Computed tomography scan (Also called CT or CAT scan.) A diagnostic imaging procedure that uses a combination of x-rays and computer technology to produce cross-sectional images (often called slices), both horizontally and vertically, of the body. A CT scan shows detailed images of any part of the body, including the bones, muscles, fat, and organs. CT scans are more detailed than general x-rays.

Computer controlled system Computer system plus its controlled function.

Computer related system Computerized system plus its operating environment.

Computer system A group of hardware components and associated software designed and assembled to perform a specific function or group of functions.

Computer vision syndrome (CVS) The complex of eye and vision problems related to near work that are experienced during or related to computer use. Its symptoms include eyestrain, dry or burning eyes, blurred vision, headaches, double vision, distorted color vision, and neck and backaches. The condition is caused by various internal and external factors. Treatment options may include prescription glasses and/or vision therapy.

Computerized system A process or operation integrated with a computer system.

Concavity (welding) A condition in which the surface of a welded joint is depressed relative to the surface of the tube or pipe. Concavity is measured as a maximum distance from the outside or the inside diameter surface of a welded joint along a line perpendicular to a line joining the weld toes.

Concentration polarization The phenomenon in ultrafiltration (UF) in which solutes form a dense, polarized layer next to the membrane surface eventually blocking further flow. UF systems counteract this by continuously flushing the solute away from the membrane surface.

Concept Mapping Theory A concept map is a diagram of a client's condition, assessment, and treatments. It can help the nurse develop interventions for treating the client as well as monitor the progress the client makes as a result of the interventions performed.

Concept mapping allows the nurse to work on critical thinking skills by determining the priority needs of the client and the relationship of the data documented on the concept map. Concept mapping is "an innovative approach to planning and organizing nursing care".

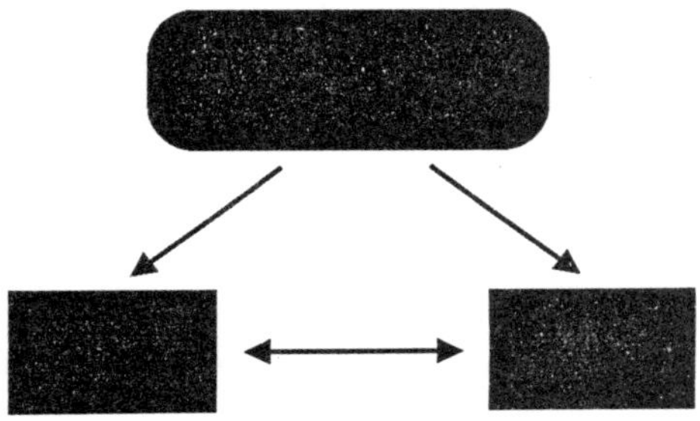

Fig. Concept mapping theory

Concurrent process validation Establishing documented evidence that a process does what it purports to do based on information generated during actual implementation of the process.

Condensate Distillate just after it has been cooled from steam into the liquid state.

Condenser The heat exchanger used in distillation to cool steam in order to convert it from the vapor to the liquid state.

Conductivity The reciprocal of resistivity (C=1/R). A measure of the ability to conduct an electric current. Since ionized impurities increase the conductivity of water, it is also an accurate measure of ionic purity. Conductivity is normally expressed in micromhos/cm (µmho/cm) or microsiemens/cm (µS/cm). To measure it, current is passed between two electrodes a fixed distance apart.

Cone A receptor cell which is sensitive to light and is located in the retina of the eye. It is responsible for color vision.

Configurable software Commercial, off-the-shelf software that can be configured to specific user applications without altering the basic program.

Configuration The three-dimensional shape or form of a macromolecule.

Confluence (of the sinuses) (Confluens sinuum, torcular herophili) An area where the dural venous sinuses (superior sagittal, straight sinus, right and left transverse sinuses) converge near the internal occipital protuberance.

Conformation The characteristic three-dimensional shape (tertiary structure) of a macromolecule.

Congenital Exsisting at birth. referring to certain mental or physical traits or peculiarities, malformations, diseases, which may be either hereditary or due to some influence occuring during gestation even up to the moment of birth.

Congenital problem Congenital problem—Problem present at birth.

Congregate Housing Dormitory-like settings where people live in the same building, occupy private rooms or apartments, and share some meals. Care is usually mostly custodial, with emergency medical assistance readily available. Some congregate housing may be rent-subsidized Section 8 housing.

Conization of the cervix Conization of the cervix—Surgical procedure performed on premalignant and malignant conditions of the cervix. A large biopsy of the cervix is taken in the shape of a cone.

Conjoined twins Conjoined twins-Twins connected at the body; they may share vital organs. Also called Siamese twins.

Conjugated Linoleic Acid (CLA) CLA occurs naturally in whole milk and red meat. A collective term used to designate a mixture of positional and geometric isomers of the essential fat linoleic acid. It is actually a fat, derived from linoleic acid (an essential fatty acid). Studies have shown that CLA can increase lean body mass and decrease fat, inhibit the growth of tumors and enhance immune function. CLA is found naturally in beef, cheese and whole milk.

Conjugated protein A protein containing a metal or an organic prosthetic group or both. Hemoglobin is a conjugated protein.

Conjunctivitis An inflammation of the conjunctiva, the transparent layer covering the inner eyelid and the white portion (sclera) of the eyeball. Conjunctivitis can be caused by a virus, bacteria, or fungus (infectious conjunctivitis, or "pink eye", may be contagious); by allergies to pollen, fabrics, animals, or cosmetics (allergic conjunctivitis); or by air pollution or noxious fumes such as swimming pool chorine (chemical conjunctivitis). Symptoms include red or watery eyes, blurred vision, inflamed inner eyelids, scratchiness in the eyes, or (with infectious conjunctivitis) a puss like or watery discharge and matted eyelids. Conjunctivitis is usually treated with antibiotic eye drops and/or ointment.

Consensus A decision by consensus is a decision in which all the group members find a common ground. It means that everyone understands the decision and can explain why it is best. It means that everyone can live with the decision.

Consent decree The result of a serious violation of regulations and related safety and quality standards. A company must agree to a series of measures aimed at bringing its manufacturing standards in compliance with regulations. Until agreed-upon conditions are met, a company may be forbidden to distribute its products in interstate commerce, except for those products deemed essential for the public health.

Conserved sequence A base sequence in a DNA molecule (or an amino acid sequence in a protein) that has remained essentially unchanged throughout evolution.

Constipation Hard, dry stools that are difficult to pass in a bowel movement, or having fewer than three bowel movements per week.

Constructed response questions A method of written examination in which examinees are required to construct their responses as opposed to selecting them from a set of options.

Consultant Pharmacist Pharmacist who is contracted by the nursing home to do drug regimen reviews and provide other services.

Contaminant Any unwanted or undesired component in a process fluid or controlled environment.

Contamination The undesired introduction of impurities of a chemical or microbiological nature, or of foreign matter, into or onto a raw material, intermediate, or API (Active Pharmaceutical Ingredient) during production, sampling, packaging or repackaging, storage or transport.

Contig Group of cloned (copied) pieces of DNA representing overlapping regions of a particular chromosome.

Contig map A map depicting the relative order of a linked library of small overlapping clones representing a complete chromosomal segment.

Continence One of the Activities of Daily Living (ADLs). The ability to control bowel and bladder function, use ostomy or catheter receptacles as needed, and apply diapers and disposable barrier pads as needed.

Continuing Care Retirement Community A campus-style community with housing which ranges from independent cottages or apartments, to assisted living facilities, to nursing home beds, allowing residents to stay within the campus as their care needs change. CCRCs often require large entrance fees, which may or may not be refundable to the residents if they leave. Generally, CCRCs only admit residents who are able to live independently, and provide residents with access to appropriate on-campus services as their care needs change. The CCRC may promise to cover care costs for life via a Life Care Contract, or may guarantee access to other services or offer priority consideration if services are needed. The terms of these agreements may or may not provide some amount of free or discounted care.

Continuing medical education (CME) A continuous process of acquiring new knowledge and skills throughout one's professional life. As undergraduate and postgraduate education is insufficient to ensure lifelong physicians' competencies, it is essential to maintain the competencies of physicians, to remedy gaps in skills, and to enable professionals to respond to the challenges of rapidly growing knowledges and technologies, changing health needs and the social, political and economic factors of the practice of medicine. Continuing medical education depends highly upon learner motivation and self-directed learning skills.

Continuity of Care The provision of midwifery care during the antepartum, intrapartum and postpartum periods, to a client by a midwife known to the woman, including 24-hours availability of care. Although the Manitoba Midwifery Regulation defines continuity of care as providing care to the same woman through at least four antepartum visits, labour and birth, the newborn examination and at least one postpartum visit, this is the minimum requirement. The expectation is that the midwife would see a woman more frequently. No more than four midwives should be involved in the care of an individual woman. Each woman must have a primary midwife, or a "shared primary care" midwife who is responsible for coordinating her care.

Continuous fermentation A process in which sterile medium is added without interruption to the fermentation system with a balancing withdrawal (or "harvesting") of broth for product extraction. The length of fermentation can be measured in weeks or months. Commercial applications of continuous fermentation are limited in number, with ethanol production by yeast the most important example.

Continuum of care A description of the wide variety of long term care needs and services, from those for people who retain a significant ability to live independently with minimal assistance, to services for people who are severely ill, bedfast, or even comatose.

Contraceptive prevalence rate (CPR) Percentage of women of reproductive age who are using (or whose partner is using) a contraceptive method at a given point in time. In practice the CPR is generally reported on women who are currently married or in union, which should be stated accordingly.

Contract manufacturer A company holding an agreement requiring the performance of some aspect of API manufacturing.

Contraction The rhythmic squeezing of the heart muscle that causes blood to be pumped out of the heart chambers and into the body. This contraction produces a heartbeat.

Contraction stress test Contraction stress test-Response of fetus to uterine contractions to evaluate fetal well-being.

Contralateral Affecting or pertaining to the opposite side.

Control area A building or portion of a building within which the exempted amounts of hazardous materials may be stored, dispensed, handled, or used.

Control group The group of subjects in a controlled study that receives no treatment, receives a standard treatment, or receives a placebo.

Control Panel A program that comes with Windows 98 that enables you to make settings for many Windows 98 actions, such as changing network, keyboard, printer, and regional settings. Some programs (including many video card drivers) may add sections to the control panel for you to use to configure that program.

Control parameters Those operating variables that can be assigned values and are used as control levels.

Control serum Serum used as a standard for clinical chemistry lab tests. Most often produced from outdated whole blood plasma. Most often turbid and difficult to filter.

Controlled area An area constructed and operated in such a manner that some attempt is made to control the introduction of potential contamination, and the consequences of accidental release of living organisms. The level of control exercised should reflect the nature of the organism employed in the process. At a minimum, the area should be maintained at a pressure negative to the immediate external environment and allow for the efficient removal of small quantities of airborne contaminants.

Controlled Substance A drug, substance or immediate precursor included in schedules I to V of the Controlled Substance Act (e.g., morphine, acetaminophen with codeine, oxycodone).

Conus medullaris The cone-shaped terminal part of the spinal cord. Located at lower border of the first lumbar vertebra.

Conventional drugs New compounds made up by chemical synthesis or fermentation. These are termed by the FDA as NCEs (new chemical entities). The FDA rates conventional drugs with important therapeutic gain as 1-A drugs, for priority review. For example, AIDS drugs are conventional drugs approved for AIDS or AIDS-associated conditions.

Conventional flow cleanroom A room supplied with filtered air with no specified requirement for uniform airflow patterns or velocity. Airflow patterns are usually turbulent.

Convergence The ability to use both eyes as a team and to be able to turn the eyes inward to maintain single vision up close.

Convergence excess (CE) A clinical condition in which the eyes have a tendency to turn excessively inward when viewing an object at a near distance. Symptoms may include visual fatigue while reading or using a computer, occasional blurred or double vision, and inability to comprehend or concentrate while reading. Clinical signs include: greater esophoria at near than distance, high AC/A ratio, and a high lag of accommodation. Can be improved with vision therapy and/or glasses.

Convergence insufficiency (CI) (clinical condition) The inability of the eyes to turn inward and/or sustain an inward turn. Symptoms include eye strain with reading and using a computer, headaches, loss of comprehension, difficulty concentrating, blurred or double vision, and eye fatigue. Clinical signs include: near point of convergence of greater than 4 inches (10 cm), greater exophoria at near than at distance, and low AC/A ratio. Vision therapy is an effective treatment option.

Converted data Any original data that has been entered into a user-developed application (spreadsheet, database, report, etc.) for manipulation, evaluation, or review.

Convexity A condition in which the surface of a welded joint is extended relative to the surface of the tube or pipe. Convexity is measured as a maximum distance from the outside or inside diameter surface of a welded joint along a line perpendicular to a line joining the weld toes.

Copper Active in the storage and release of iron to form hemoglobin for red blood cells.

Copy A command on the Edit menu that adds data (text or pictures) to the clipboard, while leaving the original data unchanged. Used often with the 'paste' command.

Coracoid process A projection of bone that originates from the upper part of the neck of the scapula and overhangs the shoulder joint.

Cord Accident A general term for many problems with the umbilical cord, including prolapse, a knot tied in the cord, or any failure of the cord to provide oxygen and nutrients to the baby.

Cord Prolapse A condition when the umbilical cord falls through the cervix and possibly even into the vaginal canal, usually during labor or when water breaks. Delivery or cesarean is usually performed immediately.

Corn steep liquor An ingredient in the culture medium for producing penicillin. A natural nitrogenous material that is a by-product of the corn milling industry.

Cornea The transparent, blood-free tissue covering the central front of the eye (over the pupil, iris, and aqueous humor) that initially refracts or bends light rays as light enters the eye. Contact lenses are fitted over the cornea.

Coronal Plane (Frontal Plane) A verticle plane running from side to side; divides the body or any of its parts into anterior and posterior portions.

Coronal suture This calvarial (vault) synostosis is the coronal plane between the frontal and parietal bones.

Coronal view Longitudinal section passing through the body at right angles to the median plane, in a "frontal" or "facing" orientation. This is the plane of the coronal suture of the skull - and vice versa.

Coronary angiogram A procedure in which catheters are passed into the heart and coronary arteries. Radiopaque dye (x-ray dye) is injected so that x-ray pictures of the heart and arteries may be taken.

Coronary arteries The arteries which originate from the root of the ascending aorta and supply the cardiac musckle of the atria and ventricles with blood.

Coronary artery bypass graft (CABG) An operation performed to circumvent blocked coronary arteries and deliver blood to areas of the heart receiving insufficient blood flow.

Coronary artery disease (CAD) The formation of blockages or atherosclerotic lesions within coronary arteries which result in restricted blood flow.

Coronary sinus The end portion of the cardiac vein which empties into the right atrium.

Corpora quadrigemina Term applied to the four protuberances on the dorsal surface of the midbrain; the two superior and two inferior colliculi.

Corpus callosum A large commissural bundle of fibers interconnecting the two cerebral hemispheres. It is subdivided into a rostrum, genu , body and a splenium.

Corpus luteum Corpus luteum—Area in the ovary where the egg is released at ovulation. A cyst may form in this area after ovulation. Called a corpus luteum cyst.

Corrosive A chemical that causes visible destruction or irreversible alterations in living tissue by chemical action at the site of contact. This term shall not refer to action on inanimate surfaces.

Corrosive liquid A liquid which when in contact with living tissue, will cause destruction or irreversible alteration of such tissue by chemical action. Examples include acidic, alkaline, or caustic materials.

Corrugated Having a ripple-like distortion.

Cortex The outer layer of a body or organ structure. From the Latin word for "bark". (Like the "cortex" of the kidney or brain.).

Cortex cerebral The superficial layer of gray matter that covers the cerebral hemispheres. It varies in thickness from 1.5 (striate cortex) to 4.5 (motor cortex) mm in thickness and consists of from 3 to 6 horizo ntal layers of cells.

Corticosteroids This is a family of drugs used to treat numerous autoimmune and inflammatory conditions. They are also used to treat severe allergic reactions and to prevent rejection after an organ transplant.

Cortisol A catabolic hormone that is released and increases in response to stress when the body is subjected to trauma such as intense exercises, including weight training. Excess cortisol is known to increase catabolism (protein breakdown in muscles). Cortisol leads to muscle breakdown through promoting a release of muscle amino acids for transport to the liver, where the amino acids are coverted into glucose.

Cosmid Artificially constructed cloning vector containing the cos gene of phage lambda. Cosmids can be packaged in lambda p0hage particles for infection into E. coli: this permits cloning of larger DNA fragments (up to 45kb) that can be introduced into bacterial hosts in plasmid vectors.

Cost benefit analysis Comparison of all the costs and benefits of a given activity or program expressed in monetary terms. It is used for the allocation of funds in health care services. This form of analysis permits one to measure the costs for reaching particular objectives. In the case of health programs, benefits are often difficult to express in monetary terms, and furthermore, benefits may extend beyond the achievement of the desired effect, which makes such evaluation difficult.

Cost Report Reports provided to Medicare Intermediaries and state Agencies by nursing homes and other healthcare providers. They are prepared on mandated forms, and there are extensive rules specifying which costs are allowable, and where and how these costs are to be reported. Costs reported may be used as the basis for "cost-based reimbursement."

Cost based reimbursement Provider reimbursement rates which are set based on facility-specific costs as reported on the facility's Cost Reports.

Cost containment Measures taken to control or restrict medical care expenditures or to reduce the rate of their growth. This includes a broad range of cost control mechanisms e.g. limiting budgets, cost-sharing, regulation of supply of services and staff, patients' waiting lists, exclusion of certain people from entitlement to services, standard costing, privatization, and managed competition.

Cost effectiveness analysis A method for evaluating the relationship between the cost and the effectiveness of an activity or to compare similar or alternative activities to determine the relative degree to which they will produce the desired objectives or outcomes. The degree of effectiveness is understood to be the extent to which a given activity or program contributes to attaining the objectives of reducing the dimension of a problem or improving an unsatisfactory situation. The preferred action is the one that requires the least cost to produce a given level of effectiveness. In the health care field, the cost is expressed in monetary terms but the consequences may be expressed in physical units such as healthy life-years gained, the number of cases of disease detected or the improvement in health status of a population.

Cost efficiency analysis A method for evaluating program or activity efficiency such as the extent to which resources are being used as productively as possible. In health care, it measures medical services provided in relation to their cost. This enables comparison between different health care providers.

Costophrenic angle Point of junction between the costal and diaphragmatic pleurae.

Costophrenic sulcus (recess) The space, or potential space, between the ribs ("costo-") of the lateral chest wall and the diagphragm ("phrenic").

Covariant Changing with another variable: exhibiting a tendency to change in conjunction with another statistical variable.

Cover test A test of eyeball alignment in which each eye is covered with an occluder (eye cover) and then uncovered to observe eye movements.

COVTT certified optometric vision therapy technician To be certified an individual must be employed by a Fellow (FCOVD), provide documentation of 2000 hours or 2 years of direct clinical experience in vision therapy; or 1000 hours of clinical experience if the individual holds an AA degree or higher with emphasis in the behavioral sciences. Submit written answers to a series of Open Book Questions dealing with various aspects of vision function, testing and therapy. Pass an extensive written and oral examination evaluating the candidate's knowledge and clinical abilities in behavioral vision, vision development and vision therapy. COVTTs must obtain at least 6 hours of continuing education annually in functional / developmental / behavioral vision care.

COX-2 inhibitors This is the newest class of non-steroid anti-inflammatory drugs, used to rein in inflammatory processes. They work by blocking the COX-2 enzyme, which is involved in triggering inflammation.

CP (cyclic polarization) An electrochemical test (ASTM G61) for metals that measures the point at which pitting corrosion begins. CP uses an electrolytic cell to directly measure the corrosion rate. By using the test piece as the working electrode, initiation of localized corrosion is shown by the potential at which the current density increases rapidly. This point is called the "pitting potential". The lower the current density at this point, the more resistance to pitting corrosion. The current density is measured in micro-amps per square centimeter.

CPU CPU stands for Central Processing Unit and is often, simply called, the processor. The CPU is a microchip that is installed on a motherboard and acts as the computer's brain—performing calculations and coordinating the hardware components.

Cranial autonomic ganglia Groups of nerve cell bodies located outside the brain and associated with cranial nerves III, VII, IX and ,X. They represent the location of postganglionic prasymapthetic neurons.

Cranial nerve ganglia Groups of nerve cell bodies located outside the brain and associated with certain of the cranial nerves. They represent the location of cell bodies of sensory neurons.

Cranial nerve lesion An injury from any of a number of causes to a cranial nerve, its nuclei of origin or termination and/or its supranuclear projections that results in some pathological alteration in its function.

Cranial nerve nuclei Groups or columns of nerve cells within the brainstem representing the sites of origin and termination of the various cranial nerves.

Cranial nerves Twelve pairs of nerves that originate in the brain and provide sensory and motor innervation to regions of the head, neck, throax and abdomen.

Cranial nerves(7/8) The twelve pairs of "nerves" that are directly connected to the brain. They are the nervi olfactorii(I), opticus(II), oculomotorius(III), trochlearis (IV), trigeminus (V), abducens (VI), facialis (VII), vestibulocochlearis (VIII), glosso-pharyngeus (IX), vagus (X), accessorius (XI), and hypoglossus (XIII). The olfactory "nerve" and the optic "nerve" are actually post-synaptic tracts with glial cells like astrocytes and oligodendrocytes, rather than Schwann cells.

Craniosacral therapy A manual procedure for remedying distortions in the structure and function of the craniosacral mechanism - the brain and spinal cord, the bones of the skull, the sacrum, and interconnected membranes. It is used to treat chronic pain, migraine headaches, TMJ, and a range of other conditions.

Cranium The part of the skull (8 bones) which encloses and protects the brain. It excludes the 14 bones of the face.

Crash The failure of a hardware component, software application, or the computer itself. A crash can affect the program you are using, the operating system, or the entire computer, and often results in the need to restart the computer.

Creatine & ATP ATP is the molecule that releases the energy for contraction of muscles, the breakdown and synthesis of proteins and all other reactions requiring energy. In short, ATP is the energy molecule powering all of our movements. By giving off its energy through its high energy phosphate bond, ATP is reduced to ADP. The problem is that the amount of ATP that is stored in our cells is limited. Depending on the intensity of the activity, ATP supplies can be used up by converting to ADP within seconds. So how do athletes run or workout for long periods. We can do that because there are three way to replenish ATP. 1.

You can restore ATP using energy derived from the oxidation of fats and carbohydrates. This is a slow process that occurs in the mitochondria. 2.

You can restore ATP through lactic acid, which is utilized to produce energy, which turns ADP back into ATP.

3. Through Creatine Monohydrate, which helps creatine phosphate create more ATP from ADP within seconds. It is a short term, high energy backup for ATP. It does not need carbohydrates, fats or oxygen to recharge ATP.

Creatine (monohydrate) A muscle fuel that is extracted naturally from meat and fish, or synthesized in the lab. Once it is in the muscles, creatine combines with phosphorous to make Creatine Phosphate (CP), a high powered chemical that rebuilds the muscles ultimate energy source, Adenosine Triphosphate (ATP). CP powers your muscles for high intensity exercise for short periods only, consequently, athletes who compete in power and sprint event will have an advantage if they take supplemental creatine. More CP in the muscle cell translates into a greater resistance to fatigue. Also, CP helps with the transfer of energy in the muscle cells, thus speeding up the action, which may enhance performances that are aerobically taxing. Reports says people who take creatine supplements may recover from intense activity faster and experience less postexercise muscle soreness.

Creatine is a naturally occurring compound in the muscle tissue and when converted in the muscle tissue to phosphocreatine during exercise can provide sudden bursts of energy. Insufficient amounts of phosphocreatine could result in a fatigued feeling in the muscle. The Creatine Monohydrate Powder provides enough energy to delay to onset of fatigue. Creatine Monohydrate is a synthesized metabolite that is the powerful energizer providing instant energy and strength with better endurance and helps to maintain optimal levels of ATP production during intense exercise.

Creatine (titrate) Titrated creatine is less expensive than effervescent creatine, but has the same total solubality and absorbability. The result is free-ionized, soluble creatine. Titrated creatine acheives the process by titrating, or changing, the pH of the water when it's stirred in. The altered pH solution enables more than 95 percents of the creatine to go into solution, so you get dissolved creatine.

Creatinine A waste product that is filtered from the blood by the kidneys and expelled in urine.

CREST One of two types of scleroderma, an autoimmune disorder characterized by thickening of the skin. Unlike the more severe form of scleroderma called progressive systemic sclerosis, which affects internal organs, CREST is limited to the skin of the hands and face. CREST stands for Calcinosis, Raynaud's phenomenon, Esophageal involvement, Sclerodactyly and Telangiectasia.

Cricoid cartilage The cartilage that forms the lower and back portion of the larynx, just above the trachea.

Crista galli A midline cocks come-like projection of the ethmoid bone into the anterior cranial fossa to which the falx cerebri attaches anteriorly.

Critical A material, process step, or process condition, test requirement, or any other relevant parameter is considered critical when non-compliance with predetermined criteria directly influences the quality attributes of the API (active pharmaceutical ingredient) in a detrimental manner.

Critical area An area where (sterile) product or contact surface is exposed, normally Class 100 (e.g., Point of Fill).

Critical device A device that directly ensures that a GMP Critical Parameter is maintained within predetermined limits (e.g., terminal HEPA filter, point of use filter). A malfunction of such a device would place product quality directly at risk.

Critical instrument An instrument that measures a GMP Critical Parameter, used to monitor and document that parameter.

Critical parameter A GMP or product quality parameter (e.g., differential pressure, unidirectional airflow pattern) that must be maintained within predefined limits to ensure product SISPQ (Strength, Identity, Safety, Purity, or Quality).

Critical point The combination of pressure and temperature at which the gas and liquid phases of a substance become indistinguishable.

Critical process step For sterile products, this normally is an activity where product or product contact parts are exposed to the surrounding environment.

Critical step(s) The point or points in the process which, if not carried out properly or if contaminated, will not allow drug substances to be made such that they will meet their intended characterizations and impurity profiles.

Critical surface The part of the working surface to be protected from particulate contamination. It is within the Critical Zone.

Critical system A structural, mechanical, or electrical system that can impact the processing parameters and attributes of the finished product or regulatory study. Critical systems may include utilities, process equipment, and systems.

Crohn's disease A chronic illness that causes irritation in the digestive tract. It occurs most commonly in the ileum (lower small intestine) or in the colon (large intestine). It is a form of inflammatory bowel disease.

Cross contamination The measurable and detrimental contamination of a material or product with another material or product.

Crossing over The breaking during meiosis of one maternal and one paternal chromosome, the exchanging of corresponding sections of DNA, and the rejoining of the chromosomes. This process can result in an exchange of alleles between chromosomes.

Crown to rump length Crown-to-rump length-Measurement from the top of the baby's head (crown) to the buttocks of the baby (rump).

Cruciate ligaments The "cross-shaped" ligaments situated in the knee joint between the femoral condyles and the proximal tibia (tibial spines) that form a cross-shaped structure.

Crude birth rate (CBR) The number of live births in a given period per 1,000 people in the same period. Usually expressed per year.

Crus cerebrii Another name for basis pedunculi of the cerebral peduncle.

Crus of diaphragm The fibromuscular bands originating from the upper three or four lumbar vertebrae and inserting into the central tendon of the diaphragm.

Cryogenic liquid A fluid that has a normal boiling point below -150°F (-101.1°C).

Cryotherapy During an operation probes are placed in the prostate. The probes are then frozen which kills the prostatic cells.

Cryptography The mathematical science of deliberately scrambling and unscrambling information. Information is protected by being transformed (encrypted) into an unreadable format, called cipher text. Only those who posses a secret key can decypher (or decrypt) that message into plain text.

Crystalline lens Transparent disc located behind the iris which changes shape to focus on objects at different distances from the eye.

CSF (cerebrospinal fluid) This is the fluid that surrounds and protects the brain and spinal cord. It is made primarily by the choroid plexus and is absorbed by the arachnoid villi and granulations of the dural sinuses and veins.

CT Computerized tomography. An imaging device that uses computation to produce an image from multiple individual measurements of X-ray attenuation ("absorption"). Modern CT machines with multiple detector arrays can make 4-8-16 slices simultaneously.

Ctrl A special key on most computer keyboards that, when used in combination with another key, allows the user to easily access special controls. For example, Ctrl+S saves a file in most Windows programs.

Ctrl+Alt+Del A common PC hotkey combination. Pressing the Ctrl, Alt, and Del keys simultaneously in a DOS environment would automatically restart (warm boot) the computer. In Windows98, the combination brings up the "close program" dialog box which allows users the choice of shutting down a specific program (usually one that has crashed), or restarting the computer.

Cuboid A cube-shaped bone in the foot.

Cul de sac A blind pouch.

Culture medium Any nutrient system for the artificial cultivation of bacteria or other cells; usually a complex mixture of organic and inorganic materials. current good manufacturing practices (cGMP's)

Cuneate tubercle A swelling on the dorsal surface of the medulla oblongata that marks the location of the underlying cuneate nucleus.

Cuneiforms A wedged-shaped bone in the foot.

Cuneus A region of the occipital lobe of the brain located on the medial surface of the cerebral hemisphere between the parieto-occipital and calcarine sulci.

Curb to Curb A common designation for Paratransit services. The transit vehicle picks up and discharges passengers at the curb or driveway in front of their home or destination. In curb-to-curb service the driver does not assist the passenger along walks or steps to the door of the home or other destination.

Curriculum An educational plan that spells out which goals and objectives should be achieved, which topics should be covered and which methods are to be used for learning, teaching and evaluation.

Cursor A blinking character that indicates the location of the next input on the display screen. The cursor indicates where you are working in a document or program. A pointing element (usually an arrow or hand) in graphical user interfaces that is controlled by a mouse or some other pointing device. Also called a pointer.

Cut A command on the Edit menu that adds data (text or pictures) to the clipboard by removing it from its original document or position in that document.

CVS (Chorionic Villus Sampling) (CVS): A procedure performed via the cervix between the 8th and 12th week of pregnancy to detect genetic defects in the fetus. Cells taken from the chorion - a layer of embryonic tissue surrounding the fetus - are analyzed for chromosomal abnormalities.

Cyanosis A bluish discoloration of the skin and mucous membranes due to an excessive concentration of reduced (deoxygenated) hemoglobin in the blood.

Cycloplegic refraction One method available to eye doctors to determine the eye's refractive error and the best corrective lenses to be prescribed if needed. The eye is dilated with the muscles of accommodation (eye focusing muscles) being temporarily paralyzed with specialized eye drops or spray (Atropine, Homatropine, Cyclogyl, or Mydriacyl). This is a good method for non-responsive or non-communicative patients such as young children. The technique of retinoscopy is used with this method.

Cylinder lens An ophthalmic lens that has at least one non-spherical surface. Used to correct astigmatism. The values are typically from -0.75 to -1.25. The cylinder measurement is given with a "-" sign. (Please note that the sign for myopia (nearsightedness) is also "-".).

Cyst A lump filled with either fluid or soft material, occurring in any organ or tissue; may occur for a number of reasons but is usually harmless unless its presence disrupts organ or tissue function.

Cyst(o) (prefix) Bladder. e.g. cystitis - inflammation of the urinary bladder.

Cystectomy Surgical removal of the bladder.

Cystic duct The connection between the neck of the gallbladder and the common bile duct.

Cystic fibrosis An inherited disease in which thick mucus clogs the lungs and blocks the ducts of the pancreas.

Cystic Fibrosis Cystic Fibrosis Cystic fibrosis is the most common genetic disease among Caucasian people. Children with cystic fibrosis have problems with lung secretions and they also have problems with enzymes that break down material in the bowel.

Cystitis Cystitis-Inflammation of the bladder.

Cystocele A herniation of bladder into vagina.

Cystogram A radiograph of the bladder opacified (filled with radiopaque contrast).

Cystoscopy A flexible scope is inserted into the urethra and then into the bladder to determine abnormalities in the bladder and lower urinary tract.

Cytogeneticist One who studies human chromosomes and their abnormalities.

Cytokine A protein that acts as a chemical messenger to stimulate cell migration, usually toward where the protein is released. Interlukins, lymphokines, and interferons are the most common.

Cytolysis The dissolution of cells particularly by destruction of their cell membrane.

Cytomegalovirus infection Cytomegalovirus (CMV) infection-Group of viruses from the herpesvirus family.

Cytopathic Damaging to cells.

Cytopathologist A medical specialty dealing with examination and diagnosis of cells.

Cytoplasm The protoplasmic contents of the cell outside the nucleus in which the cell's organelles are suspended.

Cytosine (C) A pyrimidine occurring as a fundamental unit or base of nucleic acids.

Cytostatic agents Therapeutics that inhibit cell division and growth. This term can refer to machinery, such as those that would freeze cells.

Cytotoxic Poisonous to cells.

Cytotoxicity The ability of a substance or compound to cause a cytotoxic effect.

D

D value The time under a stated set of exposure conditions (temperature in an autoclave) required to reduce a microbial population by a factor of 90% (e.g. from 10,000 to 1,000).

D&C D&C (dilatation and curettage) – Surgical procedure in which the cervix is dilated and the lining of the uterus is scraped.

D5W (5 D/W) One of the most prevalent of LVPs . Five percent dextrose in water. Presence of dextrose presents significant filtration problems. Usually requires activated charcoal pretreatment.

Dalton The unit of molecular weight, equal to the weight of a hydrogen atom.

Data The raw material of information. Refers mostly to the information entered into, and stored within a computer or file.

Data Integrity The validity of data and their relationships. For electronic records to be trustworthy and reliable, the links between raw data, metadata, and results must not be compromised or broken. Without data integrity, it is not possible to regenerate a previous result reliably.

Data migration The process of translating data from one system to another when a company replaces the current computing systems with a new one. CFR 21 Part 11 mandates that data migration implementation create accurate and complete copies of the records when they are moved to a new system.

Data Processing Operations performed on data to provide useful information to users.

Database A collection of data organized so that various programs can access and update the information.

DD An acronym for "Darling Daughter" used when talking about your own child.

DDC (direct digital control) A collection of control units (analog and discrete) connected into a data highway, usually with a host or alarming/recording computer attached.

De minimis release The release of viable microbiological agents or eukaryotic cells that does not result in the establishment of disease in healthy people, plants, or animals; or in uncontrolled proliferation of any microbiological agents or eukaryotic cells.

Dead leg An area of entrapment in a vessel or piping run that could lead to contamination of the product. In a piping system, a non-flowing pocket, tee, or extension from a primary piping run that exceeds a defined number of pipe diameters from the ID of the primary pipe. Denoted by the term L/D or L/A, where L is equal to the leg extension perpendicular to the normal flow pattern or direction, A is the annular gap width, and D is equal to the ID (or inside dimension) of the extension or leg. In some existing standards, the dimension L is measured from the centerline of the primary pipe. For bioprocessing systems, an L/D of 2:1 is achievable with today's component technology for most valving and piping configurations.

Debug The process of testing a program in order to find mistakes and eliminating them, before the program is made available to users.

Decontamination A process that reduces contaminating substances to a defined acceptance level.

Decussation A location in the brain where nerve fibers cross the midline (ie. decussation of te superior cerebellar peduncle).

Deep Extending well inward from an outer surface.

Deep lymph NODES Small masses of lymphatic tissue that connect lymph vessels in the deep fascia.

Deep tissue bodywork General term for a range of therapies that seek to improve the function of the body's connective tissues and/or muscles. Among the conditions treated are whiplash, low back and neck pain, and degenerative diseases, such as multiple sclerosis.

Default Settings or options the computer automatically adopts if the user does not specify any.

Default Directory Found in programs that are required to save information to the hard drive or disk drives such as word processor documents or spreadsheets. This is the location the program will save the files in. Usually the default directory can be chosen by the user in the program options menu.

Defecation The act of passing a bowel movement.

Defibrillation The stopping of a fast heart rate by delivering a high-energy electrical shock to restore the heart's normal rhythm. Electrical current is used to restore the heart's natural pacemaker function which resumes a normal heartbeat. The shock is administered through electrodes placed on the chest wall (external defibrillation) or in the heart (internal defibrillation).

Defibrillator An internal or external device that can deliver an electric shock to stop extremely rapid and irregular heartbeats and return the heart to normal rhythm.

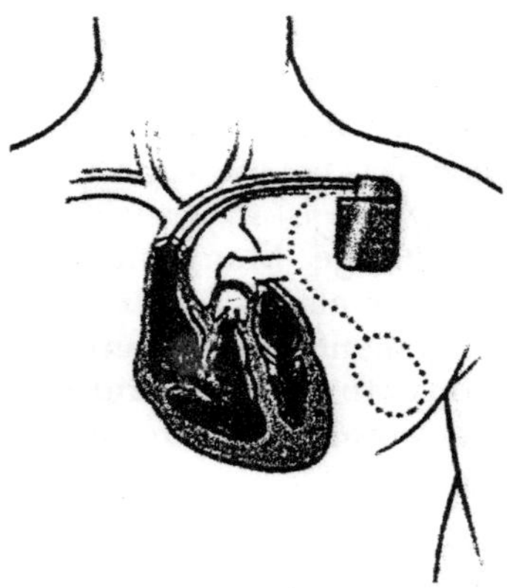

Fig. Defibrillator

Deflagration An exothermic reaction, such as the extremely rapid oxidation of a combustible dust or flammable vapor in air, in which the reaction progresses through the unburned material at a rate less than the velocity of sound. A deflagration can have an explosive effect.

Degrading Deterioration of a surface finish so that pieces of the finish (or substrate) material large enough to be visible to the unaided eye, dislodge without any direct physical contact and fall from the surface of the material.

Dehydration When the bloodstream and the cells of the body contain less fluid than normal, often due to vomiting or diarrhea. The body's mineral balance may also be affected.

Deionization Removing dissolved ions from solution by passing the solution through a bed of ion exchange resin, consisting of polymer beads that exchange hydrogen ions for cations and hydroxyl ions for anions in solution. The ionic impurities remain bound to the resins and the hydrogen and hydroxyl ions combine with each other to form water.

Delete A key on the keyboard that erases information on the screen.

Deletion map A description of a specific chromosome that uses defined mutations - specific deleted areas in the genome - as "biochemical signposts", or markers for specific areas.

Delirium An acute or sudden state of confusion. It is not the same as dementia or senility, which is an irreversible gradual chronic change. Many individuals with dementia can also get delirium. This often results in a significant sudden change in their confusion or function. Delirium is an urgent medical condition, not a psychiatric problem.

Deliveries attended by skilled health personnel Percentage of deliveries attended by skilled health personnel irrespective of outcome (live birth or fetal death).

Demand A need or desire for a product or service. Price, availability and quality of the product all affect demand. Demand for health services is often difficult to assess and surveys of willingness to pay may be necessary to estimate its scope or extent.

Demand Response The type of Paratransit service where individual passengers can request transportation from a specific location to another specific location at a certain time. Transit vehicles providing demand-response service do not follow a fixed route, but travel throughout the community transporting passengers according to their specific requests. These services usually, but not always, require advance reservations.

Dementia The loss of cognitive or intellectual function. This term describes a group of symptoms that encompass a loss of intellectual ability, mental processes, vocabulary, abstract thinking, judgment, memory loss, and physical coordination that interfere with daily activities. The symptoms can be brought on by degenerative diseases like Alzheimers, Huntington's and Parkinson's diseases, vascular diseases, stroke, metabolic disorders like thyroid, liver kidney dysfunction, certain vitamin deficiencies, AIDS, drugs and alcohol, or psychiatric disorders. Some dementing disorders may respond to treatments, others do not.

Demineralization Sometimes used interchangeably with deionization, it refers to the removal of minerals and mineral salts using ion exchange. Water softening is a common form of demineralization.

Denaturation The loss of the native structure of a macromolecule resulting, from heat treatment, extreme pH changes, chemical treatment, etc. It is accompanied by loss of biological activity. For example, proteins may be denatured by heat, pH extremes, or addition of agents such as urea or guanidinium hydrochloride.

Dendrite The highly branched tree-like process of a neuron that serves as a receptive field and conducts impulses toward the cell body.

Denial of Payment for New Admissions A penalty that must be imposed when a facility is not in substantial compliance within 3 months after being found out of compliance. Denial of payment and State Monitoring must be imposed when a facility has been found to have provided substandard quality of care on three consecutive standard surveys.

Density Refers to a diskette's data capacity. Double density (DD) disks hold twice as much information as single density, and high density (HD—today's standard) hold about twice as much as double density.

Dent A typical stainless steel interior surface anomaly that refers to a large, smooth-bottomed depression whose diameter or width is greater than its depth and which will not produce an indication.

Dentate gyrus A slender gyrus with a scalloped appearance that runs along the hyppocampal sulcus; a component of the hippocampal formation. Like the hippocampus it consists of 3 cellular layers whose proce sses do not extend beyond the hippocampal formation.

Dentate nucleus The largest and most lateral of the cerebellar nuclei. It is located deep within the white matter of cerebellum and is shaped like a crumpled purse with its hilus directed medially.It is associated functionally with the neoce rebellum.

Denticulate ligament Condensation of spinal pia mater that laterally anchors the spinal cord along its length to the dura-arachnoid sleeve.

Dentistry, wholistic Wholistic dentists are licensed dentists who bring an interdisciplinary approach to their practice, often incorporating such methods as homeopathy, nutrition and acupuncture into their treatment plans. Most wholistic dentists emphasize wellness and preventive care and avoid silver-mercury fillings.

Depo Provera A synthetic hormone given in larger doses as a form of birth control that works about three months, or a smaller dose to help stimulate periods in a woman whose cycle is not ending.

Depth perception The ability to judge relative distances of objects.

Depth perception test A test to measure the ability of the vision system to discern the relative distances of various objects. (Also called a "Stereopsis Test").

Depyrogenation The removal or destruction of endotoxins.

Derma, dermat(o) (prefix) Skin. e.g. dermatitis - inflammation of the skin.

Desalination The removal of dissolved salts from brine to produce potable water.

Descending aorta The protion of the aorta from the arch to its division in the abdomen into the common iliac arteries.

Descending colon The part of the colon between the left colic flexure ("splenic flexure") and the sigmoid colon (at the pelvic brim).

Desiccant Chemical salt used to dehumidify air, to control moisture in materials contacting that air.

Desiccators Closed containers, usually made of glass or plastic, with an airtight seal used for drying materials.

Design condition The specified range or accuracy of a controlled variable used by the designer to determine performance requirements of an engineered system.

Design specification A specification that defines the design of a system or system component.

Desktop The main workspace in a graphical user interface such as Windows or Macintosh Systems. Users open and work with files and programs on the desktop, and can store files and shortcuts there as well. The user can also customize the look of the desktop with images or wallpaper and custom icons.

Determinant Any factor, event, characteristic, or other definable entity that brings about change in a health condition or other defined characteristic.

Detonation An exothermic reaction characterized by the presence of a shock wave in a material that establishes and maintains the reaction. The reaction zone progresses through the material at a rate greater than the velocity of sound. The principal heating mechanism is one of shock compression. Detonations have an explosive effect.

Deuteromycetes Molds that cannot reproduce by sexual means. Some pathogenic fungi such as Trichophyton, which causes athlete's foot, belong to this family.

Developmental delay Developmental delay—Condition in which the development of the baby or child is slower than normal.

Developmental Disability (DD) A severe chronic disability that has its origin in childhood and results in limitations in such areas as language, self-care, mobility, learning, economic self-sufficiency and independent living. Definitions define childhood as occurring before age 22; some states use other definitions. The definition includes both mental and physical impairments; states may differ in whether physical impairments in the absence of mental impairment is defined as a developmental disability. The specific definition used in each situation will affect the supports available to an individual.

Developmental disorder When a delay in an individual's normal development has occurred.

Developmental vision analysis More comprehensive than a routine eye exam, examination will evaluate all of the patient's visual abilities such as visual acuity, eye focusing skills, eye teaming skills, eye tracking skills, visual motor skills, and visual perceptual skills.

DHEA (Dehydroepiandrosterone) A hormone made by the adrenal glands used by the body to make male (androgen) and female (estrogen) hormones; possible positive effects on mood and energy on older individuals (40+) whose production of DHEA has declined. As been referred to as the 'Fountain of Youth' hotmone bacause it declines rapidly as we age, and supplementation with this hormone reverses many of the ravages associated with aging. Studies show that men with the highest DHEA levels have better cardiovascular health.

DHL vaccine A tri-valent vaccine. Also, the most common veterinary vaccine that has a combination of viral and bacterial vaccines. Used for distemper, hepatitis (canine), and leptospira.

Dia (prefix) Through; between; ss. e.g. diarrhea - fecal matter flowing through the bowel.

Diabetes A disorder in which the body cannot convert foods properly into the energy needed for daily activities. There are two main types of diabetes. Type I, or insulin-dependent, is the more severe for of the disease. Type II, or adult onset, is the more common form and accounts for more than 85% of all cases. Diabetes cannot be cured, but it can be controlled by regulating the diet, getting regular exercise, and in some cases taking medication or insulin.

Diabetes mellitus A common form of diabetes in which the body cannot properly store or use glucose (sugar), the body's main source of energy.

Diagnosis The process of determining health status and the factors responsible for producing it; it may be applied to an individual, family, group or community. The diagnosis should take into account etiology, pathology, and severity of the clinical state.

Diagnostic A substance or group of substances used to identify a disease by analyzing the cause and symptoms.

Diagonal band (of broca) A association bundle of fibers located immediately rostral to the optic tract and forming the posterior border of the of the anterior perforated substance. It interconnects the paraterminal gyrus and subcallosal area (septal area) and septal nuclei with the hippocampus and lateral olfactory area.

Dialog Box An interactive message box; a temporary window on the screen that contains a set of choices whenever the executing program needs to collect information from the user.

Dial-Up Networking A feature of Windows 95 and 98 and UNIX based systems that enables the user to connect to other computers or the Internet over a phone line using a modem and a set of communication protocols.

Dialysis The separation of low-molecular weight compounds from high molecular weight components by diffusion through a semipermeable membrane. Frequently utilized to remove salts, introduce salts, remove biological effectors such as nicotinamide adenine dinucleotides, nucleotides phosphates, etc. from polymeric molecules such as protein, DNA, RNA, etc. Commonly used membranes have a molecular weight cutoff around 10,000 but other membrane pore sizes are available.

Diaphragm The muscle and membrane separating the abdominal and thoracic cavities of the body. Major inspiratory muscle. (also the source of meat for "fajitas" - aka "skirt steak").

Diaphragma sellae Horizontal partition of dura mater which roofs over the sella turcica (hypophysial fossa) enclosing the pituitary stalk and separating the pituitary gland from the ypothalamus.

Diaphragmatic Relating to the diaphragm.

Diaphragmatic crura Those muscle fibers of the diaphragm which cross in front of the esophagus creating an opening in the diaphragm for the passage of the esophagus and aorta.

Diaphysis The shaft of a long bone between the two "metaphyses"; tube of compact bone surrounding the marrow cavity.

Diarrhea Increase in frequency of stools compared to normal, or looser bowel movements than usual. Causes include infections of the digestive system, medicines such as antibiotics, malabsorption, and irritable bowel syndrome.

Diastasis recti Diastasis recti—Separation of abdominal muscles.

Diathermy Deep-heat therapy that uses high-frequency electric currents to produce heat in body tissues. Physical therapists and sports physicians use diathermy to treat arthritis, bursitis, and fractures. It also may help treat gynecological diseases and sinusitis.

Diatom Any minute, unicellular or colonial algae of the class Bacillariophyceae having siliceous cells walls consisting of two overlapping symmetrical parts.

Diatomaceous earth, diatomite, kiselguhr (DE) Fine silicaceous powder used as a filter aid.

Diencephalon Subdivision of the forebrain (prosencephalon) located between the telencephalon (end brain) and the mesencephalon (mid brain). It consists of the thalamus, hypothalamus, subthalamus and epithalamus and has important sensory, motor, endocrine , and visceral functions.

Dietary supplement A product intended to supply nutrients and other healthful substances that may be lacking in a diet. Term used to apply only to vitamins, minerals, and proteins. Herbs are now classified as dietary supplements, and the definition also includes amino acids, glandulars (processed animal glands), enzymes, fish oils, and various extracts, such as flower essences. While their labels may not make any claims to cure, prevent, treat, or mitigate a disease, they can claim to help a structure or function of the body. Unlike food additives and prescription and over-the-counter drugs, dietary supplements do not require FDA approval to be sold on the market.

Diffuse Not definitely localized or limited; spread widely through a tissue or substance.

Diffusion The random thermal motion of particles, which causes them to flow from a region of higher concentration to one of lower concentration until they are uniformly distributed.

Digestion How the body breaks down food and uses it for energy, cell repair, and growth. Starts in the mouth, continues in the stomach and small intestine, and is completed in the large intestine. The liver and pancreas add enzymes and juices that aid in this process.

Digestive tract The organs that are involved in digestion; including the mouth, salivary glands, esophagus, stomach, pancreas, liver, gallbladder, small intestine, and large intestine.

Digital Refers to information processing techniques that convert the actual data into binary (or machine language) code for more efficient transmission and storage. To retrieve the information, the binary code must be converted back to an analog signal.

Digital certificate An attachment to an electronic message used for security purposes. The most common use of a digital certificate is to verify that a user sending a message is who he or she claims to be and to provide the receiver with the means to encode a reply.

Digital representation Biometric parameters such as a fingerprint or retinal pattern are turned into data that a computer understands: the digital representation of the biometric. The pattern in the biometric divides it into a grid of boxes, and a zero or a one, depending on whether the box is filled in, marks each box.

Digital signature An electronic signature based upon cryptographic methods of originator authentication, computed by using a set of rules and a set of parameters such that the identity of the signer and the integrity of the data can be verified.

Dilatation (dilation) Gradual opening of the narrowed coronary artery by cracking and compressing the narrowing or obstructing plaque.

Dilution Lowering the concentration of a solution by adding more solvent.

Dilution factor The ratio of solvent to solute by volume.

Diopter (D) A measurement of the refractive (light bending) power of a lens or a prism (pd). The strength of prescription glasses and contacts are measured in these units. For example a lens that is 0.50 diopter (D) is very weak, where as a lens that is 10.0 diopter (D) is very strong.

Diphtheritic membrane A thin coating on the surface of an epithelial lined organ (e.g. intestine) that is composed of necrotic cellular debris, inflammatory cells and fibrin.

Diploic space The medullary space between the dense cortical bone of inner and outer tables of the flat calvarial bones of the skull, composed of cancellous bone and bone marrow.

Diploid A full set of genetic material, consisting of paired chromosomes one chromosome from each parental set. Most animal cells except the gametes have a diploid set of chromosomes. The diploid human genome has 46 chromosomes.

Diplophase A phase in the life cycle of an organism where the organism has two copies of each gene. The organism is said to be diploid.

Diplopia A single object is perceived as two rather than one; double vision.

Direct impact system An engineering system that may have a direct impact on product quality.

Direct observations or performance audits A traditional approach for giving a firsthand assessment of skills and performance with immediate feedback to the student. The student is observed performing a complete history and examination which provides the best possible opportunity for the observer to make multiple judgments over a period of time in a variety of clinical situations. Use of observation checklists, training the raters and agreed-upon standards increase reliability and validity of these methods over the use of global rating forms which require additional resources. This approach has an advantage over most new methods.

Direct obstetric death Those deaths resulting from obstetric complications of the pregnant state (pregnancy, labour and puerperium), from interventions, omissions, incorrect treatment, or from a chain of events resulting from any of the above.

Direct occlusion Covering the non-amblyopic eye.

Directionality/laterality Directionality relates to the awareness of the relationship of one object in space to another / laterality relates to the internal awareness of the two sides of the body. Directionality/Laterality can also be called spatial relations.

Directionality/laterality disorder A condition in which an individual has poor development of left/right awareness. Symptoms of this disorder include confusion of right and left direction and letters and/or numbers reversals. Vision therapy is a helpful treatment option.

Director of Nursing (DON) No, not the Godfather type of DON A DON oversees all nursing staff in a nursing home, and is responsible for formulating nursing policies and monitoring the quality of care delivered, as well as the facilities compliance with government regulations relating to nursing care.

Directory In MS-DOS, an area set aside on a disk to organize files into groups. A directory can contain other directories, called subdirectories, which further organize data. In Windows, a listing of all the files and directories on a drive or in a specified directory. Typing the "DIR" command at the DOS command prompt will give you a list of files in the current directory.

Disability A limitation in the performance of roles and tasks that society expects an individual to perform. The expression of a gap between a person's capabilities and the demands of an environment.

Disability Model A type of Long Term Care Insurance which pays benefits directly to the insured when the individual becomes disabled, whether or not long-term care expenses are incurred. The insured has the freedom to spend the disability payment on whatever services he/she deems appropriate.

Disaster Any event (i.e. fire, earthquake, power failure etc.), which could have a detrimental effect upon an automated system or its associated information.

Disc and disc space The space between the vertebrae, formed from a fibrous ring (the annulus) and a central "cushion" (nucleus pulposis).

Discharge The exit of a resident or patient from a facility or program. A discharge may be to another facility or program, to the resident's home, or could be a death. Payors vary in how they reimburse for days of discharge.

Discharge Planner A person responsible for the assessment, referral, and discharge planning of a resident (patient).

Discipline based approach Teaching of the individual classical medical disciplines such as anatomy, biochemistry, pathology, surgery or community medicine as separate educational building blocks. It is expected that this approach lays the foundation for contact with patients which tends to occur later, after completion of the basic science course. In this approach, it is left to the student to put together the knowledge gained in each discipline to form an overall picture of medicine.

Discoloration (welding) Any change in surface color from that of the base metal. Usually associated with oxidation occurring on the weld and heat affected zone (HAZ) on the outside diameter and inside diameter of the weld joint as a result of heating the metal during the welding. Colors may range from pale bluish-gray to deep blue, and from pale straw color to a black crusty coating.

Disease A general term used to refer to any departure from health in which a patient suffers. It can be defined as disorder of bodily function or destructive processes in organs, organs' systems or in an organism with recognizable signs and symptoms, and in many cases a known cause. The words disease, illness and sickness are used often interchangeably but are not synonymous. Rather, whereas disease relates to a physiological or psychological dysfunction, an illness is the subjective state of a patient who feels unwell and sickness encompasses a state of social dysfunction, such as the role that the individual assumes when ill.

Disease modifying anti-rheumatic drugs (DMARD) A powerful class of drugs used as a second line of defense to treat persistent inflammatory processes. These drugs can be prescribed in conjunction with more traditional non-steroidal anti-inflammatory drugs (NSAID). DMARDs slow down the biological processes that cause the persistent inflammation.

Disinfection Process by which viable microbiological agents or eukaryotic cells are reduced to a level unlikely to produce disease in healthy people, plants, or animals. These processes may use chemical agents, heat, ultraviolet light, etc. to destroy most (but not necessarily all) of the harmful or objectionable microorganisms, pathogens, and potential pathogens. Disinfection does not necessarily result in sterilization.

1. "High level disinfection" inactivates fungi, viruses, and bacteria. High-level chemical disinfectants maybe ineffective against bacterial spores if they are present in large numbers. Extended exposure times may be required.

2. "Intermediate level disinfection" destroys fungi, some viruses (lipid and most non-lipid medium-size and small viruses), mycobacteria, and bacteria.

3. "Low level disinfection" kills vegetative forms of bacteria, some fungi, and some medium-size and lipid-containing viruses. Low-level disinfectants do not reliably kill bacterial spores, mycobacteria, or small or non-lipid viruses.

Disk Refers to the most common form of data storage that uses disks of magnetized materials to save data.

Disk Drive A device used to read data from and write data to a disk.

Diskette The actual term for a floppy disk.

Dispense To deliver a prescribed drug to an ultimate user, including the compounding, packaging, and labeling necessary to prepare the prescribed drug.

Dispensing The pouring or transferring of any material from a container, tank or similar vessel, whereby vapors, dusts, fumes, mists or gases may be liberated to the atmosphere.

Dissimilation The breakdown of food material to yield energy and building blocks for cellular synthesis.

Dissolved solids The amount of nonvolatile matter dissolved in a water sample, usually expressed in parts per million (PPM) by weight.

Distal Away from or farthest from the trunk or the point or origin of a part (example, the hand is located at the distal end of the forearm).

Distance acuity The eye's ability to distinguish an object's shape and details at a far distance such as 20 feet (6 meters).

Distention Swelling or bloating, usually referring to the abdomen.

Distillation The process of separating water from impurities by heating until it changes into vapor and then cooling the vapor to condense it into purified water.

Diuretic Any agent or compound that increases the flow of urine from the body. They can range from herbal teas to powerful drugs that flush out electrolytes and water. They are classed based on the location and mechanism of action in the kidneys. Athletes use diuretics to eliminate water weight to further emphasize their muscular definitions. Most bodybuilding and fitness federations have banned the use of diurectics and test for them.

Divergence EXCESS (DE) (clinical condition) The eye's tendency to drift out relative to the direction of a distant object being viewed. Symptoms include: double vision at distance, headaches, eyestrain, nausea, dizziness, and blurred vision. Clinical signs include: exophoria greater at distance than near, high AC/A ratio, and reduced positive fusional vergence at distance. Can be improved with vision therapy.

Divergence insufficiency (DI) (clinical condition) The eye's tendency to turn more inward than necessary when viewing a distant object. Symptoms include: double vision, headaches, eyestrain, nausea, dizziness, and blurred vision. Clinical signs: esophoria greater at distance than near, low AC/A ratio, and reduced negative fusional vergence at distance. Treated with corrective lenses and vision therapy.

Divergence The ability to use both eyes as a team and be able to turn the eyes out toward a far object.

Diverticulitis Occurs when one or more small pouches in the large intestine (called a diverticulum) become irritated or infected.

Diverticulum A small pouch in the wall of the large intestine, which usually do not cause a problem unless it becomes irritated or infected.

Division This is a feature that is only available to ePIP clients that belong to a larger corporation. A Division is a unique group of facilities within your corporation that has been defined as part of a Classification. Divisions are mutually exclusive within each classification. Once a Division has been created, it can be set a Report Set parameter when requesting reports.

Dizygotic twins Dizygotic twins-Twins derived from two different eggs. Often called fraternal twins.

DMAE (Dimethyl-amino-ethanol) Supplement reported to minimize buildup of lipofuscin (age spots) in the brain. Plays a participatory role in acetycholine synthesis. DMAE has been shown to stimulate vivid, lucid dreams, suggesting possible sleep pattern enhancement.

DMSO (dimethyl sulfoxide) Solvent capable of passing through body tissues, approved by the FDA to treat one medical condition, interstitial cystitis (an uncommon bladder inflammation). Proponents & manufacturers claim that DMSO heals a wide range of problems (including bruises, pimples, herpes) and relieves pain from conditions such as muscle strains. They credit DMSO with the ability to kill bacteria and fungi, improve circulation, and stimulate the immune system. DMSO produces strong garlic breath in users, even when used topically or intravenously.

DNA (deoxyribonucleic acid) The molecule of which the genetic material is composed. It consists of two chains joined together as a double helix. Each chain is composed of a polymer of nucleotides (consisting of a nitrogenous base, a deoxyribosesugar ring, and a phosphate group) joined together by phosphodiester bonds between the 5'-phosphate of one nucleotide and the 3'-hydroxyl of the next. The two chains run in opposite directions and are held together by hydrogen bonds between the bases in equivalent positions in the two chains. There are various forms of double helical DNA. They are:

1. B-DNA (first described by Crick and Watson) is a right-handed helix with 10.6 base pairs per turn and is probably the main form of cellular DNA.

2. A-DNA is also a right-handed helix but is somewhat skewed and contains about 11 base pairs per turn. It is the form taken By DNA-RNA hybrid double helixes.

3. Z-DNA is a left-handed helix with 11 base pairs per turn. It is favored by regions rich in guanine cutosine base pairs and probably occurs infrequently in cellular DNA.

DNA array Spots of DNA arranged on a slide support such as glass or silicon "DNA chip" (or microarray), used for screening, sequencing, genetic mapping, and so on.

DNA hybridization DNA Hybridization (e.g., hybridization): The binding of complementary sequences of DNA through specific base-pairing of Adenine with Thymine and Guanine with Cytosine.

DNA Probe A segment of DNA specifically designed to be complementary to a target sequence of chromosomes, genes or gene sequences. The synthetic piece of DNA is coupled with a fluorescent indicator, or tag, so that the chromosomes or genes it binds (or hybridizes) to can be directly visualized.

DNA replication The use of existing DNA as a template for the synthesis of new DNA strands. In humans and other eukaryotes, replication occurs in the cell nucleus.

DNA vector A DNA vehicle for transferring generic information from one cell to another.

DNAse (deoxyribonuclease) An enzyme that degrades DNA.

DNP (2,4 dinitrophenol) The first weight loss drug ever offered to the public, around 1933. DNP is a yellow crystalline sold that's slightly soluabl;e in water. After being injected, it increases the metabolism an average of 30% over baseline in less than a minute, returning back to normal anywhere from 6 to 48 hours. However, DNP has way too many side effects, including blinding people, and if you take too much of it, it can cook you to death from the inside. You can lose weight with it, but it is highly dangerous. Street Names for DNP include Hexalon. DNP is now classified as a poison.

Doctor of Osteopathy (DO) A physician licensed by state law to practice osteopathic medicine.

Document A file created using an application. For example, you might create a text document using a word processing application (such as Word) or a picture document using a graphic application (such as Paint Shop Pro).

Documentation Written or pictorial information describing, defining, specifying, and/or reporting of certifying activities, requirements, procedures or results.

Domain A name by which a computer connected to the Internet is identified. A typical domain name looks like this: www.ibm.com. The "www." refers to the fact that this computer is connected to the World Wide Web; the middle portion of a domain name is usually the name of the company that owns the computer—in this case,IMB ; the final portion of a domain name tells you what kind of site is served by this machine—in this case, '.com' means this is a commercial site (other types of sites are: .edu—education, .org—non-profit organization, .net—Internet service provider).

Dominant allele A gene that is expressed, regardless of whether its counterpart allele on the other chromosome is dominant or recessive. Autosomal dominant disorders are produced by a single mutated dominant allele, even though its corresponding allele is normal.

Dominant eye The eye that "leads" it partner during eye movements. Humans also have dominant hand, foot, eye, and side of the brain (not necessarily all on the same side).

DOMS (Delayed onset muscle soreness) The pain and soreness you feel a few days after a heavy workout.

Door to Door A form of Paratransit service which includes passenger assistance between the vehicle and the door of his or her home or other destination. A higher level of service than curb-to-curb, yet not as specialized as Adoor-through-door@ service (where the driver actually provides assistance within the origin or destination).

DOP (dioctyl phthalate) A mono-dispersed test aerosol of sub-micron particles, generated to challenge (evaluate integrity) of HEPA filters for HVAC.

Dorsal Being or located near, on, or toward the back or posterior part of the human body.

Dorsal cavity The smaller of the two main cavities is called the dorsal cavity. As its name implies, it contains organs lying more posterior in the body. The dorsal cavity, again, can be divided into two portions. The upper portion, or the cranial cavity, houses the brain, and the lower portion, or vertebral canal houses the spinal cord.

Dorsalis pedis artery The continuation of the anterior tibial artery, that branches into the lateral and medial tarsal, arcuate, and deep plantar arteries.

Dorsum sellae The posterior bone margin of the pituitary fossa, that is the superior limit of the sphenoid bone. The dorsum sellae forms the boundary between the middle and posterior cranial fossae in the midline.

DOS Acronym for Disk Operating System.

Dosage form he form in which the drug is delivered to the patient. This could be parenteral, topical, tablet, oral (liquid or dissolved powder), suppository, inhalation, transdermal, etc.

Dosage group A group of subjects in a clinical trial receiving the same dosage (amount) of a drug being tested.

Dot Matrix Printer A type of printer that prints by striking wires or fine rods, within a matrix or array of dots, on an ink-coated ribbon against a piece of paper to form letters and numbers.

Dot Pitch An indication of the image quality of a monitor, it is the measurement of the distance between two phosphor dots of the same color on a monitor. The finer the dot pitch, the better the image quality (a dot pitch of .28 or smaller is generally considered good).

Dots Per Inch A measurement of resolution for printers and monitors. It refers to the number of dots these devices can produce in a linear inch. Also called DPI. More dots per inch means a better-quality output.

Double blind test Used in Clinical Trials, this is a method to ensure that any one party cannot improperly influence the test. The product (either in a single strength dosage or in multiple dosages) and the placebo are packaged and given a code name known to only the initiating party. These are then sent to another party who gives the coded packages yet another code name or number, and makes a matrix of the previous name/ number to the new name/number. This is then sent to the physician who administers these to the patient. At the end of the test, the physician provides records of which patient received which code name/number product. This is then cross-referenced to the intermediate matrix to determine the original code name/number. The results of the treatment are then correlated to determine the efficacy of the drug. The structure of DNA as proposed by Watson and Crick. It consists of two right-handed helical polynucleotide chains coiled around the same axis. The two chains are anti-parallel with their 3rd to 5th internucleotide phosphodiester bonds running in opposite directions. Under most conditions, the coiling of the chains is such that if the ends are held still, as in circular DNA or in a large chromosome, the chains cannot be separated except by cleavage of one of the strands.

Double click To depress and release a mouse button twice in quick succession. (In Windows, "double-click" usually refers to the left mouse button).

Down Syndrome A congenital disease caused by an extra copy of chromosome 21 (trisomy 21).

Download To copy or move a file from another computer or disk onto another.

Downtime The period of time a computer, or other piece of equipment is out of order or shut down for maintenance.

Drag and Drop "Drag and drop" describes a particular action you can make with the mouse. Click an object, such as a folder, then hold down the mouse button as you drag the object to a new location. You drop the object by releasing the mouse button. Drag and drop can be used to easily move, print, delete, or embed an object or file into another.

Drag To move an object on the screen from one place to another by clicking it with the mouse, holding the mouse button down, and pulling it to where you want it to be.

DRAM Dynamic Random Access Memory. The type of random access memory used in most PCs.

Dream therapy Mental activity associated with the rapid-eye-movement period of sleep. Generally consists of visual images and may reflect bodily disturbances or external stimuli. In primitive and ancient cultures, dreams played an extensive role in myth and religion. Freud emphasized dreams as keys to the makeup of the individual and distinguished between the experienced content of a dream and the actual meaning of the dream. Jung held that dreams are not limited to the personal unconscious but may also be shaped by archetypes that originate in the collective unconscious of the human species.

Dressing One of the Activities of Daily Living (ADLs). The ability to put on and take off all garments and medically necessary braces, corsets, elastic stockings or garments or artificial limbs or splints usually worn and to fasten and unfasten them.

Dreyfus Model of Skill Acquisition Based on the work of Drs. Hubert and Stuart Dreyfus, both professors at the University of California at Berkeley. This is a situational model of skill acquisition. It is the development of skilled know how. The model states that a person passes through five stages of qualitatively different perceptions of his/her task and/or mode of decision-making as his/her skill improves. It is neither expected nor possible for all individuals to proceed in a linear fashion. Skill according to this model is based on innate ability, experience and environment.

Drive Bay A slot inside your computer where a disk drive is mounted.

Driver A set of software that contains instructions that allows the computer to communicate with its peripheral devices.

Drop Down List A dialog box item showing only one entry until its drop down arrow is clicked.

Drug (medicinal) product The dosage form in the final immediate packaging intended for marketing.

Drug Any substance intended for use in the diagnosis, cure, mitigation, treatment, or prevention of disease or other conditions in persons. Any substance other than a device or food intended to affect the structure or any function of the body of persons.

Drug Irregularity A drug that is given without a medical reason; in an excessive or inadequate dose or duration of therapy; where side effects indicate that a dose modification or drug discontinuation is indicated, or inadequate monitoring for effect or manufacturer's recommendations for laboratory monitoring. This therapy results in potential negative outcome or is not achieving the stated objectives of the prescriber. The consulting pharmacist should address this potential drug therapy problem at the time of their drug regimen review.

Drug product A finished dosage form, for example, tablet, capsule, solution, etc., that contains one or more APIs (Active Pharmaceutical Ingredients) generally, but not necessarily, in association with inactive ingredients. The term also includes a finished dosage form, which does not contain an API but is intended to be used as a placebo.

Drug Regimen Review (DRR) The review of drugs being used by a resident (patient) to determine effect and potential for harmful effects.

Drug therapy Various drugs are used to alleviate symptoms of some mental illnesses. Lithium is used in alleviating symptoms of manic depression. Tranquilizers are used to reduce anxiety. All drugs have side effects, such as Ritalin, which is prescribed for hyperactive children, and can retard physical growth.

Drug Utilization Review (DUR) The study of drug use patterns in a facility.

Dry air Air from which all water vapor and contaminants have been removed. Its composition by volume is:

1. Nitrogen 78.08%
2. Oxygen 20.95%
3. Argon 0.93%
4. Carbon Dioxide 0.03
5. Other gases 0.00003

Dry Heat sterilization Sterilization utilizing a heating oven or continuous tunnel (gas or electric heated), as opposed to steam sterilization in an autoclave, usually used for glassware and metal parts. In depyrogenation temperatures of 250°C result in sterilization and the inactivation of endotoxin present on the surface of the equipment.

Dual Registration To be registered as both an RN and an RPN.

Dual chamber pacemaker A pacemaker that monitors and paces a chamber of the upper heart and a chamber of the lower heart at the same time. A dual-chamber pacemaker usually has two leads one located in the right atrium and the other located in the right ventricle.

Dual chamber pacing To pace and/or sense heart rhythm in both the atrium and the ventricle.

Duction test A test of the eye's ability to turn inward or outward while maintaining single, binocular vision with the gradual introduction of progressively stronger base-in or base-out prisms.

DumpSlang term referring to the transfer of data from one location to another. (e.g., in order to print, a program may 'dump' a file to the printer buffer).

Duodenal bulb The portion of the duodenum that forms the superior flexure with the pylorus.

Duodenal ulcer An open sore in the duodenum (first part of the small intestine).

Duodenum The first part of the small intestine, nearest to the stomach.

Dura mater The outermost tough fibrous covering of the brain and spinal cord. Also referred to as the Pachymeninx.

Durability The ability to withstand the rigors of the environment without degrading or requiring repair.

Durable Medical Equipment Equipment that lasts for several years, like wheelchairs, scooters, hospital beds, oxygen tanks, and other equipment, as contrasted with consumable medical supplies, such as diapers and dressings, which are not considered DME.

Dural septae Folds of dura mater that reflect off the surface of the skull and incompletely divide the cranial cavity into compartments.

Dust Dusting Deterioration of the finish at the surface so it is easily loosened from the surface by light physical contact (such as wiping one's hand across the surface), mechanically induced air movements or naturally occurring air movements.

DVD Digital Versatile Disc (also called Digital Video Disc and DVD-ROM). New data technology similar to Compact Discs and CD-ROMs, but with a much higher capacity and the ability to read and write data to discs.

Dynamic conditions Environmental conditions of a manufacturing room occupied by the normal number of workers appropriately garbed and with production equipment in operation. However, dynamic conditions for some dusty operations, such as aseptic powder filling, may be measured in the absence of product.

Dys (prefix) Difficult; bad; abnormal.

e.g. dysplasia - abnormal formation.

e.g. dyspnea - shortness of breath; difficulty breathing.

Dyseidetic Poor sight recognition of words. Dyseidetic is a subtype of dyslexia. Children with this form of dyslexia have trouble analyzing and remembering written symbols. They continue to confuse the orientation. For example, they will write numbers and letters backwards long after other children have mastered these skills. They often confuse letter sequences in reading, and in spelling often get all the letters but in the wrong sequence (spelling "dose" for "does", "on" for "no", etc.). Their visual memory for words is poor, and after learning a new word they may fail to recognize that same new word later in the sentence. They have trouble learning to read and spell phonetically irregular words. For example, they may read " laugh" as "log" and spell it as "laff", both of which are phonetically consistent. Their spelling will have many mistakes, but will be phonetically consistent and one can usually tell what the word was they were trying to spell. When they are attempting to read an unknown word they will usually attempt to sound it out and do so very slowly.

Dysgenesis Defective embryonic development.

Dyslexia A specific language-based disorder. The individual has difficulty with letter or word recognition, spelling, reading, writing, and sometimes naming pictures of objects. Dyslexia varies in degree from mild to very sever. It is caused by an inability of the brain's language centers to decode print or phonetically make the connection between the word's written symbols and their appropriate sounds. Dyslexia is not caused by a vision disorder. Children often are of normal or above normal intelligence. Dyslexia cannot be cured and will never be outgrown. Appropriate teaching methods can be taught to help those with dyslexia overcome their weakness. The Dyslexia Determination test which is used by many optometrists who specialize in vision related vision problems investigates if the patient has one of the three forms of dyslexia: Dyseidetic - poor sight recognition of words, Dysphonesia- inability to "sound out" words, and Dysphoneidesia - a combination of characteristics from both types. Vision therapy is NOT considered a direct treatment for dyslexia.

Dysphagia Difficulty swallowing food or liquid.

Dysphoneidesia Inability to "sound out" words and poor sight recognition of words. Dysphoneidesia is a subtype of dyslexia. Its characteristics are a combination of the other two forms of dyslexia: Dysphonesia and Dyseidetic.

Dysphonesia Inability to "sound out" words. Dysphonesia is a subtype of dyslexia. Children with this form of dyslexia have difficulty sequentially analyzing and remembering what and where the sounds are in words. The resulting phonemic processing problems make it difficult to sound out new words, learn phonics, and make them dependent on their sight vocabulary. When they come to an unknown word they will often substitute a word using context clues. For example, "pony" for "horse", even though the substituted word doesn't look or sound anything like the original word. When spelling unknown words it is often difficult to determine what the original word is. For example, they may write "fmlue" for "familiar" or "lap" for "lamp". They cannot learn phonics because they cannot process where the sounds are. Their short term sequential auditory memory can be poor and result in repeating "8167" as "8671", or remember to go to their room but forgetting to get the item requested.

Dysplasia Dysplasia—Abnormal, precancerous changes in the cells of the cervix.

Dystopia Displacement.

Dysuria Dysuria—Difficulty or pain urinating.

E

E coli (escherichia coli) A fast growing, Gram-negative bacteria commonly found in the body with a comparatively simple structure. The genetic make up of E. coli is the best known of any organism, having been widely studied during the development of genetic engineering. It has been used extensively as the host cell for novel proteins made by rDNA technology.

E health A term that refers to all forms of electronic health services provided over the Internet. It includes all educational, information and commercial services and products offered by professionals, non-professionals, businesses and consumers. Based on the unique capabilities of Internet, E-Health is enabling the delivery of clinical services that previously have been domain of telemedicine and telehealth. E-health differs from telemedicine and telehealth in that it is not "professional-centric" and is motivated by the financial gain, whereas telemedicine and telehealth are not. As it is Internet-based, E-health is making the provision of health care more efficient.

EACH Extended Aged Care at Home The EACH program is a very small, limited capacity program which enables frail aged people to remain in their homes, supported by high level care through an approved service provider.

Ear candling Also called Ear Coning. Involves placing the narrow end of a specially designed hollow candle at the entry of the ear canal, while the opposite end is lit. Primarily used for relieving wax build up and related hearing problems, ear candling is also used for ear infections and sinus infections.

Eating One of the Activities of Daily Living (ADLs). The ability to consume food that has already been prepared and made available, with or without the use of adaptive utensils. Necessary skills include reaching for, picking up and rasping a utensil and cup; getting food on a utensil and bringing food, utensil and cup to mouth; manipulating food on plate; and cleaning face and hands as necessary following meals.

ECA Stack A thermagenic supplement blend of Ephedra, Caffeine and Aspirin that is popular among fitness and bodybuilding cultures. It is said that these three ingredients give a synergistic effect together which give better results than any one on its own.

Eccentric fixation The deviating eye does not use the central foveal (center of the retina that produces the sharpest eyesight) area for fixation. Commonly, individuals with amblyopia and some individuals with strabismus will have this visual adaptation.

In esotropia, the eccentrically located retinal point used for fixation is usually in the nasal retina. In exotropia, the eccentrically located retinal point used for fixation is usually in the temporal retina. Vision therapy is a treatment option for those with amblyopia and/or strabismus. It is not a treatment option for an individual with a fovea that has been destroyed.

Ecchymosis A purplish patch caused by extravasation of blood into the tissues differing from petechiae only in size.

Echincea Herb with immune protective properties, shown to have some benefit protecting against colds and flu. It can be used as a preventive measure to protect the body against the natural stress the immune system suffers in heavy training.

Eclampsia Eclampsia-Convulsions and coma in a woman with pre-eclampsia. Not related to epilepsy.

Ecology The study of the interrelationships between organisms and their environment.

Ectasis (suffix) To stretch; dilate. e.g. bronchiectasis - dilatation of bronchi. The noun form is ectasia

Ectodermal germ layer Ectodermal germ layer—layer in the developing embryo that gives rise to developing structures in the fetus. These include skin, teeth and glands of the mouth, the nervous system and the pituitary gland.

Ectomy (suffix) Excision. e.g. cholecystectomy - excision of the gallbladder.

Ectopic pregnancy Ectopic pregnancy—Pregnancy that occurs outside the uterine cavity.

EDC EDC (estimated date of confinement)-Anticipated due date for delivery of the baby. Calculated from the first day of the last Period counting forward 280 days.

EDD EDD (estimated date of delivery)-Anticipated due date for delivery of the baby. Calculated from the first day of the last Period counting forward 280 days.

Edema Excessive swelling during pregnancy, which can be a sign of complications, such as preeclampsia.

Edematous Swollen.

Edge failure A control parameter value that, if exceeded, may result in adverse effect on state of control and/or fitness for use of the product.

EDO RAM Extended Data-Out RAM. EDO RAM is about 10 per cent faster than regular RAM. EIDE Enhanced Intelligent Drive Electronics. The protocol used to connect specific hardware devices, such as disk drives, to the computer. EIDE is newer, faster, and more versatile than its predecessor, IDE.

Educational or instructional objectives Statements that describe what learners should be able to master. A major aim is the acquisition of facts, concepts and principles. Developing instructional objectives involves learning the fundamentals and vocabulary of each discipline and developing a logical progression of concepts in each discipline. Resources and materials are more effectively deployed when instructional objectives are explicit. It is important to assure that objectives are measurable and that they delineate a specific level of competence. One can and should distinguish between knowledge, skill and attitude objectives.

Effacement Effacement—Thinning of cervix that happens toward the end of your pregnancy or just before labor begins.

Effectiveness A measure of the extent to which a specific intervention, procedure, regimen, or service, when deployed in the field in routine circumstances, does what it is intended to do for a specified population. In the health field, it is a measure of output from those health services that contribute towards reducing the dimension of a problem or improving an unsatisfactory situation.

Efficiency An ability to perform well or achieve a result without wasted energy, resources, effort, time or money. Efficiency can be measured in physical terms (technical efficiency) or terms of cost (economic efficiency). Greater efficiency is achieved where the same amount and standard of services are produced for a lower cost, if a more useful activity is substituted for a less useful one at the same cost or if needless activities are eliminated.

Effluent The output or discharge from a process, such as a wastewater treatment process.

Egg protein Source of protein with high Protein Efficiency Ratio, usually in egg white form (albumin) when used in protein powder to avoid cholesterol in egg yolk. Egg protein is the standard by which all other proteins are measured because of its very high ration of indispensable amino acids (also called essential amino acids because they must be supplied to the body from food or supplements) to dispensable amino acids.

Ejection fraction (left ventricular: LVEF) The percentage of blood filling the left ventricle during each heartbeat that flows out of the ventricle into the body's circulatory system. This reading is a direct measure of the "pumping" capability of the heart. Damaged/diseased hearts may have an ejection fraction below 50%.

Elastin An albuminoid, or scleroprotein present especially in yellow elastic fibrous tissue.

Elastomer Long chain co-polymers or terpolymers (two or three different monomers in one chain) that contain adequate crosslinks among individual chains. Fluorinated elastomers are more stable than hydrocarbon or silicon elastomers because C-F bonds are approximately 30% stronger than C-H bonds. There are five major FDA compliant elastomers used in the pharmaceutical and biopharmaceutical industries: EPDM (ethylene-propylene-diene rubber), fluororelastomers (FKM), platinum-cured silicon (pt-Si), and finally Kalrez parts using compounds KLR-6221 and KLR-6230, which are perfluoroelastomers.

Elastomeric material A material that can be stretched or compressed repeatedly and, upon immediate release of stress, will return to its approximate original size.

Elbow joint The large joint for the upper extremity, between the distal humerus and the proximal radius and ulna. Fx Radius/Ulna Fx Elbow.

Elder Abuse Elder abuse is defined by state laws which vary considerably about what constitutes the abuse, neglect, or exploitation of the elderly. Abuse is often categorized as physical, sexual, emotional, financial, neglect, and/or abandoment. Most often it is defined as an action taken by someone who is trusted by an elder that causes harm.

Elective Abortion Elective abortion usually refers to a D&C surgery performed to end a pregnancy around 7-9 weeks, even as late as 15 weeks. Sometimes an elective abortion is performed (depending on where you live) in early pregnancy via a drug called RU486, which will also end the pregnancy.

Elective program An educational program where students are given the opportunity to select subjects or projects of their own choice, not covered by obligatory medical courses. This enables students to pursue individual aspirations, provides students with increased responsibility to further their own learning, and facilitates career choice by providing an opportunity to explore various areas of interest.

Electrical area classifications Facilities, or portions of facilities are classified electrically according to the type of material present and its flammability and/or explosive potential. Each area classification carries with it specific requirements for the construction requirements found within that space to guard against sparking. The Class of an area refers to the type of material; the Division of the area refers to whether that material is normally found in that area or not.

Electrical code Electrical Groups Electrical groupings are based on the characteristics of the materials involved. These include the following: 1. Class I, Group A: Atmospheres containing acetylene.

2. Class I, Group B: Atmospheres containing hydrogen, fuel and combustible process gases containing more than 30 percent hydrogen by volume, or gases or vapors of equivalent hazard such as butadiene, ethylene oxide, propylene oxide, and acrolein.

3. Class I, Group C: Atmospheres such as ethyl ether, ethylene, or gases or vapors of equivalent hazard.

4. Class I, Group D: Atmospheres such as acetone, ammonia, benzene, butane, cyclopropane, ethanol, gasoline, hexane, methanol, methane, natural gas, naphtha, propane, or gases or vapors of equivalent hazard.

5. Class II, Group E: Atmospheres containing combustible metal dusts, including aluminum, magnesium and their commercial alloys, or other combustible dusts whose particle size, abrasiveness, and conductivity present similar hazards in the use of electrical equipment.

6. Class II, Group F: Atmospheres containing combustible carbonaceous dusts, including carbon black, charcoal, coal, or coke dusts that have more that 8 percent entrapped volatiles, or dusts that have been sensitized by other materials so that they present an explosion hazard.

7. Class II, Group G: Atmospheres containing combustibles dusts not included in Group E or F, including flour, grain, wood, plastic, and chemicals.

Electrocardiogram (ECG/EKG) A method of recording the electrical impulses given off by the heart as it beats. This may be done while resting or exercising.

Electrocautery The use of electrical currents to stop bleeding during surgery.

Electrode Transmits or receives electrical impulses from one point to another.

Electrodialysis (ED) A membrane separation method used for the separation of charged molecules from a solution by application of a direct current. The membranes contain ion-exchange groups and have a fixed electrical charge. This method is very effective in the concentration of electrolytes and proteins.

Electrogram (EGM) A picture of the electrical activity of the heart as sensed from within the heart. This is different from an ECG, which is a picture of your heart's electrical activity sensed from the surface of your skin.

Electrohydraulic Lithotripsy (EHL) This technique uses a special probe to break up small stones with shock waves generated by electricity. Through a flexible ureteroscope, the physician positions the tip of the probe 1 mm from the stone. Then, by means of a foot switch, the physician projects electrically generated hydraulic shock waves through an irrigating fluid at the stone until it is broken into small fragments. These can be passed by the patient or removed through the previously described extraction methods. EHL has some limitations It requires general anesthesia, and is generally not used in close proximity to the kidney itself, as the shock waves can cause tissue damage. Fragments produced by the hydraulic shock also tend to scatter widely, making retrieval or extraction more difficult.

Electrolytes Minerals in the bloodstream and in the cells of the body, such as sodium (salt), potassium, and calcium. Electrolytes must remain in proper balance for the body to function normally.

Electromagnetic field Invisible lines of force that are the result of the use of electricity, such as anything plugged into an outlet or operated by a battery.

Electromagnetic interference (EMI) Produced by an electromagnetic field — if strong enough, it may interfere with the operation of an AICD system. This happens only on very rare occasions.

Electron microscopy (EM) A technique for visualizing material that uses beams of electrons instead of light rays and that permits greater magnification than is possible with an optical microscope. Electron microscopes have been used to examine the structure of viruses and bacteria, to identify and classify pollen grains, etc.

Electronic record Any combination of text, graphics, data, audio, pictorial, or other information representation in digital form that is created, modified, maintained, archived, retrieved, or distributed by a computer system.

Electronic signature or e sig According to FDA, an electronic signature is a computer data compilation of any symbol or series of symbols executed, adopted, or authorized by an individual to be the legally binding equivalent of the individual's handwritten signature.

Electrophoresis The migration of electrically charged proteins, colloids, molecules, or other particles when dissolved or suspended in an electrolyte through which an electric current is passed. The most important use of electrophoresis is in the analysis of blood proteins. Since the proportion of these proteins varies widely in different diseases, electrophoresis can be used for diagnostic purposes. Electrophoresis is used to study bacteria and viruses, nucleic acids, and some types of smaller molecules, including amino acids.

Electrophysiology (EP) test or study An observation and measurement of the electrical impulses running through the heart as it beats. This test can help a doctor to recognize abnormal heart rhythms, to determine the origin of arrhythmias and to determine how well medicines are working. A doctor may also use the test to observe the implantable defibrillator to see how well it functions during an abnormal heart rhythm.

Electropolishing Also known as "chemical machining" and "reverse plating", electropolishing is an electrochemical process far superior to any available mechanical process for the removal of minute surface imperfections in stainless steel. It levels and brightens the material surface by anodic dissolution in an electrolyte flowing solution with an imposed electrical current. When the proper combination of electrolyte current & temperature is attained, the high points of surface irregularities, or high current density areas, are selectively removed at a greater rate than the remainder of the surface, resulting in improved surface smoothness. During electropolishing, the polarized surface film is subjected to the combined effects of gassing (oxygen) that occurs with electromechanical metal removal, saturation of the surface with dissolved metal, and the agitation and temperature of the electrolyte.

Electrostatic fluidized bed A container holding powder coating material which is aerated from below so as to form an air-supported expanded cloud of such material which is electrically charged with a charge opposite to the charge of the object to be coated. Such object is transported through the container immediately above the charged and aerated materials in order to be coated.

ELISA (enzyme linked immunosorbent assay) A test to measure the concentration of antigens or antibodies.

Ellinghausen's medium A complex medium for growing Leptospira. Contains numerous salts, nutrients, and BSA (bovine serum albumin).

Elute To separate one solute from another by washing. Elution may include the removal by means of a suitable solvent of one material (absorbed material) from another (adsorbent) that is insoluble in that solvent.

Em, en, in (prefix) Into. e.g. encyst - to enclose in a cyst or sac.

E-Mail Electronic Mail, one of the most popular features of the internet. E-Mail allows users to send messages and files to one another, via modems almost instantly.

Embedded Object Data stored in a document that originated from another application. Differing from a linked object, this type of object doesn't have its own file on the disk. However, it runs its source application for editing when you double-click it. For example, a Paint Shop Pro graphic embedded in a Word 97 document.

Embolism The sudden blocking of an artery by a clot of material (embolus). The process of the formation of an embolus.

Embolus A clot, usually part or all of a thrombus, carried by a larger vessel and forced into a smaller vessel, thus obstructing blood flow.

Embriology The study of the early stages in the development of an organism. In these stages a single highly specialized cell, the egg, is transformed into a complex, many-celled organism resembling its parents.

Embryo Embryo—Organism in the early stages of development.

Embryonic period Embryonic period—First 10 weeks of gestation.

Emesis (suffix) Vomit. e.g. hematemesis - vomiting blood.

Emia (suffix) Blood. e.g. lipidemia - excess lipid in the blood.

Emissary veins Veins which pierce the skull and connect the dural venous sinuses with the extracranial veins.

Emmetropia Normal vision, no correction needed.

Emulation A technique that allows a piece of software or hardware to 'act' like another in order to cooperate with otherwise incompatible products. A very common use of emulation is using a printer with certain types of software.

Encopresis Constipation and intestinal obstruction (blockage) lead to an involuntary leakage of loose stool.

Encryption A technique of scrambling transmitted data, using special software, so that only a party with the ability to unscramble the message has access to it.

Endemic A disease present in a community or among a group of people; used to describe a disease prevailing continually in a region.

Endergonic reaction A chemical reaction with a positive standard free energy change, an "uphill" reaction.

Endo (prefix) Within. e.g. endocardium - the inner lining of the heart. e.g. endometrium - the mucous membrane lining of the uterus.

Endocardial lead A long, thin insulated wire that runs from a pulse generator through a vein into the heart. The lead transmits signals from the heart to the pulse generator and transmits therapy from the pulse generator to the heart.

Endocardial The inside surface of the heart. Endocardial leads are inserted into the heart through the veins.

Endocervical canal The portion of the uterine cavity that lies within the cervix - the passage that connects the vaginal canal with the main uterine cavity (lumen).

Endocrine glands The glands that secrete their products (hormones) into the blood that then carries them to their specific target organs. Endocrine glands are the pituitary, thyroids, adrenals, pancreas, ovaries (in females), and testes (in males). Endocrine glands are found in some invertebrates as well as in vertebrates.

Endocrine hormones The products secreted by the endocrine glands. These help control long-term processes, such as growth, lactation, sex cycles, and metabolic adjustment. The endocrine system and the nervous system are interdependent and are often referred to collectively as the neuroendocrine system. For example, the juvenile hormone, found in insects and annelids, affects sexual maturation. There is currently great interest in the possible use of such hormones in the control of destructive insects.

Endocrinology Medical Specialty dealing with diseases of the glands and hormones.

Endodermal germ layer Endodermal germ layer-Area of tissue in early development of the embryo that gives rise to other structures. These include the digestive tract, respiratory organs, vagina, bladder and urethra. Also called endoderm or entoderm.

Endometrial Biopsy A test for progesterone where a bit of the lining is taking from the uterus to check if the lining is "in phase," or at the proper point of development for that part of the cycle.

Endometrial cycle Endometrial cycle—Regular development of the mucous membrane lining the inside of the uterus. It begins with the preparation for acceptance of a pregnancy and ends with the shedding of the lining during a menstrual period.

Endometrium Endometrium—Mucous membrane that lines inside of the uterine wall.

Endonuclease An enżyme that cleaves its nucleic acid substrate at internal sites (other than the terminal bonds) in the nucleotide sequence.

Endorphins Endogenous opiates having morphine-like effects consisting of small polypeptides such as enkephalin and leu-enkephalin and longer polypeptides such as alpha-, ß-, and gamma-endorphins. They bind to opiate receptors in the brain. Endorphins induce analgesia when injected intraventricularly but not when administered peripherally, presumably because of their inability to cross the blood/brain barrier. The amino acid sequence of the endorphins is short enough to allow the gene sequences coding for them to be synthesized.

Endorsement Acknowledgement that the clinicians practice meets the criteria for the level of practice being applied for in the opinion of the endorser.

Endoscope A small, flexible tube with a light and a camera lens at the end, used to examine the inside of the digestive tract. It can also be used to take tissue samples for testing from inside the digestive tract.

Endoscopic Referring to procedures performed inside the body through small incisions or within the lumen of an organ with the aid of a special camera.

Endoscopic retrograde cholangio-pancreatography (ERCP) A test using endoscope to send dye through the digestive tract. The dye shows up on x-ray and gives the physician a look at the bile and pancreatic ducts.

Endoscopy A test that uses an endoscope to examine the inside of part of the digestive tract.

Endospore A highly heat and chemical resistant dormant inclusion (spore) occurring within the substance of certain genera of bacteria, mainly Bacillus and Clostridium.

ENDOTAK An implantable lead system used to sense heart rhythms and deliver energy to the heart.

Endothelial cells A layer of flat cells that line the tumor blood vessel structure.

Endothelium The cells or membrane lining organs.

Endotoxin A poisonous complex molecule (lipopolysaccharide) that forms an integral part of the bacterial (gram-negative bacteria) cell wall and is only released when the integrity of the wall is disturbed. Certain organisms may release endotoxins (e.g. E. coli) during biosynthesis of a recombinant

DNA product, thus necessitating purification steps to ensure their removal. In water treatment, it most often refers to pyrogens.

Endotracheal tube (ET) An airway catheter (tube) that is inserted into the trachea to assist breathing and ventilation of the lung. ET tubes are used with mechanical ventilation for critical patients.

Enema A liquid placed into the rectum to either clear stool out of the large intestine, or to examine the large intestine with an x-ray (barium enema).

Energy field work Practitioners look for weaknesses in the energy field in and around the clients body and seek to restore its proper circulation and balance. Energy channeled through the practitioner is directed to strengthen the body's natural defenses and help the client's physical, mental, emotional and/or spiritual state.

Engorgement Engorgement-The term for the full, sometimes painful feeling when your milk "comes in". The fullness is caused not only by the milk, but also by swollen tissues and extra blood volume in the breasts.

Enhanced documentation Collection of Engineering, Quality Control, and Regulatory Affairs documents, which will be required for the operation, validation, maintenance, and regulatory compliance of a pharmaceutical plant.

Enter A key on the keyboard that, when pressed, instructs the computer to do something with the data just typed in. In word processing applications, the Enter key is analogous with the 'return' key on a typewriter.

Enter(o) (prefix) Intestine. e.g. enteritis - inflammation of the intestine.

Enterocele Herniation of small bowel into vagina.

Enthalpy A thermodynamic property that indicates the total energy in a sample of dry air and water vapor, measured in Btu/lb dry air. Dry air at zero degrees Fahrenheit and atmospheric pressure is designated as zero enthalpy.

Entry level Following the completion of orientation, including all competencies, clinicians will begin their practice becoming comfortable with patient care management, systems and resources. When the clinician has consistently demonstrated entry level behavior the manager/director will recognize them as practicing at the Entry level. This level must be achieved within three to twelve months of hire.

Enzyme Any of numerous proteins or conjugated proteins produced by living organisms and functioning as complex biochemical catalysts. They not only promote reactions but also function as regulators making sure the organism does not produce too much or too little of any chemical substance. Although all enzymes are proteins, many contain additional non-protein components essential for catalytic activity. Such enzymes are termed haloenzymes. The protein part of this enzyme is termed an apoenzyme and the non-amino acid part is termed a coenzyme.

Enzyme linked immunosorbent assay (ELISA) A blood test used to detect bacteria that can cause ulcers known as Helicobacter pylori (or H. pylori).

Enzyme therapy A form of therapy that employs supplements of plant and animal enzymes to improve digestive function and other conditions. During digestion, the body's own digestive enzymes are not the only ones at work; the enzymes present in raw fruits and vegetables also contribute to the breakdown of food in the stomach. Enzyme therapy advocates supplementation to reduce the work that the body has to do, and because plant enzymes are destroyed in cooking. Since enzymes can't be synthetically manufactured, supplements are derived from plants or from animal tissues. Some practitioners inject liquid enzymes to treat cancer and multiple sclerosis. Enzyme supplements are available over the counter, singly or in combination, in capsule, tablet, powder, and liquid form.

Ependyma Single uninterrupted layer of ciliated squamous to columnar epithelial-like cells that line the cerebral ventricles and central canal of the spinal cord.

Ephedra / Ephedrine The active ingredient in the Oriental herb Ma Huang (Ephedra sinensis); this chemical has been proven to be both a powerful energizer and weight loss aid. Ephedrine is a powerful thermogenic agent: It releases norepinephrine, a brain neurotransmitter than exerts a stimulating effect. This same neurotransmitter signals the sympathetic nervous system, which is called into play during a 'fight or flight' response. Body temperature rises and promotes the breakdown of fat cells for fuel.

Use ephedrine for short periods only. Cycling ephedrine can help you avoid side effects as well as improve results of your hard training. Ephedrine, taken with caffeine, can increase each other's ability to induce lipolysis (fat burning). Ephedrine acts at your body's nerve junctions, changing the release and activity of norepinephrine as well as acting on your beta-2 adrenergic receptors.

Epi (prefix) Upon; over. e.g. epibulbar - situated upon the eyeball.

Epicardial The outside surface of the heart. Epicardial leads are placed on the heart during open-chest surgery.

Epicardium The inner layer of the serous pericardium which is in contact with the heart.

Epidemic A disease attacking many people in a community simultaneously; distinguished from endemic, since the disease is not continuously present but has been introduced from outside.

Epidemiology The study of the patterns of human disease, health and behaviours.

Epidural A regional anesthetic used for pain relief by some women in labor. It is injected into the dural space in your spine, and the anesthetic takes effect from your chest down. About 80-85% of women who have it report satisfactory pain relief from it. The others report anything from "windows" of pain to no relief at all. If you have an epidural, you will lose all motor control from your chest down, and be required to be on the fetal monitor continuously. You will also have to have an IV. Some women develop a fever that is related to the epidural, which means antibiotics are added to their IV. Some women find their labors pick up once they have an epidural and are able to relax, others find their labors slow down and they end up having pitocin added to their IV to augment their labor.

Epidural block Epidural block—Type of anesthesia. Medication is injected around the spinal cord during labor or other types of surgery.

Epidural space Narrow space situated between the dura mater and the bony skull or vertebral column.

Epiglottis (literally above the glottis) The cartilagenous structure which overhangs the larynx - it acts like a flap valve to prevent food entering the airway when swallowing. Epiglottitis

ePIP ePIP is the electronic version of CHSRA's Provider Initiative Project (PIP)/ORYX initiative. It allows members of the PIP/ORYX initiative to submit MDS data electronically to CHSRA for analysis, and to view, print or download QI reports based on the data submitted. ePIP also provides members with many new features including the ability to run specialized reports and Report Sets, as well as access to a great deal of QI related information.

Episiotomy Episiotomy—Surgical incision of the vulva (area behind the vagina, above the rectum). Used during delivery to avoid tearing or laceration of the vaginal opening and rectum.

Epithalamus The postero-dorsal part of the diencephalon located above the thalamus at the point where the cerebral aqueduct joins the third ventricle. Consists of the habenular nuclei, pineal body, subcimmissural organ, posterior and habenular commissures.

Epithelium The layer(s) of cells between an organism or its tissues or organs and their environment (skin cells, inner linings of lungs or digestive organs, outer linings of kidneys, etc.).

Epitympanic recess The upper portion of the tympanic membrane, above the level of the tympanic membrane.

EPO (erythropoietin) A glycoprotein hormone that stimulates the production of red blood cells. It is a commercialized product of recombinant DNA technology.

Epoxy These materials are based on the reactive oxirane group, which are characterized by the attachment of one oxygen atom to two different adjacent carbon atoms. Standard epoxy resins are the reaction product of bisphenol A and epichlorohydrin. Curing of epoxy resins generally occurs at ambient temperatures and is achieved by the chemical reaction of the epoxy with a second reactant such as amines, polyamines, amine products, or other reactants. Cure can occur at higher temperatures when reacted with anhydrides, carboxylic acids, phenol or novolac (phenol-formadehyde) thermoplastic resins. These reactants are sometimes referred to as catalysts, which is a misnomer.

Equine Of, pertaining to, or characteristic of a horse, such as equine hormones.

Equipment suitability The established capacity of process equipment and ancillary systems to operate consistently within established limits and tolerances.

Equity A state of being fair or equal; equity in health implies the ideal that everyone should have a fair opportunity to attain his or her full health potential. More pragmatically, it implies that no one should be disadvantaged by being prevented from achieving this potential. The term inequity refers to differences in health, which are not only unnecessary and avoidable but, in addition, are considered unfair and unjust.

ERCP Endoscopic Retrograde Cholangio-Pancreatography- An examination of the common bile duct and pancreatic duct performed with a specially designed endoscope and X-ray.

Erector spinea muscle Intermediate muscles of the back that produce extention in the vertebral column. It originates from the sacrum, iliac crest, and spines of the lumbar and eleventh and twelfth thoracic vertebrae, splitting into the iliocostals, longissimus, and spinalis muscles.

Ergogenic aids Any nutrients that improve athletic performance.

Eroded Having a shallow or superficial ulceration.

Erythrocyte The red blood cell consisting largely of hemoglobin and carrying nearly all the oxygen contained in the blood. Erythrocytes are biconcave discs that are manufactured in the bone marrow.

Erythrocyte Sedimentation Rate (ESR) A test that measures the rate at which red blood cells settle in unclotted blood. The ESR may be used to evaluate patients with unexplained symptoms or a deterioration of health when: an inflammatory, neoplastic (cancer in its earliest stages), or infectious disease is suspected and a specific diagnosis is not made effectively by other means

Erythromycin An antibiotic that binds to the 50S subunit of prokaryotic ribosomes and inhibits translocation of mRNA along the ribosome.

Esc The escape key. Used to exit or stop a program immediately, or to cancel what is being done at that moment and return to a previous screen. The effects of the escape key are usually controlled by the software and, are different with various programs.

Escherichia coli (Also known as E. coli.) A bacteria that can cause infection of the large intestine. E. coli is found in rare or undercooked meat, and can also be spread by using dirty cooking utensils or through contaminated water.

Esophageal atresia During pregnancy, the baby's esophagus does not develop properly, and ends before reaching the stomach. Food cannot pass from the mouth into the stomach.

Esophageal hiatus The defect in the diaphragm through which the esophagus passes from the thorax into the abdomen.

Esophageal manometry A test that measures the muscle tone in the esophagus.

Esophageal pH monitoring A test used to monitor the amount of acid in the esophagus, which helps evaluate gastroesophageal reflux disease (GERD).

Esophageal stricture A narrowing in the esophagus, often caused by irritation from long-term presence of acid in the esophagus with chronic gastroesophageal reflux disease (GERD).

Esophagectomy Removal of the esophagus.

Esophagitis Inflammation of the lining of the esophagus.

Esophagogastroduodenoscopy (EGD) A test using an endoscope to look at the inside of the esophagus, stomach, and upper part of the small intestine. Tissue samples can also be taken to test for diseases.

Esophagus The musculomembraneous tube connecting the pharynx to the stomach.

Esophoria (Eso) (clinical condition) A tendency of the eyes to want to turn more inward than necessary when an individual is viewing an object at near or at distance, which may cause the individual to experience eyestrain and other symptoms. Symptoms of basic esophoria include: eyestrain, headaches, blurred or double vision, apparent movement of print, and difficulty concentrating on and comprehending reading material. Clinical signs of basic esophoria include: AC/A ratio is normal, equal esophoria at distance and near, and normal near point of convergence. Sometimes esophoria is caused by a refractive error such as hyperopia (farsightedness), and glasses or contacts can correct the problem alone. However, sometimes vision therapy is needed to to help re-train the eyes to function more appropriately.

Esotropia (ET) (clinical condition) A condition in which an eye is turned either constantly or intermittently inward toward the nose. Esotropia is a type of strabismus. It is caused by a reduction in visual acuity, reduced visual function, high refractive error, traumatic brain injury, oculomotor nerve lesion, or eye muscle injury. Treatment options may include one or more of the following: glasses or contacts, bi-focal lenses, prisms, vision therapy, surgery, or Botulinum Toxin Type A (Oculinum, Botox) injections. In some cases, esotropia is caused by a refractive error such as hyperopia (farsightedness), and glasses or contacts alone may allow the eyes to straighten. Vision therapy is most appropriate when there are small degrees of misalignment. Surgery, to re-position or shorten the eye muscles, may be required for high degrees of misalignment. If surgery is required, a combination of surgery and vision therapy often yields the best results.

Essays or open ended questions An assessment method, distinguished from short-answer questions by the scope, the length of required answers, and the relative lack of specific cues for recall. Essay questions typically deal with larger issues and are based on information that is spread out over a number of learning sources. Students' answers should reflect both how much is known about a topic and how well organized knowledge of the subject is. As essay questions and answers are comparatively complex, more abilities are displayed than with other question types. They may be used to assess knowledge of basic and clinical science and its application to clinical problems. They provide information about the respondent perceptions, reasoning abilities, attitudes, feelings, and experiences. Because such questions typically require extensive knowledge as well as analytical and writing skills, they perhaps are best suited for deciding who the top students in a course are. The essential weakness of essay questions is that they can be ambiguous, difficult to grade reliably and require scorers with relevant knowledge and training.

Essential A nutritional term applied to vitamins, minerals, and amino acids; refers to anything that the body does not manufacture and that must be obtained through the diet.

Essential amino Acids Amino acids that cannot be synthesized by human and other vertebrates and must be obtained from the diet.

Essential Fatty Acids (EFA) They include Linoleic Acid, Omega-3 Fatty Acids, and Monounsaturated fats. These are considered the 'good' fats. They cannot be made by the body and must be supplied by our diet. You need approxiamately 2% of your daily calories as EFA's. By consuming plenty of EFAs, you supply your body with the appropriate precursors to form cell membranes and regulatory eicosanoids.

EST (expressed sequence tag) ethical pharmaceutical A controlled substance for the diagnosis or treatment of disease.

Estimated date of confinement Estimated date of confinement.

Estimated date of delivery Estimated date of delivery.

Estrogen Hormones responsible for the development of female sex characteristics; produced by the ovary.

Ethics The branch of philosophy that deals with distinctions between right and wrong and with the moral consequences of human actions. Examples of ethical issues that arise in medical practice and research include informed consent, confidentiality, respect for human rights, and scientific integrity.

Ethmoid sinus The paranasal sinus located within the ethmoid bone, between the orbits, below the brain, and above the nasal cavity.

Ethylene oxide (ETO) A toxic compound used in gaseous form as a sterilizing agent, usually as a 10% mixture with carbon dioxide or 12% mixture with freon (referred as 12-88). Sterilization using ETO leaves residual chemicals such as ethylene chlorohydrin and ethylene glycol.

Etiologic agent A disease-causing organism or toxin.

Etiology The causative agent in a lesion.

Eukaryote An organism that carries its genetic material physically constrained within a nuclear membrane, separate from the cytoplasm. All animal and plant cells except bacteria, viruses, and bluegreen algae are eukaryotic. Eukaryotes are five to ten times larger than prokaryotes in diameter.

Eustachian tube A hollow cartilagenous tube connecting the tympanic cavity (middle ear) and the nasopharynx. An open tube can equilibrate the pressure in the middle ear. Yawning opens the tube to allow the ears to "pop!" when changing altitude.

Eutectic Of, pertaining to, or formed at the lowest possible temperature of solidification for any mixture of specified constituents. A common term used to describe metal alloys.

Evaluation A process that attempts to systematically and objectively determine the relevance, effectiveness, and impact of activities in light of their objectives. Evaluation can be related to structure, process, or outcome. One can distinguish these various types:

Formative individual evaluation provides feedback to an individual (usually a learner) in order to improve that individual's performance. This type of evaluation identifies areas for improvement and provides specific suggestions for improvement serving as an educational tool.

Summative individual evaluation measures whether specific objectives were accomplished by an individual in order to place a value on the performance of that individual. It may certify competency or lack of competency in performance in a particular area.

Formative program evaluation provides information in order to improve a program's performance. It usually takes the form of surveys of learners to obtain feedback about and suggestions for improving a curriculum. Quantitative information such as ratings of various aspects of the curriculum can help identify areas that need revision. Qualitative information, such as responses to open-ended questions about program strengths and weaknesses, as well as suggestions for change, provide feedback in areas that may not have been anticipated and provide ideas for improvement. Information can also be obtained from faculty or other observers, such as nurses and patients.

Summative program evaluation measures the success of a curriculum in achieving learner objectives for all targeted learners, its success in achieving its process objectives, and/or its success in engaging, motivating, and pleasing its learners and faculty. In addition to quantitative data, summative program evaluation may include qualitative information about unintended barriers or unanticipated effects encountered in program implementation.

Formative evaluations generally require the least amount of rigor, whereas summative individual and summative program evaluation for external use (e.g., certification of competence) requires the greatest amount of rigor. When a high degree of methodological rigor is required, the measurement instrument must be appropriate in terms of content, reliability, validity, and practicality.

Evaluation, 360-degree A method used to assess interpersonal and communication skills, professional behaviors, and some aspects of patient care and systems-based practice. Usually, evaluators completing rating forms in a 360-degree evaluation are superiors, peers, subordinates, and patients and their families. Most 360-degree evaluation processes use a surveyor questionnaire to gather information about an individual's performance on several topics, such as teamwork, communication, management skills, and decision-making. Most 360-degree evaluations use rating scales to assess how frequently a behavior is performed. The ratings are summarized for all evaluators by topic and also overall to provide feedback. Such feedback is more accurate when the evaluation is intended to give formative feedback rather than summative. Reproducible results are easily obtained when several evaluators rate examinees; a greater number of faculty and patients are needed for a greater degree of reliability.

Evaporator Apparatus used in distillation to heat a liquid and create a phase change from the liquid to the vapor state. A steam boiler is an evaporator.

Evidence based Care The conscientious, judicious and explicit use of current best evidence in providing information to individual clients and supporting those clients in making informed decisions about their care. Evidence-based care de-emphasizes intuition and unsystematic clinical experience and stresses that clinical decision-making requires examination of evidence from clinical research. Evidence-based care requires the midwife to search literature efficiently and to apply critical thinking skills in evaluating the clinical literature.

Ex(o) (prefix) Out of; away from; outside of.

e.g. exophytic - projecting out from a surface.

Excipient A more or less inert substance added in a prescription drug compound as a diluent or vehicle or to give form or consistency when the remedy is given in a pill form; simple syrup, aromatic powder, honey, and various elixirs are examples of excipients.

Excrete Remove waste from the body.

Exergonic reaction Referring to a chemical reaction that takes place with release of negative standard energy to its surroundings, a "downhill" reaction.

Exfiltration Leakage of air out of a room through cracks in doors and pass-throughs through material transfer openings, etc. due to a difference in room pressures.

Exhaustion Occurs when absorbents, such as activated carbon or ion exchange resins, have depleted their capacity by using up all active sites. Ion exchange resins may be regenerated to reverse the process.

Exogenous DNA DNA originating outside an organism.

Exon The proteincoding DNA sequence of an eukaryotic gene.

Exonuclease An enzyme that cleaves nucleotides sequentially from free ends of a linear nucleic acid substrate.

Exophoria (Exo) (clinical condition) A tendency of the eyes to want to turn more outward than necessary when an individual is viewing an object at near or at distance, which may cause the individual to experience eyestrain and other symptoms. Symptoms of basic exophoria include: eyestrain, headaches, blurred or double vision, apparent movement of print, and difficulty concentrating on and comprehending reading material. Clinical signs of basic exophoria include: normal AC/A ratio, equal exophoria at distance and near, and decreased near point of convergence. Vision therapy is an effective treatment option.

Exotic organism A biological agent where either the corresponding disease does not exist in a given country or geographical area, or where the disease is the subject of prophylactic measures or an eradication program undertaken in the given country or geographical area.

Exotoxins Proteins produced by bacteria that are able to diffuse into a medium through the bacterial cell membrane and cell wall. They are generally more potent and specific in their actions than endotoxins.

Exotropia (XT) (clinical condition) A condition in which an eye is either constantly or intermittently turned outward toward the ear. Exotropia is a type of strabismus. It may also be called divergent strabismus, wandering eye, or wall eye(s). It is caused by a reduction in visual acuity, reduced visual function, high refractive error, traumatic brain injury, oculomotor nerve lesion, or eye muscle injury. Treatment options may include one or more of the following: glasses or contacts, bi-focal lenses, prisms, vision therapy, surgery, or Botulinum Toxin Type A (Oculinum, Botox) injections. Vision therapy is most appropriate when there are small degrees of misalignment. If surgery is required, a combination of surgery and vision therapy often yields the best results.

Expansion Card A circuit board that plugs into a computer and gives it additional specialized functions (e.g. advanced graphics, video, sound, modem).

Expansion Slot A socket on the main board of a computer where expansion cards are inserted.

Experience The transformation of preconceived notions, expectations and/or theory by means of encounters with actual clinical situations.

Expiration date The date placed on the container/labels of an API (Active Pharmaceutical Ingredient) designating the time during which the API is expected to remain within established shelf life specifications if stored under defined conditions, and after which it should not be used.

Explorer A program that comes with Windows 95 and 98 that helps you view and manage your files (Replaces the "File Manager" in older Windows programs, such as 3.1).

Explosion resistance A type of construction used to house solvents in sufficiently large quantities, to qualify the space electrically as an explosion potential area. Typically the internal walls, ceiling, and floor are constructed of material strong enough to withstand a specified intensity of explosion, and at least one wall has explosion relief devices that direct the explosion outwardly. In a single story arrangement, or if the explosion resistant area is on the top floor, the roof may also have devices that can be used to relieve the explosion.

Explosive A chemical that causes a sudden, almost instantaneous release of pressure, gas and heat when subjected to sudden shock, pressure, or high temperatures, or a material or chemical, other than a blasting agent, that is commonly used or intended for the purpose of producing an explosive effect.

Exposed or open process The drug substance is exposed to the room environment during processing.

Express To translate the genetic information stored in the DNA into protein.

Expression system A host organism combined with a genetic vector (such as virus or circular DNA molecule called a plasmid) that is loaded with a gene of interest. The expression system provides the genetic context in which a gene will function in the cell - that is, the gene will be expressed as a protein.

Expressive therapies Use the arts to promote physical & mental health and personal growth. Examples of expressive therapies include art therapy, dance therapy, drama therapy, music therapy, poetry, and psychodrama.

Extended Class A class of registration that's currently available to RNs who have successfully demonstrated competence to practise as primary health care nurse practitioners. They are able to practise with extended scope in assessment, diagnosis and health care management.

Extended Survey A survey conducted within 14 days of a finding of substandard care during a standard survey.

Extension An unbending movement around a joint in a limb that increases the angle between the bones of the limb at the joint.

External acoustic (Auditory) canal The opening in the external surface of the temporal bone, behind the condyle of the mandible and in front of the mastoid air cells that conducts air and sound toward the tympanic membrane.

External auditory meatus The opening for the passage from the external ear toward the tympanic membrane. Also called the External Auditory Canal.

External Beam Radiation therapy A 25-28 treatment protocol that utilizes External Beam Radiation. Approximately 6800-7400 rads of radiation energy is delivered to the Prostate. There can be some radiation effect on surrounding tissues.

External capsule The thin association fiber layer of white matter immediately overlying the lateral convex surface of the putamen.

External iliac artery Artery which originates from the common iliac and branches into the inferior epigastric and deep circumflex iliac arteries.

External iliac vein The continuation of the femoral vein, beginning at the level of the inguinal ligament, and joining the internal iliac vein at the sacroiliac articulation to form the common iliac vein.

External oblique muscle Muscles that run from the lower eight ribs at the costal cartilages to the crest of ilium and linea alba, that are responsible for flexing and rotating the torso and vertebral column.

Extracorporeal Shock Wave Lithotripsy (ESWL) Extracorporeal shock wave lithotripsy uses highly focused impulses projected from outside the body to pulverize kidney stones.

Extractables Undesirable foreign substances that are leached or dissolved by water or process streams from the materials of construction used in filters, storage vessels, distribution piping, and other wetted surfaces.

Extraocular muscles The muscles attached to the outside of the eyeball which control eye movement. Each eye has six muscles (lateral rectus, medial rectus, superior oblique, inferior oblique, superior rectus, and inferior rectus) that are coordinated by the brain.

Extrapyramidal Symptoms (EPS) Abnormal movements of the mouth or tongue, pill rolling, tremors, rigid movements, mask-like face, constant movement of legs or body, tics, blinking, pacing, eyes rolled up, drooling.

Extreme capsule Thin layer of association fibers between the claustrum and cortex of the insula.

Eye hand coordination The ability of our eyes to guide our hands, also called visual motor integration.

Eye trac (equipment) An electronic testing and recording system of eye movements as in reading.

Eye tracking The ability of the eyes to smoothly and effortlessly follow a moving target.

F

Face presentation Face presentation—Baby comes into the birth canal face first.

Face velocity The velocity obtained by dividing the air quantity by the component face area (NEBB).

Facial artery A branch of external carotid that branches into the ascending palatine, tonsillar, submental, inferior labial, superior labial, septal, lateral nasal, angular, and glandular arteries.

Facility General term used for any type of nursing home or intermediate care facility for the mentally retarded.

Facility Admission Profile (FAP) The proportion of residents (patients) who have a given condition (e.g., pressure ulcer) upon admission to a facility. The FAP reflects the facility's resident (patient) population admitted over a 12-month period and is intended to capture the admitting characteristics of individual facilities. The FAP is used as a form of risk adjustment for some QMs.

Facility flexibility A qualitative measure of the number of different products that can be produced in a facility or area of a facility.

Facility of accommodation A measure of the ease and speed of the eye(s) to change focus.

Facility user The end user of a facility, often called the Owner, represented by operating, maintenance, and quality control personnel.

Factor VIII (hemophilia factor) Also known as antihemophilic factor or AHF (Brinkhous) in the clotting of blood, Factor VIII is a labile protein of the blood-clotting system that assists in the conversion of Factor IX into plasma factor X (Stuart factor). Deficiency of factor VIII is associated with classic hemophilia A, a hereditary, sex-linked, hemorrhagic tendency that occurs almost exclusively in men; clotting time is prolonged, less thromboplastin is formed, and the conversion of prothrombin is diminished.

Faculty development Because faculty members may be experts in their subject but may not have received special training in educating others, faculty development programs exist to enable these teachers to acquire the necessary professional knowledge, skills, attitudes and tools. It is an essential component for obtaining high reliability and validity of applied assessment on a day-to-day basis. It also enhances ongoing formative evaluation so that students are given feedback to help them improve continuously. Faculty development activities can be organized as series of special workshops, readings, or individualized feedback sessions. Since teaching is considered a very important aspect of a physician's work, such educational programs are often viewed as a form of Continuing Medical Education.

Faculty ratings questionnaires Questionnaires completed by faculty members that are used in the assessment of student deficiencies and achievements as well as professional behavior and competence. They provide indirect, inexpensive measures of clinical skills attainment and real-life students' performance. However, Faculty-Ratings Questionnaires are subject to rating biases.

Failure to thrive A condition that occurs when a baby does not gain weight and grow normally; caused by many factors, including disease or poor nutrition.

Falciform ligament (of Liver) An extension of the coronary ligament of the liver that attaches the liver to the diaphragm and separates the right and left lobes of the liver.

Fallopian tubes These muscular tubes connect from the uterus (upper lateral cornu) to the peritoneal cavity in the area of the ipsilateral ovary. During Ovulation, the tubes carry the ova (eggs) from the ovary and into the uterus.

False labor False labor—Tightening of uterus without dilatation of the cervix.

False vocal CORD A fold of mucous membrane in the larynx that separates the vestibule from the laryngeal ventricle, all above the true vocal cords (glottis).

Falx cerebri Sickle-shaped fold of dura mater that extends vertically in the midline between the two cerebral hemispheres.

F. Cerebelli: Sickle-shaped fold of dura mater that extends vertically between the cerebellar hemispheres along the posterior midline of the posterior cranial fossa.

FAQ (Frequently Asked Questions)+A1594. Usually found on the internet and new software, FAQs are helpful resources that contain the answers to the most frequently asked questions about a topic.

Fascia The tough connective tissue that surrounds muscles and holds them in place.

Fasciculus Bundles of nerve fibers (tract) within the central nervous system which have a common origin, course, and termination, and function.

Fastigial nuclei Paired cerebellar nuclei located on either side of the midline deep within the white matter of the cerebellar vermis. Associated with the vestibulocerebellum.

Fastigium The mid-dorsal apex of the fourth ventricle that extends into the medullary substance of the cerebellum.

Fasting blood sugar Fasting blood sugar-Blood test to evaluate the amount of sugar in the blood following a time period of fasting.

Fat Macronutrient that is a source for long term energy and energy storage (as adipose tissue); necessary for absorption and transport of fat-soluble vitamins and constituant of hormones and cell membranes.

One gram of fat equals nine calories. There are 455 grams in one pound. So nine calories times 455 grams equals 4,025 calories per pound of fat. So, technically, you need to lose 4,025 calories to lose one pound of fat.

Fats One of three main types of foods, along with proteins and carbohydrates. Provides the body with a source of energy. Needs bile in order to be digested properly and utilized for energy.

Fax A method of digitally copying a document then converting the copy to an analog signal to be transmitted to a remote location using standard phone lines. Because faxing isn't exact, what is received at the other end is rarely a perfect copy, and usually just a "reasonable facsimile thereof" (thus the term facs—er, fax).

FDA form 483 The official form of notification prepared at the conclusion of an inspection (without review by FDA management) listing observations of perceived violations of Good Manufacturing Practices that may constitute violations of law in the opinion of an inspector. Originally intended to inform companies of possible product adulteration, they must be replied to satisfactorily and/ or corrective action taken in order to alleviate any offensive notification and avoid action from the FDA (i.e., plant shut-down). Accessible through the Freedom of Information Act to competitors, potential customers, and the media; 483s can lead to withholding of product approvals, may come into play in due diligence phases of acquisitions and mergers, and can potentially cost companies money.

Fecal fat test Assesses how well the body can break down and absorb fat. A fat free diet is eaten for two to three days, and then stool samples are collected and examined for the amount of fat they contain.

Fecal occult blood test Checks for occult (hidden) blood in a random stool sample.

Fed batch fermentation The most common operating mode for rDNA fermentation. After an initial partial charge of media to the fermenter and seed transfer, sterile media is added at measured rates during the balance of the fermentation cycle. Cell mass and broth are withdrawn only at the end of the cycle.

Fee For Service Programs where services are paid for based on actual utilization of services, using payment rates set for units of care provided, such as daily nursing home rates. For each service, a fee is paid. Contrast this to managed care programs which pay for services on a capitated basis.

Fee Schedule A schedule of standard rates for specific services provided. Providers set their own fee schedules of rates they charge to private or self-pay residents. Fee schedule reimbursement is based upon units of service provided, which may be visits or encounters, or the number of items provided (as with medical supplies or medical equipment.)

Feedback loop A central concept in industrial controls in which the value of a process variable is compared with the desired value (setpoint), and any discrepancy (error) is converted into a modified output signal.

Feedwater The water entering a treatment process.

Fellow of the college of optometrists in vision development (FCOVD) Individual who is a licensed optometrist for a minimum of three years and directly involved in vision therapy for a minimum of 2 years, has completed a guided study program, submitted evidence of 100 hours of continuing education in functional vision (and vision therapy), and passed rigorous written, oral, and clinical examinations. Fellows are Board Certified in Vision Development and Therapy and must obtain at least 15 hours of continuing education annually in functional / developmental / behavioral / rehabilitation vision care.

Femoral artery A continuation of the external iliac that branches into the superficial epigastric, superficial circumflex iliac, external pudendal, deep femoral, and descending geniculate arteries.

Femoral condyles (medial and lateral)Two articulating surfaces located on the distal end of the femur and articulate with the proximal head of the tibia.

Femoral head The round ball-shaped proximal end of the Femur that articulates with the socket formed by the ischium, pubis, and acetabulum (joined together by the triradiate cartilage).

Femoral vein The continuation of the popliteal vein that becomes the external iliac at the inguinal ligament.

Femur The proximal bone of the lower extremity. It is the largest bone in the body. AKA "thigh bone".

Feng shui An ancient Chinese practice of configuring home or work environments to promote health, happiness, prosperity. Feng shui consultants may advise clients to make adjustments in their surroundings, from color selection to furniture placement, to promote a healthy flow of chi, or vital energy.

Fermentation The process of growing microorganisms within an enclosed tank (fermenter) under controlled conditions of aeration, agitation, temperature, and pH. The different types organisms used as a basis for fermentation are:

1. Bacteria (E. coli)
2. Yeasts
3. Molds
4. Chinese Hamster Ovary (CHO) cells
5. Kidney cells
6. Vaccines to viruses.

Fermenter A tank or vessel used for carrying out fermentation. There are various choices of fermenters, depending on whether cells are suspended in the medium or attached to some type of support:

1. In suspension reactors
2. Attached growth reactors
3. Stirred-tank reactors
4. Airlift fermenters
5. Packed bed reactors
6. Two-chamber reactors
7. Hollow-fiber reactors

Fertilization Fertilization-Joining of the sperm and egg.

Fertilization age Fertilization age—Dating a pregnancy from the time of fertilization. 2 weeks earlier than the gestational age.

Fetal anomaly Fetal anomaly—Fetal malformation or abnormal development.

Fetal calf serum The liquid portion remaining after natural coagulation of blood drawn from the heart of an unborn calf. Because of the absence of gamma globulin, fetal calf serum is a good tissue culture serum.

Fetal death (deadborn fetus) Death prior to the complete expulsion or extraction from its mother of a product of conception, irrespective of the duration of pregnancy. The death is indicated by the fact that after such separation, the fetus does not breathe or show any other evidence of life, such as beating of the heart, pulsation of the umbilical cord, or definite movement of voluntary muscles.

Fetal Demise Death of the baby in utero, diagnosed via ultrasound

Fetal goiter Fetal goiter—Enlargement of the thyroid in the fetus.

Fetal monitor Fetal monitor—Device used before or during labor to listen to and record the fetal heartbeat. Can be external monitoring (through maternal abdomen) or internal monitoring (through maternal vagina) of the baby inside the uterus.

Fetal period Fetal period—Time period following the embryonic period (first 10 weeks of gestation) until birth.

Fetal growth retardation Fetal-growth retardation (IUGR)—Inadequate growth of the fetus during the last stages of pregnancy.

Fetus Fetus—Refers to the unborn baby after 10 weeks of gestation until birth.

Fever Also known as pyrexia, a human body temperature above the normal 98.6°F (37°C).

Fiber The more insoluble the fiber is (fiber that does not dissolve in water), the better it is for you. Insoluble fiber reduces the risk of colon cancer and high blood pressure. Fruit fiber seems to be more beneficial then vegetable or cereal fibers, probably because fruits are loaded with Pectin, an insoluble fiber. As a rule, the higher the insolubility, the fewer the calories. Corn bran is the best, followed by wheat bran, and then oat bran. It is best to eat fiber after you work out to avoid intestinal discomfort.

Fibrin A plasma protein that, in its aggregated state, is the major component of a blood clot. It is produced from fibrinogen, a soluble precursor, by the action of the proteolytic enzyme, thrombin.

Fibrinogen In the clotting of blood it is known as Factor I. The plasma protein that becomes converted to a clot at the end of the coagulation process. Present in plasma; absent in serum.

Fibromyalgia Fibromyalgia is a chronic disorder that causes widespread musculoskeletal pain, fatigue, and multiple tender points in localized areas, such as the neck, spine, shoulders, and hips. The syndrome is marked by concurrent symptoms including sleep disturbances, morning stiffness, irritable bowel syndrome, anxiety, and other symptoms.

Fibula The thin bone of the lower leg. The large bone is the Tibia.

Fifth Disease Fifths Disease is an illness commonly acquired by small children resembling the flu with a rash across their cheeks. Most adults have been to exposed to this disease already and are immune, but a pregnant woman who has never been exposed to this disease may pass it on to the fetus, causing (in very rare cases) complications or fetal death.

Figure ground The ability to recognize distinct shapes from their background, such as objects in a picture, or letters on a chalkboard.

File A computer file is similar to a paper document holding related information. For example, each computer program or document is stored in a separate file, designated by its own filename.

File Extension The final part of an MS-DOS filename that denotes the file format. The extension is usually three to four letters set apart from the rest of the file name by a period. Examples of file extensions are: .gif, .html, .doc, .txt, .wav, wpd and so on.

File Format File format refers to files' type based on a files' structure, layout or how a particular file handles the information contained within that file. A files' format is usually indicated by the three or four letter file extension in the MS-DOS filename. All of these file formats handle different information (sounds, words, images) in different ways.

File Transfer Protocol Also called FTP. FTP is the standard protocol for uploading and downloading files to the internet, for instance for building a webpage.

Filename A name, specified by either the user, programmer, or software, comprised of alphanumeric characters, to identify a file and its contents. Different programs and operating systems have their own naming rules. A basic MS-DOS filename contains up to eight letters or numbers, followed by the file's three- or four-letter file extension, in this format: "filename.ext". Windows95 and 98 allow users to specify a filename of up to 255 characters.

Fill and finish (parenteral drugs) Preparation of parenteral drugs, either LVPs or SVPs, demands the highest level of contamination control, because the human body's normal defenses against infection are bypassed when parenteral medications are introduced either intramuscularly (I.M.) or intravenously (I.V.) directly into the body. The processing of raw materials into finished dosage forms must comply at all times with cGMPs and must be able to support process validation. Mechanical design should include HVAC Classifications considered essential to attain global regulatory acceptance. The desire for increased levels of sterility assurance has led the FDA to promote the use of terminal sterilization for aseptically filled products. The FDA has stated that terminal sterilization processing is the method of choice unless the manufacturer can show that it is detrimental to the product. Terminal sterilization may be accomplished using autoclaves that apply overpressure to balance the pressures that are developed across the inside and outside of the containers. Because of product sensitivities, biologics, and blood products are not appropriate applications for terminal sterilization

Filters Filtering centrifuges accommodate a range of liquid-solid separations. The two batch types, basket and peeler centrifuges, can separate almost any liquid-solid slurry. For continuous operation, there are pusher and conical centrifuges.

a) Pusher - with a horizontal axis, the pusher centrifuge operates at a constant fixed speed. It has a perforated bowl, generally with a bar-type screen. One end of the bowl is open while the opposite end is closed with a reciprocating diaphragm, or disc, which rotates with the bowl.

b) Conical - the standard conical centrifuge consists of a cone with a small closed end and a large open end to which is attached a coarsely woven drainage screen, topped with a filter screen or perforated plate. A compartmentalized casing surrounds the bowl. There are two variations of the basic conical centrifuge: the tilting conical centrifuge and the conveyor conical type.

Filtration Removal of suspended matter from a fluid by passing it through a porous matrix that prevents particles from getting through, usually by entrapment on or in the filter matrix.

Filum terminale Thread-like filament of pia mater within the lumbar cistern extending from the end of the spinal cord to the coccyx.

Fimbria Efferent fiber bundle arising from the hippocampus and continuing as the fornix.

Final bulk product The final drug product after chemical or biological processing and purification, ready for concentration, drying, and filling into containers prior to dispensing and final filling.

Fine motor skills The ability to coordinate hand and finger movements.

Finished product A medicinal product that has undergone all stages of production, including packaging in its final container.

Firmware A combination of hardware and software with the programming written directly into read-only memory (ROM).

FISH (fluorescent in situ hybridization) A physical mapping approach that uses fluorescein tags to detect hybridization of probes with metaphase chromosomes and with the less condensed somatic interface chromatin.

Fissile material A radioisotope that could undergo a nuclear fission reaction and is usually found at reactor sites or as part of a nuclear weapon.

Fissure Certain deep clefts (sulci) which separate various parts of the central nervous system (ie. lateral fissure of Sylvius, primary fissure etc.) .

Fissures A crack in the lining or surface of an organ such as in the anus.

Fistula An abnormal, tube-like passage from a hollow organ to the surface, or from one organ to another.

e.g. esophageal fistula - a communication between the esophagus and some portion of the respiratory tract.

Fixation The ability to direct and maintain steady visual attention on a target. Fixations are a form of pursuits.

Fixation disparity (FD) Over-convergence or under-convergence, or vertical misalignment of the eyes under binocular (both eyes) viewing conditions small enough in magnitude so that fusion is present.

Fixed Route Transit services where vehicles run on regular, pre-designated, pre-scheduled routes, with no deviation.

Typically, fixed-route service is characterized by printed schedules or timetables, designated bus stops where passengers board and alight and the use of larger transit vehicles.

Flag QIs flag when they reach the threshold or a set point at which the likelihood of a problem is sufficient to warrant further investigation. A QI will flag if it is ranked at the 90th percentile or above. In the case of sentinel health events, if even one resident is in the numerator, the QI will flag. It should be noted that CMS uses the 75th percentile as its threshold for LTC surveys.

Flaggelae Thin, helical filaments attached to the surface of bacterial and eukaryotic (e.g. sperm, protozoa) cells. They are motile structures containing microtubules (composed of proteins called tubulin) that enable cells possessing them to move.

Flammable liquid A liquid having a closed cup flash point below 100°F (37.8°C). Flammable liquids do not include compressed gases or cryogenic fluids. Flammable liquids are subdivided as follows: 1. Class I-A - Liquids having a closed cup flash point below 73°F (22.8°C) and having a boiling point below 100°F (37.8°C).

2. Class I-B - liquids having a closed cup flash point below 73°F (22.8°C) and having a boiling point at or above 100°F (37.8°C).

3. Class I-C - liquids having a closed cup flash point at or above 73°F (22.8°C) and below 100°F (37.8°C).

Flammable solid A solid substance, other than one which is defined as a blasting agent or explosive, that is liable to cause fire through friction or as a result of retained heat from manufacture, which has an ignition temperature below 212°F (100°C), or which burns so vigorously or persistently when ignited that it creates a serious hazard. Flammable solids include finely divided solid materials which when dispersed in air as a cloud could be ignited and cause an explosion.

Flavonoids A group of compounds widely distributed in plants which have a characteristic molecular structure. They have been found to have many beneficial activities, such as anti-inflammatory and anti-carcinogenic properties.

Flaws Metallic flaws are unintentional irregularities that occur at one place or at relatively infrequent or widely varying intervals on the surface. Flaws include such defects such as cracks, blowholes, inclusions, pits, checks, ridges, scratches, and other surface abnormalities.

Flaxseed Oil Flaxseed is an excellent source of the omega-3 fatty acid alpha-linolenic acid (an EFA). Supplementing with flaxseed oil has been shown to lower cholesterol, decrease heart disease, increase satiety and improve cell integrity.

Flexion A bending movement around a joint in a limb that decreases the angle between the bones of the limb at the joint.

Flexner report, The report researched, written and published by Abraham Flexner (1866-1959) in 1910 for the Carnegie Foundation and entitled "Medical Education in the United States and Canada" is known today as the Flexner Report. It triggered much-needed reforms in the standards, organization, and curriculum of North American medical schools. At the time of the Flexner Report, many medical schools were proprietary schools operated more for profit than for education. Flexner proposed that medical schools operate instead in the German tradition of combining strong biomedical sciences with hands-on clinical training. The report caused many medical schools to close down. It remains one of the most important publications on medical education in the 20th century.

Abraham Flexner was not a doctor, but a secondary school teacher and principal for 19 years in Louisville, Kentucky. He did graduate work at Harvard University and the University of Berlin and joined the research staff of the Carnegie Foundation for the Advancement of Teaching. In 1930, Flexner founded the Institute for Advanced Study at Princeton University and served as its first director. Albert Einstein joined the Institute in 1933. Flexner was one of the great educators of the 20th century. Modern medical education and medicine in North America owes a large debt to him.

Floaters Also known as spots, are usually clouded or semi-opaque specks or particles within the eye that are seen in the field of vision. The eyes are filled with fluid which maintains the shape of the eye, supplies it with nutrition and aids in the focusing of light. Often, particles of protein or other natural materials are left floating or suspended in this fluid when the eye is formed before birth. If the particles are large or close together, they cast shadows which make them visible. This is particularly true when nearsightedness occurs or becomes more severe. In most cases this is normal but floaters can also be caused by certain injuries, eye disease or deterioration of eye fluid or its surrounding structures.

Floc Mass having a fluffy or wooly appearance.

Flocculation A technique for liquid/solids separation. Cationic or anionic polyelectrolytes (e.g. polyacrylamides) are added to highly colloidal water causing coagulation and subsequent settling. The phenomena could be charge neutralization or a bridging effect between separate particles.

Flocculent Having downy or flaky shreds.

Floor of orbit The inferior portion of the bony cavity that contains the eyeball, made up of the maxilla, zygomatic, and palatine bones.

Floor of sella The inferior portion of the sella turcica (pituitary fossa).

Floppy One of several types of magnetic storage media. The term "floppy" refers to any disk that is made of a flexible material, such as Mylar, instead of some type of metal. Almost all floppy disks used now are 3 ½ inch (which hold a maximum of 1.44 megabytes). The smaller, higher capacity disks have become the industry standard, with their older, larger counterparts disappearing into obscurity.

Florence Nightingale's Theory of Nursing Nightingale's theory of nursing described the relationship between the person and the environment. She saw the environment as serving a key factor in the prevention of disease and in the restoration of health in the presence of disease. In the context of sickness her theory proposed that nursing's role was to establish for the patient the optimum environment in which nature could act to bring about healing. Nightingale refers to this need for the nurse to achieve an optimum healing environment with the following:

"nursing...ought to signify the proper use of fresh air, light, warmth, cleanliness, quiet and the proper selection and use of diet".

Nightingale believed that the presence of disease and its associated symptoms represented a reparative process, "...an effort of nature to remedy a process of poisoning or of decay"

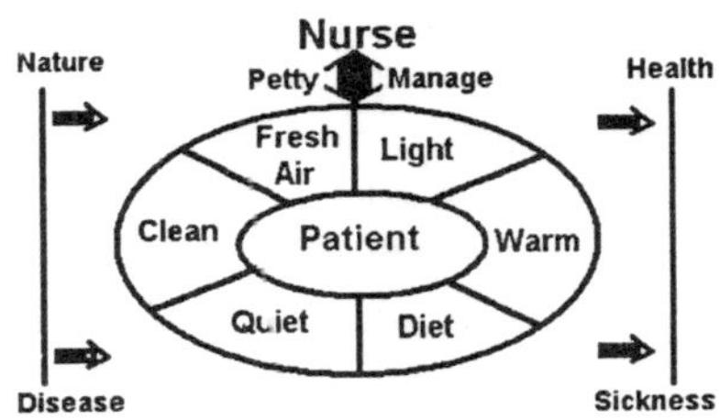

Fig. Florence Nightingale's Theory of Nursing

Flow cytometry Analysis of biological material by detection of light-absorbing or fluorescing properties of cells or subcellular fractions (i.e., chromosomes) passing in a narrow stream through a laser beam. An absorbance or fluorescence profile of the sample is produced. Automated sorting devices, used to fractionate samples, sort successive droplets of the analyzed stream into different fractions depending on the fluorescence emitted by each droplet.

Flow decay Measuring the decline in flow rate through a filter to establish a Silt Index for the water being filtered. The Silt Index is a measure of suspended solids and their ability to clog the filter.

Flow restrictor A flow-limiting orifice used to control flow rate or pressure drop in a liquid stream.

Flower essences Are intended to alleviate negative emotional states that may contribute to illness or hinder personal growth. Drops of a solution infused with the captured essence of a flower are placed under the tongue or in a beverage. The appropriate essences are chosen, focusing on the clients emotional state rather than on a particular physical condition.

Fluid service (piping) As defined in ASME B31.3, fluid service is a general term concerning the application of a piping system, considering the combination of fluid properties, operating conditions, and other factors, which establish the basis for design of the piping system.

1. Category D Fluid Service: A fluid service in which all the following apply: (a) the fluid handled is nonflammable, nontoxic, and not damaging to human tissues . (b) The design gage pressure does not exceed 1035 kPA (150 psi). (c) The design temperature is from -29°C (-20°F) through 186°C (366°F).

2. Category M Fluid Service: A fluid service in which the potential for personnel exposure is judged to be significant and in which a single exposure to a very small quantity of a toxic fluid, caused by leakage can produce serious irreversible harm to persons upon breathing or bodily contact, even when prompt restorative measures are taken.

3. High Pressure Fluid Service: A fluid service for which the owner specifies the use of chapter IX (High Pressure Piping) for piping design and construction.

4. Normal Fluid Service: A fluid service pertaining to most piping covered by ASME B31.3, i.e., not subject to the rules for Category D, Category M, or High Pressure Fluid Service, and not subject to severe cyclic conditions.

Damaging to human tissues for the purpose of the Code, describes a fluid service in which exposure to the fluid, caused by leakage under expected operating conditions, can harm skin, eyes, or exposed mucous membranes so that irreversible damage may result unless prompt restorative measures are taken. These measures may include, flushing with water, administration of antidotes, or medication.

Fluidized bed A container holding powder coating material which is aerated from below so as to form an air-supported expanded cloud of such material through which the preheated object to be coated is immersed and transported.

Fluorescein An orange-red compound, C20H12O5, which exhibits intense fluorescence in alkaline solution.

Fluorinated plastics Fluorinated plastics are thermoplastic paraffinic polymers where the hydrogen has been replaced by fluorine, and in some cases, chlorine. These materials are some of the more popular in the CPI because of good chemical resistance to a wide variety of aggressive chemicals, and relatively high heat resistance of 400°F to 500°F. They include FEP, PTFE, PFA, PCTFE, ETFE, PVDF, and PVF.

Fluoroscopy A radiologic procedure that functions like an X-ray TV camera.

Flux removers Chlorinated solvents with alcohols that may be sprayed from aerosol cans to remove welding flux.

Folder A collection of files. In graphical user interfaces, such as Windows and MACs, folders are the same as DOS directories. Folders can hold files and other folders for organizational purposes.

Foley catheter A catheter placed through the urethra into the bladder to drain urine and monitor the volume of urine output.

Folium One of the narrow transverse folds of the cerebellar surface.

Font A description of how to display a set of characters. The description includes the shape of the characters, spacing between characters, effects (for example, bold, italics, and underline) and the size of the characters.

Foramen A communication between two cavities such as the brain ventricles or an opening in bone for passage of vessels and/ or nerves.

Foramen magnum The large opening that connects the vertebral canal to the cranial cavity, located in the anterior and inferior portion of the occipital bone, and allows passage of CSF and connection of the medulla oblongata to the cervical spinal cord.

Foramen ovale The passage for the mandibular (3rd) branch of the trigeminal (Vth) nerve through the medial and posterior part of the greater wing of the sphenoid bone.

Foramen rotundum The opening that allows the passage of the maxillary (2nd) branch of the trigeminal (Vth) nerve through the medial part of the greater wing of the sphenoid bone.

Foramen spinosum The opening near the posterior angle of the greater wing of the sphenoid bone, posterior to the spinous process, that allows passage of the middle meningeal artery.

Foramen transversium The opening in the transverse process which allows the vertebral vessels to pass through the cervical vertebra.

Forceps Forceps—Instrument used to help remove baby from the birth canal during delivery.

Forceps major Fibers of the splenium of the corpus callosum which extend laterally and posteriorly into the occipital lobe interconnecting comparable cortical regions.

F. Minor: Fibers of the genu of the corpus callosum that extend laterally and anteriorly interconnecting comparable regions of the frontal lobe.

Foregut Pertaining to that part of the GI tract from the mouth to the duodenum.

Forfeiture State imposed fine for nursing home noncompliance with State licensure statutes or regulations .

Form constancy The ability to recognize two objects that have the same shape but different size or position. This ability is needed to tell the difference between "b" and "d", "p" and "q", "m" and "w".

Formaldehyde A colorless, highly irritating, pungent compound used in the pharmaceutical and cosmetic industries as an antimicrobial agent.

Format To magnetically prepare a disk to receive data. A diskette or hard disk must be formatted before it can be used. Formatting a diskette erases all data previously stored on it. MS-DOS and Windows format disks differently than does the Macintosh System, therefore you can rarely use a disk formatted for a Mac in a PC. Most disks can be purchased pre-formatted, so that you do not have to format them.

Fornix Efferent fiber tract that arises from the hippocampus, arches forward over the thalamus, then courses downward to terminate mainly in the mammillary body of the hypothalamus.

Forward flow test An objective and quantitative method of determining filter integrity. A test in which the filter is wetted and a predetermined constant air pressure is applied. A measurement of pure diffusional airflow through the wetted membrane is made. If the diffusional airflow across the membrane is below the maximum allowable value given, then the filter is acceptable.

Fossa A depression (ie. posterior cranial fossa).

Fouling Occurs when gelatinous coatings, colloidal masses, or dense bacterial growth form a compacted crust on membrane or filter surfaces which blocks further flow.

Fourth ventricle The cavity in the rhombencephalon located between the medulla oblongata, the pons, and the isthmus ventrally and anterior and the cerebellum dorsally and posterior.

Fovea Center of the retina that can produce the sharpest eyesight and contains the most cones. .

Fovea capitus The depression where the ligamentum teres attaches to the head of the femur, containing the vascular supply for the intracapsular portion of the femur (head and proximal neck).

Frank breech Frank breech—Baby presenting buttocks first. Legs are flexed and knees extended.

Fraternal twins Fraternal twins-Twins derived from two different eggs. Often called fraternal twins.

Free Radicals Free radicals are highly reactive molecules in the body which can destroy tissues by oxidizing cell membrane lipids and damaging DNA, the body's genetic material. Free redicals are produced through the body's normal process of metabolizing the air we breath and the food we eat, as well as exposure to tabacco smoke, excess sunlight and environmental pollutants. Antioxidants work in the body by neutralizing free radicals before the can do significant harm.

Freeware A method of software distribution where a programmer creates a program and makes it available for free.

Friable Breaks apart or crumbles easily.

Frontal horn The extension of the lateral ventricle into the frontal lobe of the brain.

Frontal lobe The portion of the anterior cerebral hemisphere from the frontal pole to the sulcus centralis (central sulcus).

Frontal sinus A paired paranasal sinus within the frontal bone that is connected to the middle meatus of the nasal cavity by the nasofrontal duct. Both functionally, and embryologically, the frontal sinus represents the most anterior ethmoid air cell.

Fume hoods Units that collect fumes from chemicals, solvents, acids, and other hazardous materials. Hoods may include HEPA filters if powders are present, or carbon filters to filter fumes from the work surface and return cleaned air to the room. Most fume hoods are 100% exhausted to outdoors. A glass, Plexiglas or acrylic front panel may be included for worker safety.

Function Keys A set of programmable keys on a keyboard (typically across the top of the keyboard),labeled F1 through F12, that perform different tasks, determined by the various software programs.

Functional description A written description of what a system is to do with sequence of operation relating activities to Critical Parameters (Why the system does what it does for GMP reasons). A non-GMP system should also have a functional specification to aid designers and software development.

Functional gene tests Biochemical assays for a specific protein, which indicates that a specific gene is not merely present but active.

Functionality Suitability for the intended purpose.

Fundus The top of the uterus. This is the landmark used by practitioners when they are measuring the size of the uterus during pregnancy. The measuring starts at the pubic bone and ends at the fundus. On average, the number of weeks of pregnancy matches the number of cm from the pubic bone to the fundus, give or take a few cm.

Fundus of stomach The portion of the stomach that lies above and to the left of the entrance of the esophagus.

Fungi Plural of fungus. Low forms of plant life unable to form protein and carbohydrates (heterotrophs) that are widespread in nature. Fungal cells are larger than bacterial cells, and their typical internal structures, such as nucleus and vacuoles, can be seen easily with a light microscope. On the basis of their mode of sexual reproduction, fungi are grouped in four classes. Phycomycetes, Ascomycetes, Deuteromycetes (Fungi Imperfectii), and Basidiomycetes. Two major groups of fungi are the yeasts and molds.

Fungicide An agent that destroys fungi.

Funiculus Refers to three broad columns of white matter within the spinal cord that contain several different ascending and descending tracts or fasciculi.

F. (Dorsal): Column of white matter located between the dorsal roots and dorsal median septum of the spinal cord.

F. (Lateral): Spinal cord white matter located between the emerging dorsal and ventral roots.

F. (Ventral): Column of spinal cord white matter located between the emerging ventral roots and ventral median fissure.

Fusiform Descriptive term applied to structures that taper at both ends (ie. muscle spindle).

Fusion The union of images from each eye into a single image. There are three degrees of fusion. 1st degree fusion is the superimposition of two dissimilar targets. 2nd degree fusion is flat fusion with a two-dimensional target. 3rd degree fusion is depth perception (stereopsis) with a three-dimensional target.

Fusion test Determines the eyes ability to unite the images from each eye into a single image.

Fusion welding Welding in which the base material is fused together without the addition of filler material to the weld.

Fusional vergence A convergence response which serves to maintain (fusion) the union of images from each eye into a single image. The eyes will turn with a slow smooth tonic movement or a fast jumping movement called phasic.

G

Gait How a person walks.

Galactocele A cyst in the breast caused by obstruction of the ductal system with debris. The cyst is usually small, filled with milk and occurs after the cessation of lactation. May result in breast abscess or infection if left untreated.

Gall bladder The reservoir for bile located between the right and quadrate lobe on the posteroinferior surface of the liver.

Gamete Mature male or female reproductive cell (sperm or ovum) with a haploid set of chromosomes (23 for humans).

Gamma Butyrolactone (GBL) A related product to GHB (Gamma hydroxybutyrate).

Gamma globulin A blood protein that plays a major role in the process of immunity. Sometimes the term "gamma globulin" refers to a whole group of blood proteins that are known as antibodies or immunoglobulins (Ig). Most often, however, it applies to a particular immunoglobulin, designated as IgG, believed to be the most abundant type of antibody in the body.

Gamma Hydroxybutyrate (GHB) GHB is a simple carbohydrate fond naturally in every cell of the human body. GHB is both a metabolite of and a precursor to an amino acid called GABA (Gamma Aminobutyric Acid). The FDA has labeled GHB has a 'date-rape' drug, and wants to ban it from the market. GHB itself does not cause a person to remain conscious, engage in sex and then forget what they did. The problems occur when you take GHB with high levels of alcohol, since both alcohol and GHB are metabolized by the same enzyme in the body.

Ganglion A collection of nerve cell bodies located outside the central nervous system serving a common function, either sensory or autonomic.

Gangrene Death of tissue caused by infection and/or lack of circulation.

Garcinia Cambogia Fruit from India that contains Hydroxicitric Acid (-HCA), an organic acid influencing carbohydrate and fat metabolism.

Garlic Can be called the 'Stinking Rose'. Studies show that garlic may lower blood cholesterol levels, lower elevated blood pressure and offer a hedge against the onset of several types of cancer. Some studies show that garlic has enhanced fat breakdown coupled with an increasd amount of brown adipose tissue (BAT), a type of specialized fat that is known to convert fat calories into heat, thereby disspating excess calories.

Gas Air that collects in the stomach and intestines as a natural result of digesting food. Passed out of the body via the rectum or the mouth.

Gas metal arc welding (GMAW) An arc welding process that produces coalescence of metals by heating them with an arc between a continuous filler metal (consumable) electrode and the work. Shielding is obtained entirely from an externally supplied gas or gas mixture. Some variations of this process are called MIG (metal inert gas) Or CO2 welding, nonpreferred terms.

Gas room A separately ventilated, fully enclosed room in which only toxic and highly toxic compressed gases and associated equipment and supplies are stored or used.

Gas tungsten arc welding (GTAW) An arc welding process that produces coalescence of metals by heating them with an arc between a tungsten (nonconsumable) electrode and the work. Shielding is obtained from a gas or gas mixture. Pressure may or may not be used and filler material may or may not be used. (This process is sometimes called TIG (Tungsten Inert Gas) welding, a nonpreferred term).

Gastric Related to the stomach.

Gastritis Inflammation of the lining of the stomach.

Gastroduodenal artery The artery which originates from the common hepatic artery and branches into the supraduodenal and posterior superior pancreaticoduodenal arteries.

Gastroenteritis Irritation or infection of the stomach and intestines. May be caused by bacteria or parasites, irritating food, stress, or emotional upset.

Gastroenterologist Medical specialist for diseases of the gastrointestinal tract.

Gastroenterology Medical specialty that deals with the digestive system.

Gastroesophageal junction The point where the stratified squamous epithilium of the esophagus meets the simple columnar epithilium of the cardia of the stomach. The GE junction may be above the diaphragm when there is a hiatal hernia. In turn, hiatal hernia may be associated with GERD (Gastroesophageal Reflux Disease).

Gastroesophageal reflux disease (GERD) Movement of food, fluids, and digestive juices from the stomach back up into the esophagus; causes irritation of the esophagus with acid, resulting in discomfort. GERD occurs when the muscle between the stomach and the esophagus, known as the lower esophageal sphincter, opens when it should stay closed, or is weak.

Gastrointestinal Relating to the digestive tract.

Gastrointestinal tract (Also called the digestive tract.) The parts of the body that break down food into small particles, allowing nutrients from food to be used for energy and growth: the mouth, esophagus, stomach, pancreas, liver, gallbladder, small intestine, and large intestine.

Gastroparesis Muscle or nerve damage in the stomach, which causes slow digestion and stomach emptying.

Gastrostomy A surgically created opening in the stomach and the abdominal muscles. A tube is passed through these openings, into the stomach, to allow for feeding of a person who cannot eat normally.

Gel A colloid, where the dispersed phase is liquid and the dispersion medium is solid.

Gel electrophoresis A DNA separation technique that is very important in DNA sequencing. Standard sequencing procedures involve cloning DNA fragments into special sequencing cloning vectors that carry tiny pieces of DNA. The next step is to determine the base sequence of the tiny fragments by a special procedure that generates a series of even tinier DNA fragments that differ in size by only one base. These nested fragments are separated by gel electrophoresis, in which the DNA pieces are added to a gelatinous solution, allowing the fragments to work their way down through the gel. Smaller pieces move faster and will reach the bottom first. Movement through the gel is hastened by applying an electrical field to the gel.

Gel polarization The phenomenon of formation of a layer of insoluble/semi-soluble material at a liquid/filter interface. It is a common occurrence with excessive linear velocity flow through filters of colloidal suspensions and macromolecular solutions.

Gelatin A derived protein formed from the collagen of the tissues by boiling in water, sometimes called an albuminoid, though it lacks the characteristic albuminoid properties. Glue, size, and isinglass are forms of gelatin.

Gene A natural unit of hereditary material that is the physical basis for the transmission of the characteristics of living organisms from one generation to another. The basic genetic material is fundamentally the same in all living organisms. It consists of deoxyribonucleic acid (DNA) in most organisms and ribonucleic acid (RNA) in certain viruses, and is usually associated in a linear arrangement that, in part, constitutes the chromosome. The average length of a gene is 1μm and thus, about one million genes could be contained in a one-meter stretch of DNA. The segment of DNA that is involved in producing a polypeptide chain, it includes regions preceding (leader) and following (trailer) the coding region as well as intervening sequences (introns) between individual coding segments (exons).

Gene amplification Increase in the normal copy number of a gene.

Gene expression The process by which a gene's coded information is converted into the structures present and operating in the cell. Expressed genes include those that are transcribed into mRNA and then translated into protein and those that are transcribed into RNA but not translated into protein

Gene family Group of closely related genes that makes similar products.

Gene mapping Determination of the relative positions of genes on a DNA molecule (chromosome or plasmid) and of the distance, in linkage units or physical units, between them.

Gene markers Landmarks for a target gene, either detectable traits that are inherited along with the gene, or distinctive segments of DNA.

Gene product The biochemical material, either RNA or protein, resulting from expression of a gene. The amount of gene product is used to measure how active a gene is; abnormal amounts can be correlated with disease causing alleles.

Gene sequencing The determination of the sequence of bases in a DNA strand. The two most widely used methods are the chain-termination method, developed by Sanger in the mid-seventies, and the chemical method developed by Maxam & Gilbert around the same time.

Gene splicing The enzymatic attachment of one gene or part of a gene to another.

Gene therapy The insertion of normal DNA directly into cells to correct a generic defect.

General binocular vision disorder Inability to efficiently utilize and/or sustain binocular vision. Symptoms include eyestrain, headaches, decreased comprehension, inability to concentrate while reading, excessive tearing, and blurred vision. A patient will have difficulty with both base-in and base-out prisms. Vision therapy is an effective treatment option.

General Class The most common class of registration for RNs and RPNs.

Generic drug A drug produced and marketed under its chemical or "generic" name (e.g. acetaminophen) as opposed to "Tylenol", a brand name for the former produced by Johnson & Johnson. A generic drug can be sold only after a proprietary drug goes off patent (i.e. when the patent runs out after 17 years). There are numerous generic drug manufacturers. While generic drugs are cheaper for consumers, they still must meet the standards of GMPs as set out by the FDA.

Genesis (suffix) Origin. e.g. spermatogenesis - formation of sperm.

Genetic code The sequence of nucleotides, coded in triplets (codons) along the mRNA that determines the sequence of amino acids in protein synthesis. The DNA sequence of a gene can be used to predict the mRNA sequence, and the genetic code can in turn be used to predict the amino acid sequence.

Genetic counseling Genetic counseling-Consultation between a couple and a specialist about genetic defects and the possibility of genetic problems in a pregnancy.

Genetic diseases Diseases that occur because a mutation in the genetic material.

Genetic engineering The selective, deliberate alteration of genes by technological means.

Genetics The scientific study of heredity: how particular qualities or traits are transmitted from parents to offspring.

Genistein A compound thought to protect you against cancer. It is found in soy based food products. It surpresses the production of stress proteins in cells, proteins that otherwise help cancer cells survive destruction by the immune system.

Genital herpes simplex BILATERAL—Herpes simplex infection involving the genital area. It can be significant during pregnancy because of the danger to a newborn fetus infected with herpes simplex.

Genitourinary problems Genitourinary problems—Defects or problems involving genital organs and the bladder or kidneys.

Genome project Research and technology development effort aimed at mapping and sequencing some or all of the genome human beings and other organisms.

Genomic library A collection of clones made from a set of randomly generated overlapping DNA fragments representing the entire genome of an organism.

Genomic sequence The order of the subunits, called bases, that makes up a particular fragment of DNA in a genome. DNA is a long molecule made up of four different kinds of bases, which are abbreviated A, C, T, and G. A DNA fragment that is 10 bases long might have a base sequence of, for example, ATCGTTCCTG. The particular sequence of bases encodes important information in an individual's genetic blueprint, and is unique for each individual (except identical twins).

Genotype The genetic composition of an organism. In karyotyping, the genotype is designated 46, XX for normal females and 46, XY for normal males. (46 refers to the total number of chromosomes: one pair of each chromosome numbers 1 through 22 plus a pair of sex chromosomes, X and Y).

Genu Refers to a number of different angled or bent structures within the nervous system resembling the knee.

G. of the Corpus Callosum: Anterior part of corpus callosum continuous with the rostrum below and the body posteriorly.

G. of the Facial Nerve(Internal): Loop of facial nerve fibers over the rostral pole of the abducent nucleus within the floor of the 4th ventricle. The elevation left by these structures on the floor of the ventricle is referred to as the faci al colliculus.

G. of the Facial Nerve (External) Abrupt bend of the facial nerve within the facial canal of the petrous temporal bone.

G. of the Internal Capsule: The point of junction between the anterior and posterior limbs of the internal capsule.

GERD Gastroesophageal reflux disease.

Germ layers Germ layers—layers or areas of tissue important in the development of the baby.

Germicidal lamps Light sources that emit ultraviolet radiation at a wavelength of 254 nanometers. These lights are commonly found in biological safety cabinets and used to inactivate bacteria, viruses and fungi which are either airborne or on exposed surfaces.

Germicide An agent that destroys microorganisms, especially pathogenic microorganisms ("germs"). Sterilants, disinfectants, and antiseptics are germicides.

Germplasm The total genetic variability, represented by germ cells or seeds, available to a particular population of organisms.

Gestational age Gestational age—Dating a pregnancy from the first day of the last menstrual period; 2 weeks longer than fertilization age.

Gestational diabetes Gestational diabetes—Occurrence or worsening of diabetes during pregnancy (gestation).

Gestational trophoblastic disease Gestational trophoblastic disease (GTN)—Abnormal pregnancy with cystic growth of the placenta. Characterized by bleeding during early and middle pregnancy.

Giardia lamblia A parasite found in spoiled food or unclean water that can cause diarrhea.

Gigabyte or GB A unit of data measurement equal to approximately one billion bytes. Hard drive manufacturers use an even number as a multiplier. In this case 1 GB would be 1,000,000,000 Bytes.

Ginkgo Biloba A herb shown to enhance mental accuity. Some research has shown that Ginkgo Biloba increases cerebral blood flow to the brain. Also, boost brain levels of adenosine triphosphate and scavenge free radicals. Combined with ginger, gingko has also been shown too reduce stress induced anxiety.

Ginseng A family of herbs with adaptogenic properties affecting energy. There are different ginsengs (Asian, American, Siberian). Some ginsengs have shown to have mental enhancing effects. Studies show that an individual ginseng component called ginsenoside Rb acts favorably in reversing memory deficits by increasing he secretion of acetychilone. Studies also suggest that ginseng extract improved learning and retention processes.

Glandulars Freeze-dried animal glands, processed into pill form and taken to provide the body an extra dose of a hormone. Typically made from cow, sheep, or pig glands, glandulars on the market include adrenal, testicular, ovary, pancreas, pituitary, prostate, and thymus products. Critics point out that these supplements are unlikely to boost gland function because digestion breaks down and inactivates the DNA in a glandular. In addition, using glandulars may encourage your own glands to reduce hormone production. Other risks include bacterial contamination of the product, and the antibiotics and pesticides present in the glands of the livestock they are taken from.

Glenoid fossa The a shallow "cup" on the lateral edge of the scapula that is the point of articulation between with the head of the humerus.

Glia Synonymous with Neuroglia.

Glitch A slang term for an unexpected problem, found in either the software or hardware, which usually does not occur in a regular pattern.

Global minimum essential (core) requirements Specification of the competencies related to knowledge, skills, professional attitudes and ethical values which students should possess at graduation, regardless of where they are trained. In medical education, this is represented as a three-tiered structure with international, national, and local layers, which reflects the competencies specific to given settings and cultures where the physician will practice in addition to universal competencies required by physicians throughout the world.

Global rating of live or recorded performance forms Ratings by faculty supervisors to assess trainees' medical knowledge, interpersonal and communication skills and patient care clinical skills which are completed retrospectively and are based on general impressions collected over a period of time. They are derived from multiple sources of information such as direct observations or interactions, input from other faculty, residents or patients; review of work products or written materials. They differ from other rating forms in that a rater judges general categories of ability and skills rather than specific skills, tasks or behaviors. The rating forms contain scales used by the evaluator to judge knowledge, skills, and behaviors listed on the form. Scoring these forms entails combining numeric ratings with comments to obtain a useful judgment about performance based upon more than one rater. Reproducibility appears easier to achieve for ratings of knowledge and more difficult to achieve for patient care and interpersonal and communication skills. To improve reproducibility, the rater should be well trained; otherwise the scores can be highly subjective and competencies may be rated similarly regardless of performance.

Globe The eyeball.

Globose nucleus Several small cell groups embedded in the white matter of the cerebellum medial to the emboliform and lateral to the fastigial nucleus.

Globus pallidus Component of the lenticular nucleus situated between the putamen and the internal capsule. The principal efferent nucleus of the corpus striatum. Also known as the paleostriatum.

Glossoepiglottic fold The folds of mucous memrane located between the tongue and epiglottis.

Glottis A synonym for the vocal cords.

Glucomannan A fiber derived from the Amorphophallus Konjac root, a perennial plant of the Araceae family. The root is low in protein, lipids (fats), calories and vitamins, but, because of its glucomannan content, it can provide many tangible bodybuilding and health advantages. Glucomannan can help mitigate insulin response to high glycemic corbohydrates, which might allow bodybuilders to add variety to low carb diets and still accrue the benefits of the regimens. Glucomannan may also help remove fat from the body.

Glucosamine Organic compound found in cartilage and joint fluid; relieves joint pain and may help in healing some joint injuries. Glucosamine is a provider of the building blocks of joints.

Glucosamine sulfate A natural amino sugar found in joint spaces. As a dietary supplement, it is said to stimulate the repair of arthritic joints by building up the protective cartilage that arthritis destroys.

Glucose (monosaccharide) Type of sugar that circulates in the bloodstream, thus the term 'blood glucose levels' or 'blood sugar'. All carbohydrates, whether simple or complex, are eventually converted to glucose in the body. Glycogen is many units of glucose together.

Glucose Tolerance Factor (GTF) GTF is thought to be a complex of chromium, nicotinic acid, and the amino acids glycine, cystein and glutamic acid (these aminos are components of gluthathione). GTF is thought to be synthesize by the liver. In many people, chromium is likely the deficient substrate for GTF formation. GTF is found in foods such as organ meats, whole gains, cheese, mushrooms and brewer's yeast.

Glucose tolerance test Glucose-tolerance test—Blood test done to evaluate the body's response to sugar. Blood is drawn at intervals following ingestion of a sugary substance. This test is often routinely given during pregnancy.

Glucosuria Glucosuria—Glucose in the urine. This is often tested for during prenatal visits and may lead to a glucose tolderance test to make you that you are not diabetic.

Glutamine An amino acid. Glutamine is the most abundant amino acid in muscle tissue. Studies are beginning to show that having extra glutamine in your body may be important to maximize muscle growth, by increasing growth hormone levels. Glutamine also is important to maintain proper health, and is shown to have anabolic and anticatabolic properties. During intense training, the signal for muscle breakdown (which is a bad thing) may be the release of skeletal muscle glutamine. That means that each time you train, your muscles release glutamine which in part triggers a catabolic state (a catabolic state is synonymous with muscle breakdown). By proving Glutamine, documented clinical studies have shown that Glutamine will have a significant impact on maintaining a positive nitrogen balance which is essential to muscular development and recovery.

Gluten A protein in grains such as wheat, oats, rye, and barley.

Gluteus maximus Muscle originating form the lateral surface of the ilium, dorsal surface of the sacrum and coccyx, and the sacrotuberus ligament, and inserting into the iliotibial tract of the facia lata, and the gluteal tuberosity of femur. It is responsible for the extension. abduction, and lateral rotation of the thigh.

Gluteus medius Muscle originating between the anterior and posterior gluteal lines at the lateral surface of the ilium, and inserting at the greater trochanter of the femur. It is responsible for abduction of the thigh.

Gluteus minimus Muscle originating between the anterior and posterior gluteal lines at the lateral surface of the ilium, and inserting at the greater trochanter of the femur. It is responsible for the abduction and medial rotation of the thigh.

Glycemic Index The glycemic Index (GI) measures only the rise in blood sugar elicited by various foods and drinks. It is not like an index of factors like nutrient density or vitamin or fiber content. The GI can help you if you want to avoid a spike in blood sugar, and insulin. If measures how much a food affects your blood sugar.

Glycerin Glycerin is a trihydric alcohol that is derived from animal fats and plants emollients. It is used in many protein bars to give the bar a soft texture and to make it easy to chew. Glycerin yields 4.32 calories per gram. Glycerin is a crystalline, viscous liquid formed when fat molecules split. It is half as sweet as sugar and is used to keep bars moist and to plasticize other foods such as fudge, gum, geltin, etc. The big question is if glycerin is a carb or is it a new 'category'. The reason that glycerin is not listed as a carbohydrate by some manufacturers is that glycerin does not effect blood glucose or insulin levels. However, the FDA states that glycerin is to be listed as a carbohydrate; thus the controversy.

Glycogen (Liver) Liver glycogen is a fuel reserve that helps maintain blood glucose levels. This is important because the brain relies on a constant supply of glucose to function properly.

Glycogen (Muscle) Muscle glycogen is extremely important for bodybuilding, since it's the primary fuel that powers anaerobic training, such as lifting weights. Glycogen that's stored in a muscle is available only to that muscle because muscles lack a certain enzyme, glucose-6-phosphatase, that's needed to release glucose into the blood. Muscles can absorb glucose without insulin, which why exercise helps prevent diabetes.

Glycogen It is a term for many units of glucose strung together. The body stores glycogen in two areas, the liver and the muscles. Only about 5 grams, or 20 calories worth of glucose flows in the blood. Liver stores about 75 to 100 grams, or 300 to 400 calories; an hour of aerobics can burn up half the liver glycogen content. The muscles store around 360 grams, or 1,440 calories. Carbohydrate loading is one technique used to increase muscle glycogen content. By not consuming enough carbohydrates, you deplete both liver and muscle glycogen reserves. While complex carbs are considered to be more desirable than simple carbs, simple carbs are more efficient after a workout for replacing muscle glycogen. Simple carbs are absorbed faster, and promote a greater insulin output. A carbohydrate drink with at least 50 grams of carb will do the trick.

GMP critical parameter A parameter that has a direct effect on product quality.

GMP facility A production facility or clinical trial materials pilot plant for the manufacture of pharmaceutical products. It includes the manufacturing space, the storage warehouse for raw and finished product, and support lab areas.

Goal A general aim, object or end-effect which one strives to achieve.

Golgi bodies Very small particles composed of membrane aggregates and responsible for the secretion of certain enzymes and macromolecules. Golgi bodies are the deposition and packaging site for many excreted products.

Gonorrhea Gonorrhea-Contagious venereal infection, transmitted primarily by intercourse. Caused by the bacteria Neisseria gonorrhea.

Good engineering practice (GEP) A combination of standards, specifications, codes, regulatory and industrial guidelines as well as accepted engineering and design methods intended to design, construct, operate, and maintain pharmaceutical and/ or biotechnology facilities taking into account not only regulatory compliance but also safety, economics, environmental protection and operability. Standards and specifications are provided by recognized sources such as established engineering and architectural contractors as well as pharmaceutical companies. Guidelines are issued by professional societies, industrial organizations, or regulatory agencies. Engineering design methods have been established throughout the engineering educational system.

Good large scale practice organism (GLSP) The National Institutes of Health (NIH) specifies physical containment levels and defines Biosafety Levels for Large Scale in their "Guidelines for Research Involving Recombinant DNA Molecules" - Appendix K - May 1999. Level of physical containment recommended for large-scale (more than 10 liters of culture) research or production involving viable, non-pathogenic, and non-toxigenic recombinant strains derived from host organisms that have an extended history of safe large scale use. Likewise, the GLSP level of physical containment is recommended for organisms that have a built-in environmental limitation that permits optimum growth in large-scale bioreactors, but limited survival if released to the environment.

Gracilis Muscle that originates at the inferior ramus of the pubis, and inserts into the medial surface of the tibial shaft. It is responsible for adduction of the thigh and flexion of the knee.

Graduate medical education (GME) In the United States, this term typically refers to residency training and fellowships; the education physicians receive after finishing medical school. In many other countries it is called specialty training or postgraduate education.

Graduate training or internship The phase of acquiring widening clinical experience through the practice of basic clinical skills and judgment. This is normally used to designate the period of hospital clerkship. The periods of undergraduate education and graduate training together comprise the doctor's basic medical education.

Grand mal seizure Grand mal seizure—loss of control of body functions. Seizure activity of a major form.

Granuloma A focal collection of activated macrophages.

Granulomatous Composed of granulomas.

Grape Seed Extract Source of proantho-cyanadins, an important antioxidant.

Graphical User Interface (GUI) The name given to an operating system or operating environment that uses pictural representations (icons) and menus, with a pointing device concept to execute commands and other tasks, rather than requiring the user to type commands. The Macintosh operating system and Microsoft Windows are examples.

Gravid Pregnant.

Gravida The number of live children you have borne. An example would be Para 4 Gravida 3 if you're pregnant for the fourth time and have three living children.

Greater curvature (stomach) The lateral and inferior border of the stomach.

Greater trochanter (femur) Process on the lateral surface of the proximal femur, the point of attachment for the gluteus medius and minimus.

Greater tuberosity (humerus) Prominence on the lateral surface of the proximal humerus. Point of attachment for the infraspinatus, supraspinatus, and teres minor muscles.

Greater wing of sphenoid Winged-shaped process of the sphenoid bone that helps form the floor and lateral walls of the middle cranial fossa and the lateral wall of the orbit.

Green Tea Perhaps more notable, recent research has shown that green tea reduces the risk of developing stomach cancer by 50% and esophageal cancer by 6-%. No one knows for sure, but scientists think that polyphenols in green tea protect health by combating free radicals.

The main constituents of green tea are polyphenols, caffeien, vitamins, minerals, amino acids and other nitrogenous compounds, it also contains small amounts of carbohydrates and lipids. Also, green tea contains polyphenols, theanine, and catechins. The greater the theanine content in green tea, the higher the price.

Grey matter The grey nervous tissue of the brain and spinal cord consisting of the cell bodies and dendrites of nerve cells rather than the myelinated axons.

Group-B streptococcal infection Group-B streptococcal infection—Serious infection occurring in the mother's vagina and throat.

Growth Hormone Known in the medical community as somatotropin. It is a powerful anabolic hormone that affects all systems of the body and plays an important role in muscle growth. It is a peptite hormone, which is composed of many amino acids (191 of them) linked together. It is rapidly metabolized by the liver and has a half-life in the blood of approxiamately 17 to 45 minutes. Because of this, detecting GH in a drug screen is very hard.

Grumose Lumpy or clotted.

GTN Gestational trophoblastic disease (GTN)—Abnormal pregnancy with cystic growth of the placenta. Characterized by bleeding during early and middle pregnancy.

Guarana Source of caffeine. Comes from the seed of a herb found in the Amazon, long popular among Brazilians for its stimulatory effects.

Guardian Legal representative, appointed by a court, to make decisions for a person not competent to make their own decisions. Generally resident (patient) guardians have all of the legal rights normally granted to competent residents (patients).

Guardianship Court-appointed person designated to act for someone who has been declared incompetent. The guardian may or may not be a family member.

Guggulsterone Guggulsterone is a ketosteroid specifically called Z-Guggulsterone. It's effect on the thyroid is that it increases the metabolic rate via stimulation of the tyroid gland. Studies indicate that Guggulsterone can result in higher levels of T4 (Thyroxine), one of the two main thyroid hormones.

Guidelines A set of steps to be taken in performing a task or implementing a policy, program or activities and the manner of doing so. Guidelines are more specific and more detailed than guiding principles, on which they are based.

Gyri Gyri—Prominent, rounded elevation found on the surface of the brain tissue.

Gyrus The convolutions on the surface of the cerebral hemispheres separated by sulci or fissures.

H

H2 blockers Medications used to treat gastroesophageal reflux disease (GERD) that decrease the amount of acid made by the stomach. The stomach lining has sites that react to a chemical normally found in the body called histamine. When histamine attaches to these sites, the stomach produces acid that aids in digestion of food. H2 blockers prevent the stomach from reacting to histamine, thereby decreasing stomach acid.

Habenular nuclei Nuclei (medial and lateral) underlying the habenular trigone and part of the epithalamus. They receive afferents from the preoptic, anterior thalamic, and septal areas via the stria medullares and sen d fibers to the brain stem interpeduncular, raphe nuclei and reticular formation.

H. Trigone: Small eminences on the dorsomedial aspect of the posterior thalamus lateral to the stalk of the pineal body formed by the habenular nuclei.

H. Commissure: Small commissural band of transverse fibers located above the stalk of the pineal body connecting the two habenular areas accross the midline.

Habit Training A behavioral technique that calls for scheduled toileting at regular intervals on a planned basis. Unlike bladder training, there is no systematic effort to motivate the patient to delay voiding and resist urge.

Habitual Aborter A woman with several unexplained spontaneous miscarriages.

Habitual abortion Habitual abortion—Occurrence of three or more spontaneous miscarriages.

HACC Home and Community Care The HACC Program is a cost-shared program between the Commonwealth and State and Territory governments. The program provides funding for a range of services which support people who are at risk of inappropriate admission to long term residential care. The Program also supports their carers. The type of services funded through the HACC Program include, but are not limited to nursing care; allied health care; meals and other food services; domestic assistance; personal care; home modification and maintenance; transport; respite care; counselling, support, information and advocacy; and assessment.

Hairpin A double helical region formed by base pairing between adjacent (inverted) complementary sequences in a single strand of RNA or DNA.

Haloenzyme An enzyme that contains a non-protein component.

Halogen One of the chlorine group (bromine, chlorine, fluorine, iodine) of elements, all univalent; they form monobasic acids with hydrogen, and their hydroxides (fluorine forms none) are monobasic acids. The radioactive element, astatine, also belongs to the halogen group.

Halophile An organism that displays accelerated growth or is dependent on high salt concentrations.

Handshake Requires the recipient of an electronic data record to acknowledge to the sender that the record has been received.

Hands On Assistance When a person always requires the physical assistance of another person to perform one or more Activities of Daily Living (ADLs), generally because they are physically unable to perform that activity.

Handwritten signature The scripted name or legal mark of an individual handwritten by that individual and executed or adopted with the present intention to authenticate a writing in a permanent form. The act of signing with a writing or marking instrument such as a pen or stylus is preserved. The scripted name or legal mark, while conventionally applied to paper, may also be applied to other devices that capture the name or mark.

Haploid A single set of chromosomes (half the full set of genetic material), present in the egg and sperm cells of animals and in the egg and pollen cells of plants. Human beings have 23 chromosomes in their reproductive cells.

Hard Copy Refers to a document printed on paper, rather than saved in "soft" form on a disk or displayed on a screen.

Hard Disk Commonly refers to a form of magnetic media that uses a hard metal disk to store data. Unlike its "floppy" counterparts, a hard disk can typically hold much more data and is much faster, but is non-removable, or "fixed" to your computer. This is typically where the computer's operating system and other software is installed. The terms "hard disk" and "hard drive" are often used interchangeably since the disk and the drive are usually contained in the same unit.

Hard Drive or Hard Disk Drive A device used to read data from a hard disk.

Hard palate The anterior (bone) portion of the horizontal partition separating the nasal cavity (above) from the oral cavity (below). The posterior half of the partition is the "soft palate".

Hardness Concentration of calcium and magnesium salts in water. Hardness originally referred to the soap-consuming power of water; as such it is sometimes also taken to include iron and manganese. "Permanent hardness" also known as "noncarbonated hardness " is the excess of hardness over alkalinity. "Temporary hardness" also known as "carbonated hardness" is equal or less than the alkalinity. Permanent hardness can cause boiler or pipe scale and failure of reverse osmosis membranes.

Hardware The physical devices that comprise a computer system.

Harm Negative effect that has occurred to a resident (patient), infringement of a 'resident's (patient's) rights, or compromising of a 'resident's (patient's) ability to meet their highest practicable level of physical, mental, or psychosocial well being.

Harvesting The separation of cells from growth media. It can be accomplished by filtration, precipitation, or centrifugation.

Haustra The indentations of mucosa in the wall of the colon - between the teniae coli - that create segments or sacculations of the colon.

Hazardous chemical reaction A reaction which generates pressure or byproducts which could cause injury, illness or harm to humans, domestic animals, livestock or wildlife.

Hazardous substance A substance which by reason of being explosive, flammable, toxic, poisonous, corrosive, oxidizing, irritant or otherwise harmful, is likely to cause injury.

Haze The abnormal appearance of a localized diminishing in brightness or luster of a surface when compared to the adjacent surfaces.

HCG Human chorionic gonadatropin (HCG)- Hormone produced in early pregnancy. Measured in a pregnancy test.

hCG levels The amount of pregnancy hormone in a woman's body. A level of 5 is considered "pregnant," although a home pregnancy test will require a level of 50-80 to be positive.

HDL High Density Lipoprotein Cholesterol. Protects against cardiovascular disease. HDLs help to shuttle cholesterol out of the blood and back to the liver, where it's degraded into bile that then can be excreted from the body.

Head of rib The posterior end of a rib, that articulates with the body of the vertebrae.

Healing touch Is practiced by registered nurses and others to accelerate wound healing, relieve pain, promote relaxation, prevent illness and ease the dying process. The practitioner uses light touch or works with his or her hands near the client's body in an effort to restore balance to the client's energy system.

Health In accordance with the Constitution of the World Health Organization (1948), health is "a state of complete physical, mental and social well-being and not merely the absence of disease or infirmity". Health is defined here as a positive concept, emphasizing social and personal resources as well as physical capabilities.

Health care Services provided to individuals or communities by a health care system or by professionals to promote, maintain, monitor, or restore health. Health care contains a broad spectrum of services and activities delivered by a team of health personnel. This contrasts with medical care, which concentrates on diagnostic and therapeutic actions performed by or under the supervision of an individual physician.

Health economics A discipline which concentrates on application of the principles and rules of economics in the sphere of health. In broad terms, it includes analysis and evaluation of health policy and the health system from an economic perspective. In particular, it includes health system planning, market mechanisms, demand for and supply of health care, micro-economic evaluation of individual diagnostic and therapeutic procedures, determinants of health and its valuation, and evaluation of the performance of health care systems in terms of equity and allocative efficiency.

Health hazard Classification of a chemical for which there is statistically significant evidence based on at least one study conducted in accordance with established scientific principles that acute or chronic health effects may occur in exposed persons. The term "health hazard" includes chemicals that are carcinogens, toxic or highly toxic agents, reproductive toxins, irritants, corrosives, sensitizers, hepatotoxins, nephrotoxins, neurotoxins, agents that act on the hematopoietic system, and agents that damage the lungs, skin, eyes or mucous membranes.

Health maintenance organization (HMO) An organization that arranges a wide spectrum of health care services which commonly include hospital care, physicians' services and many other kinds of health care services with an emphasis on preventive care.

Health maintenance services Any health care service or program that helps maintain an individual's good health. This includes all preventive medical practices such as immunizations and periodic examinations, as well as health education and special self-help programs.

Health management Systematic use of the full range of human, technical and financial resources of the health system through planning, organizing, leading and controlling the effort of members to achieve stated goals and to render optimum services at minimum cost. Health managers achieve desired goals by directing and influencing subordinates, and organizing others to perform essential tasks to ensure that the organization is moving towards its goal of improving health.

Health plan A term that has different meanings depending upon the context. "Health plan" can be used to mean an HMO; a "health benefits plan" is provided by an employer to its employees, or services offered by an insurer or third party administrator to employers and/or employees.

Health policy A set of decisions or commitments to pursue courses of action aimed at achieving defined goals of improving health. Policies usually state or imply the values that underpin the policy position. They may also specify the source of funding that can be applied to planning and implementation of policy and to relevant institutions to be involved in this process.

Health promotion The process of enabling individuals to increase control over and improve their health. It involves the population as a whole in the context of their everyday lives, rather than focusing on people at risk for specific diseases, and is directed toward action on the determinants or causes of health.

Health risks appraisal A method of describing an individual's probability of becoming ill or dying from selected causes. Starting from the average risk of death for that individual's age and sex, various lifestyle and physical factors are considered and it is determined whether the individual is at greater or lesser than average risk from the commonest causes of death for their age and sex. Health risk appraisal also indicates the reduction in risk which could be achieved by the individual's altering any of the causal factors (such as cessation of cigarette smoking).

Health services Services performed by health care professionals or by others under their direction for the purpose of promoting, maintaining, or restoring health. In addition to personal health care, health services include health protection, health promotion, and disease prevention.

Health status A general term for the state of health of an individual, group or population that reflects the degree to which a person is able to function physically, emotionally, and socially, with or without aid from the health care system.

Health system A complex of interrelated elements that contribute to health in homes, educational institutions, workplaces, public places, and communities. A health system is usually organized at multiple levels, starting at the most local level, also known as community or primary health care level, and proceeding through the intermediate (district, regional or provincial) to the central level, providing progressively more complex and more specialized care and support.

Healthy behavior The combination of knowledge, practices and attitudes that together contribute to motivate actions we take regarding our own health. Healthy behavior may promote and preserve good health. On the other hand, behaviors harmful to health such as tobacco smoking, alcohol drinking, drug abuse and lack of physical exercise may be determinants of disease.

Heart attack A myocardial infarction (MI). This occurs when an artery that feeds the heart becomes blocked. As a result, blood does not get to some parts of the heart and some of the heart tissue dies. Symptoms may include nausea, shortness of breath and pain in the chest, arm or neck.

Heart block A condition in which the natural pacemaker signals sent out by the S-A node are delayed or fail to reach the ventricles.

Heart rhythm Another term for heartbeat. You may hear your doctor refer to your rhythm as being normal or irregular, meaning there is an abnormality. A normal heart rate typically ranges from 60 to 100 beats per minute at rest.

Heartburn Heartburn-Discomfort or pain that occurs in the chest. Often occurs after eating. A common occurence during pregnancy, especially during the last triemester.

Heat A form of energy associated with the motion of atoms or molecules in solids and capable of being transmitted through solid and fluid media by conduction, through fluid media by convection, and through empty space by radiation. Two important characteristics of heat are:

1. Heat cannot be destroyed, only transferred from on body to another, or converted to another form of energy.
2. Heat always flows from the warmer to the colder substance.

Heat affected zone (HAZ) That portion of the base metal that has not been melted but whose microstructure or mechanical properties have been altered by the heat of welding, brazing, soldering, forming, or cutting.

Heat labile Able to be destroyed or altered by high temperature. Heat labile pharmaceuticals are sterilized by filtration.

Heat number An alphanumeric identification of a stated tonnage of metal obtained from a continuous melting in a foundry furnace.

Heat of vaporization The amount of heat needed to change a unit volume from a liquid to a vapor at a given pressure without a temperature change.

Heavy metals High molecular weight metal ions, such as lead. Known for their interference with many processes, and "poisoning" of catalysts, membranes, and resins.

HeLa cells An established line of human cervical carcinoma cells used to study the biochemistry and genetics of human cell growth.

Helicobacter pylori (H. pylori) Bacteria found in the stomach that can damage the lining of the stomach and upper small intestine, leading to ulcer formation.

Helix A spiral, staircase-like, structure with a repeating pattern described by two simultaneous operations, rotation, and translation. It is the natural conformation of many biological polymers.

Hellerwork A system of somatic education and structural bodywork which is based on the inseparability of body, mind & spirit, making the connection between movement, body alignment and personal awareness. During sessions, the structural balance of the body is realized through the systematic release of muscle and connective tissue to restore the body's optimal natural balance, posture and flexibility. Myofascial release, movement awareness and dialogue are the essence of the sessions enabling one to move more fluidly, and have increased stamina, strength and energy.

Help A program that gives you information about how to run Windows 95 or 98 and its programs, including how to use the Help program. Help programs are also available in most currently released programs.

Hema, hemato, haemo (british) (prefix) Blood. e.g. hematocrit - the volume percentage of erythrocytes in whole blood.

Hemangio (prefix) Blood vessel.

e.g. hemangiosarcoma - malignant tumor of a blood vessel.

Hematin An iron protoporphyrin differing from heme in that the central iron atom is in the ferric (Fe+++) rather than the ferrous (Fe++) state; the prosthetic group of methemoglobin.

Hematocrit Hematocrit-Determines the proportion of blood cells to plasma. Important in diagnosing anemia.

Hematoma A localized collection of extravasated blood, usually clotted.

Hemidiaphragm One side (one "half") of the diaphragm that separates the chest (thorax) from the abdominal cavity.

Hemoglobin The red, respiratory conjugated protein of erythrocytes, consisting of approximately 6 percent heme and 94 percent globin (a protein).

Hemolytic disease Hemolytic disease—Destruction of red blood cells.

Hemophilia A hereditary, plasma-coagulation disorder, principally affecting males but transmitted by females, and characterized by excessive, sometimes spontaneous, bleeding.

Hemopoietic Pertaining to or related to the formation of blood cells.

Hemorrhoidectomy Excision of hemorrhoid.

Hemorrhoids Hemorrhoids—Dilated blood vessels in the rectum or rectal canal. Common during pregnancy.

Hemosiderin A breakdown product of red blood cell pigments.

Hemothorax A collection of blood in the pleural cavity.

HEPA (high efficiency particulate air) filters Filters with a minimum efficiency of 99.97% for 0.3μm particle size as determined by test. The test can be by the monodispersed dioctyl phthalate (DOP) method or other equally sensitive method. When operated at design velocity, larger and smaller particles are captured at higher efficiencies. HEPA filters are made of compressed and bonded micro-fiberglass or Teflon corrugated to produce a high surface area in a small area panel of filter medium. Employed in unidirectional airflow benches, air handlers, and as terminal air supply filters in cleanrooms.

Heparin Heparin is a blood-thinning drug used to treat women suspected of certain immune causes of miscarriage. The drug cannot cross the placenta, so does not affect the baby. It should be discontinued, however, well prior to delivery since it will hamper the mother's ability to clot from labor or surgery.

Hepatic Relating to the liver.

Hepatic artery The artery which originates from the celiac trunk and branches into the right gastric, gastroduodenal, and hepatic proper arteries.

Hepatic flexure A bend in the right/superior large intestine, where the ascending colon becomes the transverse colon.

Hepatic veins Veins which receive blood from the central veins of the liver and flow into the inferior vena cava on the posterior side of the liver.

Hepatitis Inflammation of the liver that sometimes causes permanent damage; caused by viruses, drugs, alcohol, or parasites. Hepatitis has the following forms:

Hepatitis A A form of infectious hepatitis caused by the hepatitis A virus. The virus may be spread by fecal-oral contact, fecal-infected food or water, and may also be spread by a blood-borne infection (which is rare).

Hepatitis B A form of infectious hepatitis caused by the hepatitis B virus. Transmission of the hepatitis B virus occurs through blood and body fluid exposure such as blood, semen, vaginal secretions, or saliva.

Hepatitis C A form of infectious hepatitis caused by the hepatitis C virus. Transmission of the hepatitis C virus occurs primarily from contact with infected blood, but can also occur from sexual contact or from an infected mother to her baby.

Hepatitis D A form of infectious hepatitis caused by the hepatitis (Delta) virus. This form of hepatitis can only occur in the presence of hepatitis B. Transmission of hepatitis D occurs the same way as hepatitis B.

Hepatitis E A form of infectious hepatitis caused by the hepatitis E virus. This form of hepatitis is similar to hepatitis A. Transmission occurs through fecal-oral contamination. Hepatitis E is most common in poorly developed countries and is rarely seen in the US.

Hepatitis G The newest form of infectious hepatitis. Transmission is believed to occur through blood and is seen in IV drug users, individuals with clotting disorders, such as hemophilia, and individuals who require hemodialysis for renal failure.

Hepatotoxin A toxin that is destructive to parenchymal (specific tissue) cells of the liver.

Herbalism Uses natural plants or plant-based substances to treat a range of illnesses and to enhance the functioning of the body's systems. Though herbalism is not a licensed professional modality, herbs are prescribed by a range of practitioners, from holistic M.D.s to acupuncturists to naturopaths.

Hereditary Transmitted from parent to offspring; derived from ancestry.

Heredity Transfer of genetic information from parent cells to progeny.

Hernia A section of intestine or other internal organ that pushes through an opening in an abdominal muscle.

Herniorrhaphy An operation done to repair a hernia.

Hertz A measurement of timing expressed in cycles per second. It measures electrical current, sound pitch, or the clock speed of a computer's CPU.

Hetero (prefix) Dissimilar. e.g. heterocellular - composed of more than one type of cell.

Heterophoria Tendency of the eyes to deviate from their normal position for visual alignment. This condition may be observed when one eye is covered.

Heterotrophs One of two categories in which microorganisms are classified on the basis of their carbon source. Heterotrophs use organic compounds such as carbohydrates, lipids, and hydrocarbons as a carbon and energy source.

Heterotropia The eyes are abnormally turned.

Heterozygosity The presence of different alleles at one or more loci on homologous chromosomes.

Hiatal Hernia A hernia defect occurring in the area where the esophagus passes through the diaphragm from the chest into the abdomen.

High Level Care High level care provides ongoing 24 hour nursing care, as well as meals, laundry, cleaning and personal care.

High purity process systems The equipment that includes the stainless steel vessels, tube, pipe, fittings, and valves used to manufacture and transport drug products.

High Risk Pregnancy A pregnancy is considered high-risk for chromosomal abnormality(ies) when one of the following occurs: abnormal results are obtained from maternal serum screening or ultrasound, the maternal age is 35 years or older, or there is a family history of genetic disorders.

Hilar vessels The vascular pedicle for the lung, including the lymphatics, pulmonary arteries and veins.

Hip joint One of the largest joints in the body (it depends on how you measure). Each ball-and-socket hip supports about 3/8 of the total body weight.

Hippocampal formation Consists of the dentate gyrus, hippocampus, subicular cortex (part of the parahippocampal gurus) and associated nerve fibers.

Hippocampus A long cortical eminence (cornu ammonis) invaginated into the medial wall and floor of the temporal horn of the lateral ventricle. This is phylogenetically old 3 layer archicortex of which the pyramidal cell laye r is the most characteristic. Regional variations in morphology, development, and connectivity subdivide the hippocampus into sectors designated CA1 to CA4.

Hippocratic oath An affirmation usually taken by physicians about to enter the practice of medicine. It is attributed to Greek physician, Hippocrates of Cos, who is called the "Father of Medicine" (circa 460- 377 B.C). Its content reflects the ethical code of the physicians' attitudes and behavior and obligations towards patients, colleagues and society. The complete text can be found here.

Hirschsprung's disease Caused by malformation of a baby's large intestine during pregnancy. Some of the nerve cells that are normally present are missing, causing problems moving stool through the intestine. This can cause obstruction (blockage) of the intestine.

Histiocyte A large, phagocytic cell of the reticuloendothelial system; a macrophage.

Histiocytoma A common neoplasm of young dogs composed of round histiocytic cells, thought to be Langerhan's cells. Most tumors spontaneously regress.

HIV therapies Practitioners offer a range of therapies that aim to treat the human immuno-deficiency virus, AIDS, or its' symptoms. Due to the life-threatening nature of this disease, these therapies are often used as complements to conventional approaches to HIV.

Hold up volume The volume of liquid remaining in a vessel or piping system after it has been allowed to drain.

Holistic/wholistic An adjective meaning targeted to the whole person - mind, body, and spirit. Wholistic medicine considers not only physical health but also the emotional, spiritual, social, and mental well-being of the person.

Hollow fiber Refers to reverse osmosis and ultrafiltration membranes formed into small diameter (about 0.05" I.D.) tubes. The inner surface is a very thin (RO or UF) membrane skin supported by a thicker porous outer layer that gives the tube its strength. Hollow fibers are used in bundles of 1,000 or more in a single cartridge shell. Water is forced through the center (upstream surface) of each tube and purified permeate is collected from the outer wall (downstream surface).

Homans' sign Homans' sign—Pain caused by flexing the toes when a person has a blood clot in the lower leg.

Home and Community Based Services Non-medical services provided to older people still living in their own homes. These services may include case management, meals, companions, houskeeping, adult day care, senior center, and other services designed to keep people as independent as possible..

Home Care Care provided in the patient's home. A wide range of health-related services such as assistance with medications, wound care, intravenous (IV) therapy, and help with basic needs such as bathing, dressing, mobility, etc., which are delivered at a person's home. This type of care can include nurses, social workers, occupational therapists, physical therapists, and other rehabilitation services.

Home Health Agency A licensed provider which delivers medical services in patients' homes. Individual plan of care records are kept on each patient, there is supervision by a qualified professional (RN or licensed social worker), and the facilities employees receive appropriate specialized training. HHAs usually provide Registered Nurses, License

Homemaker Services Non Personal Care services delivered at home, such as shopping, laundry, light cleaning, meal preparation, transportation assistance, money management, home repairs, yard work, and personal hygiene and grooming.

Homeo, homo (prefix) Similar; same. e.g. homeotypical - resembling the normal or usual type.

Homeobox A short stretch of nucleotides whose base sequence is virtually identical in all the genes that contains it. It has been found in many organisms from fruit flies to human beings. In the fruit fly, a homeobox appears to determine when particular groups of genes are expressed during development.

Homeopathy A medical system that uses infinitesimal doses of natural substances to stimulate a person's immune and defense system. Homeopathic remedies are named for the plant or animal ingredient they are made from.

Homesharing A cost-effective living arrangement in which one or more unrelated people move into the house or apartment of an older adult. Often the person who moves in functions as a light caregiver, prepares meals, and helps with housekeeping in lieu of rent.

Homologous chromosome Chromosome containing the same linear gene sequences as another, each derived from one parent.

Homology Similarity in DNA or protein sequences between individuals of the same species or among different species.

Hormonal therapy Involves the use of anti-androgens. An androgen is a male hormone needed for the production of testosterone. By depriving the cancer cells of the testosterone they need for growth, tumors regress in size and cellular activity. Side effects include gynecomastia, the enlargement of breast tissue, hot flashes, and loss of libido (desire to have sex). Some long term hormonal therapy is associated with the loss of muscle mass, osteoporosis, and malaise (loss of energy).

Hormone A type of chemical messenger, occurring both in plants and animals, that acts to inhibit or excite metabolic activities. Its site of production is distant from the site of biological activity.

Hospice A special concept of care designed to provide comfort and support to patients and their families when a life-limiting illness no longer responds to cure-oriented treatments.

Hospice Care Supportive care provided to terminally ill patients and their families in the final 6 months (Medicare definition) of a patient's life. This care is managed and coordinated by a certified Medicare hospice provider.

Host A computer connected to the internet that allows users to connect to it.

Host vector (HV) system The host is the organism into which a gene from another organism is transplanted. The guest gene is carried by a vector, which is a larger DNA molecule, such as a plasmid, or a virus into which that gene is genetically engineered and which then propagates in the host. NIH Guidelines under Appendix E. - Certified Host-Vector Systems contains a list of derivatives host-vector systems previously classified as Host-Vector 1 Systems or Host-Vector 2 Systems, they are: Bacillus subtilis, Saccharomyces Cerevisiae, Escherichia coli, Neurospora crassa, Streptomyces, and Pseudonomas putida.

Hot can (Active can) Electrical current flows from the lead in the heart to the surface of the pulse generator.

Hotkey or **Hotkey Combination** A hotkey is a combination of keyboard strokes used by software programs to save the user some time. The hotkey combination "Ctrl+S" is commonly used to save a file. Hotkeys can also be used to access programs running on your computer, for example, in Windows the hotkey combination "Alt+Tab" will allow the user to switch to another program running in Windows.

HPLC (high pressure liquid chromatography) Sometimes called high-performance liquid chromatography, is a separation technique based on a solid stationary phase and a liquid mobile phase. Separations (into distinct bands) are achieved by partition, adsorption, or ion-exchange processes, depending upon the type of stationary phase used. Each band is then profiled as the solvent flows through a UV detector, or by fluorescence, or refractive index detectors.

HSA (human serum albumin) The main protein constituent of human serum. It has no prosthetic group and is soluble in water and dilute salt solution. It is sometimes used in the treatment of shock, hypoproteinemia, and erythroblastosis fetalis.

HTS computerized binocular home vision therapy system A computer program which is prescribed by an eye doctor. The computer program is for improving eye tracking, eye teaming, and/or eye focusing.

Human Caring All human life is equally respected and given high regard and reverence. Thus, the implementation of Human Caring requires understanding individuals' wholeness and uniqueness, not only their biological existence but also their cultural, social, and historical uniqueness. Moreover, Human Caring requires integration of concepts and theories with wisdom that has been passed on from generation to generation throughout human history.

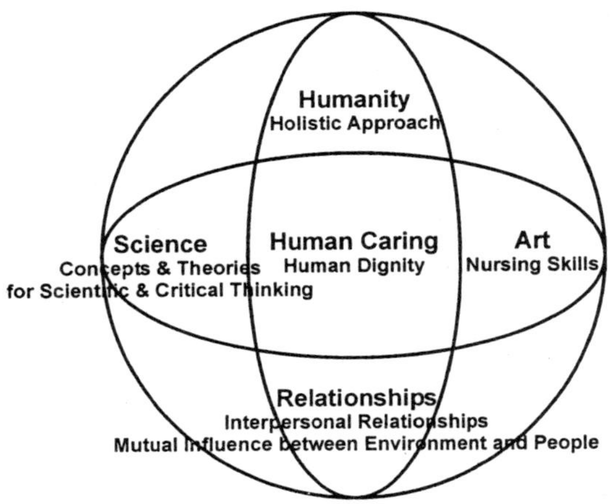

Fig. Human Caring

Human chorionic gonadatropin Human chorionic gonadatropin (HCG)-Hormone produced in early pregnancy. Measured in a pregnancy test.

Human gene therapy Insertion of normal DNA directly into cells to correct a genetic defect.

Human genome initiative Collective name for several projects begun in 1986 by DOE to:

1. Create an ordered set of DNA segments from known chromosomal locations.

2. Develop new computational methods for analyzing genetic map and DNA sequence.

3. Develop new techniques and instruments for detecting and analyzing DNA.

This DOE initiative is now known as the Human Genome Program. The national effort, led by DOE and NIH, is known as the Human Genome Project.

Human Genome The complete set of human genes - approximately 100,000 total - which together contain information covering every aspect of human physical development and function.

Human Genome Project Begun in 1990, it aims to identify, map and sequence all of the estimated 100,000 human genes by the year 2003, producing a vast database of human genetic information.

Human placental lactogen Human placental lactogen-Hormone of pregnancy produced by the placenta. Found in the bloodstream.

Humerus The large single bone of the proximal arm (upper extremity).

Hyaline membrane disease Hyaline membrane disease-Respiratory disease of the newborn.

Hybrid systems Combination of electronic and paper records, common in today's analytical labs, in which raw data is recorded electronically to reconstruct the analysis, but the final results are printed and signed on paper. FDA does not prohibit hybrid systems but has expressed some concerns about their usefulness.

Hybridization Hybridization (e.g., DNA hybridization): The binding of complementary sequences of DNA through specific base-pairing of Adenine with Thymine and Guanine with Cytosine.

Hybridoma A hybrid cell resulting from the fusion of a specific antibody producing spleen cell with a myeloma cell. The hybrid cell has the growth characteristics of the myeloma component and the antibody secreting characteristics of the spleen cell and will multiply to become a source of large quantities of pure, monoclonal antibody.

Hydatid disease From the Greek, for "watery" cyst - usually an echinococcus cyst.

Hydiltidiform mole Hydiltidiform mole.

Hydramnios Hydramnios-Increased amniotic fluid.

Hydro, hygro (prefix) Water; fluid. e.g. hydronephrosis - distension of the renal pelvis and calices with urine.

Hydrocele A painless swelling of the scrotum, caused by a collection of fluid around the testicle; commonly occurs in middle-aged men.

Hydrocephalus A condition in which there is either overproduction, obstructed circulation or impaired absorption of CSF resulting in abnormal progressive accumulation of fluid within the cerebral ventricles and/o r subarachnoid spaces, dilation of the venricles, compression of brain substance, raised intracranial pressure and consequent neurological and functional disturbances.

Hydrochloric acid Acid made by the stomach that breaks down proteins in the foods we eat.

Hydrogen breath test A test that measures the amount of hydrogen in the breath, and helps diagnose lactose intolerance. If the body is unable to digest lactose properly, it will make excess amounts of hydrogen.

Hydrogen peroxide (H_2O_2) A colorless, heavy, strongly oxidizing, unstable liquid used principally in aqueous solutions as an antiseptic, bleaching agent, oxidizing agent, and laboratory reagent. In the vapor phase, as an airborne sterilant.

Hydrolysis A chemical reaction between water and organic compounds, particularly esters, ketones, and alcohols. This reaction can lead to breakdown of some proteins.

Hydrophilic Having a strong affinity for water. Its opposite, hydrophobic.

Hydrophobic Non-wetting; water repelling.

Hydrosol The water that is obtained along with essential oil after plant materials are distilled. In distillation, plant materials are heated in water to release plant oils. The steam and vapor are channeled through a tube to a condensing coil, where they cool and return to liquid form. The essential oils float on top of the water. The hydrosol contains water-soluble plant constituents and trace amounts of essential oil. Hydrosols are sometimes used in aromatherapy together with the essential oils and may be spritzed in the air and on the face and body.

Hydrotest A pressure test of piping, pressure vessels, or pressure-containing parts, usually performed by pressurizing the internal volume with water at a pressure determined by the applicable code or to test the integrity of a process system.

Hydroureter Distension of the ureter with fluid due to obstruction. Hydroureter is often accompanied by hydronephrosis if the obstruction is in the bladder trigone or more distal.

Hydroxicitric Acid (HCA) Also known as Citrimax. Acid found in the fruit Garcinia Cambogia that affects fat and carbohydrate metabolism. Studies have shown it reduces the conversion of carbs into bodyfat. HCA competitively inhibits an enzyme kown as ATP-Citrate lyase (the major enzyme responsible for the production of fatty acid). When HCA blocks the production of fatty acids, a buildup of citrate occurs, which may cause the cell to inhibit glycolysis (breakdown of stored sugars).

Hygienic Of, or pertaining to, equipment and piping systems that by design, materials of construction, and operation provide for the maintenance of cleanliness (pyrogen free but not sterile) so that products produced by these systems will not adversely affect human or animal health.

Hygienic clamp joint A tube outside diameter union consisting of two neutered ferrules having flat faces with a concentric groove and mating gasket that is secured with a clamp, providing a nonprotruding, recessless product contact surface. Tri-clamp is a Tri-Clover proprietary name; consequently, it should not be used to describe the above-mentioned fitting unless that particular brand is used.

Hygroscopicity The affinity for absorbing water.

Hyoid bone The horse shoe shaped bone that lies above the thyroid cartilage at the base of the tongue.

Hyper (prefix) Above and beyond; excessive. e.g. hyperacidity - excessive acidity. e.g. hyperchromasia - excessive pigmentation

Hyper Link A command embedded in the contents of a HyperText document that, when accessed by a user, automatically opens a designated resource.

Hyperbilirubinemia Too much bilirubin in the bloodstream, due to liver problems. Causes a yellow color of the skin known as jaundice.

Hypercoagulability A clinical state with a variety of causes in which the blood clots more easily than normal.

Hyperemesis gravidarum Hyperemesis gravidarum—Severe nausea, dehydration and vomiting during pregnancy. Occurs most frequently during the first trimester. Extreme morning sickness.

Hyperemia Presence of an increased amount of blood in a part or an organ.

HyperlipidemiaThe condition of having an elevated level of fat circulating in the blood.

Hypermobility A condition characterized in which the pelvic floor muscles can no longer provide the necessary support to the urethra and bladder neck. As a result, the bladder neck drops when any downward pressure is applied and causing involuntary leakage. This condition is the most common cause of stress urinary incontinence.

Hyperopia Farsightedness, an individual will have difficulty seeing clearly up close. Light entering the eye focuses behind the retina when the eye is at rest and is corrected with a plus lens. Vision therapy is not prescribed for hyperopia. Children, up to about the age of 8 years, are often farsighted.

Hyperphoria A condition in which one eye has a tendency to point higher than the other eye, causing eyestrain. Sometimes improved by prisms in glasses.

Hypertension Hypertension— pregnancy-induced-High blood pressure that occurs during pregnancy. Defined by an increase in the diastolic and/or systolic blood pressure.

Hyper Text Markup Language Also called Hypertext (HTML). Hyper Text Markup Language is a document creation language used to create hyper links between documents. This language is used extensively on the World Wide Web.

Hyperthyroidism Hyperthyroidism-Elevation of the thyroid hormone in the bloodstream.

Hypertrophy An increase in the size of a cell, tissue or organ usually as a physiologic response to a stimulus.

Hypertropia Strabismus, one eye turned in an upward direction.

Hyponsis Although the condition resembles normal sleep, scientists have found that the brain wave patterns of hypnotized subjects are much closer to the patterns of deep relaxation. Hypnosis is now generally viewed as a form of attentive, receptive, highly focused concentration in which external events are omitted or disregarded. Widely used by surgeons, dentists, and psychotherapists to relieve anxiety or as an anesthetic. Used to relax a patient, reduce resistance to therapy, facilitate memory, to address stopping smoking, eating less, or fighting fears.

Hypoglossal trigone An elevation located on the floor of the fourth ventricle on either side of the caudal midline overlying the motor nucleus of the hypoglossal nerve.

Hypoglycemia A term meaning low blood sugar. It's a set of symptoms that point to irregularities in the way the body handles glucose, the sugar that circulates in the blood. Symptoms of hypoglycemia include sweating, trembling, anxiety, fast heartbeat, headache, hunger, weakness, mental confusion, and on occasion, seizures and coma. However, it occurs rarely because the body has a lot of backup systems preventing it.

Hypopharynx The portion of the pharynx, under the epiglottis, that opens into the larynx and esophagus.

Hypophoria A condition in which one eye has a tendency to point lower than the other eye. This condition may be observed when one eye is covered.

Hypophysis (cerebri) Endocrine gland (pituitary) which occupis the hypophysial fossa of the sphenoid bone. It is attached to the base of the brain (hypothalamus) by the infundibular stalk and consists of the adenohypophysial and neurohypophysial lobes, both of which are under neural control.

Hypoplasia Underdevelopment of a tissue or organ usually due to a decrease in the number of cells.

Hypotension Hypotension—Low blood pressure.

Hypothalamus A small subdivision of the diencephalon located below the thalamus on either side of the third ventricle. It is the only part of the diencephalon visible externally at the base of the brain. It is bounded by the optic chiasma anter iorly, the optic tracts laterally and the mammillary bodies caudally. It is concerned with the regulation of visceral, autonomic and endocrine function. and its destruction is incompatible with life.

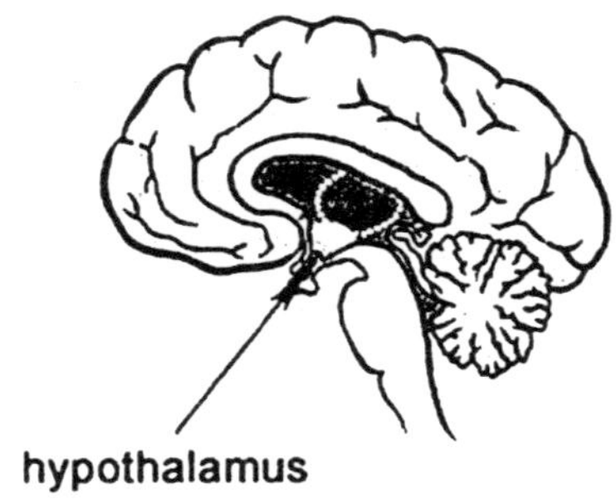

Fig. Hypothalamus

Hypothyroidism A condition of which the Thyroid gland does not produce enough Thyroid Hormone. Has several causes.

Hypotonia Abnormally decreased tonicity, tension or strength; ocular hypotony refers to low intraocular pressure.

Hypotropia Strabismus, one eye turned in a downward direction.

Hysterical amblyopia A non specific visual loss with an unknown cause. Upon examination the doctor is unable to find corroborating objective evidence of this abnormality. The most common symptom is an isolated visual acuity impairment, followed by combined visual acuity impairment and visual field constriction, and whereas an isolated visual field constriction occurred most infrequently. This vision loss may be due to anxiety or emotional repression.

Hysterosalpingogram (HSG) A radiographic procedure that uses contrast (radiopaque) material injected into the uterus and fallopian tubes. May be used to diagnose fertility problems and anomalies of the female genital tract.

I

Iasis (suffix) A process, especially a morbid one. e.g. amebiasis - the state of being infected with amebae.

IBC (intermediate bulk container) A container for storing, transporting, and handling dry materials. Normally bigger than ½ cubic meter but smaller than 3 cubic meters, dust free, able to receive and discharge a variety of materials, and capable of automation.

IBCLC International Board Certified Lactation Consultant

Icon A pictorial representation of a program or software function or feature.

IDE Intelligent Drive Electronics. IDE is the protocol that most PC disk drives use to communicate with the processor.

Identical twins Identical twins.

Idiopathic Occurring without known cause.

IDLH (immediately dangerous to life and health) A concentration of airborne contaminants, normally expressed in parts per million (ppm) or milligrams per cubic meter, which represents the maximum level from which one could escape within 30 minutes without any escape-impairing symptoms or irreversible health effects. This level is established by the national institute of occupational safety and health (NIOSH).

IGF-1 Stands for Insulin-like growth factor. An important hormone for muscle growth. Naturally produced by the body in response to exercise and is necessary for normal physiological functioning. Excess of IGF-1 may be associated with an increased risk of breast cancer, and prostate cancer.

Ileal vessels Branches of the Superior Mesenteric Artery (SMA) that form the vascular supply to the "ileum" or distal portion of the small intestine.

Ileocecal valve The valve-like structure formed by the flaps of the ileocecal opening. May prevent reflux of colonic contents into the small intestine.

Ileocolic artery The artery which originates from the superior mesenteric and branches into the anterior and posterior cecal, appendicular, colic, and ileal rami arteries.

Ileum The lower end of the small intestine.

Iliac crest The arching ridge of bone on the upper border of the ilium.

Iliac lymph nodes Lymph nodes situated along the iliac vessels.

Iliacus muscle Muscle that originates at the iliac fossa and base of the sacrum, and inserts into the lesser trochanter of the femur. It contributes to the flexion of the thigh and trunk against the lower limb.

Iliolumbar artery Artery which originates from the internal iliac and branches into the iliac and lumbar branches and lateral sacral arteries.

Iliopsoas muscle A compound muscle made up of the iliacus and psoas muscles, a flexor of the hip, inserts onto the lesser trochanter of the proximal femur. The psoas arises along the lateral border of the lumbar spine.

Ilium The superior portion of the hip or pelvic bone.

Ill sustained accommodation This clinical condition is also called Accommodative Fatigue. It is the inability of the eye to adequately sustain sufficient focusing over an extended time period. The most common sign or symptom is blurred vision after prolonged near work such as reading and using a computer. In addition, such patients often have asthenopia (eyestrain). Clinical signs include: normal amplitude of accommodation, decreased PRA, and the patient generally fails the +/-2.00 D flipper test. Plus lenses (glasses or contacts) and vision therapy are effective in treating this condition.

Immediate Jeopardy A situation in which a provider's noncompliance with one or more regulations has caused, or is likely to cause, serious injury, harm, impairment, or death to a resident (patient).

Immune globulin preparation Immune globulin preparation-Substance used to protect against infection with certain diseases, such as hepatitis or measles.

Immune response The production of antibodies (humoral response) or particular types of cytotoxic lymphoid cells (cell-mediated response) on challenge with an antigen.

Immunity The state of an organism in which protection from many infectious diseases is afforded by prior exposure to the infectious agents.

Immuno electrophoresis The separation of different antigen-antibody systems by diffusion in an agar gel; a separate precipitation band in the gel detects each system.

Immunogen A substance that is capable of causing antibody formation.

Immunoglobulin (Ig) A member of a class of proteins that functions as an antibody. The wide range of different specifities of antibodies depends on subtle differences in their structure.

Immunoglobulin (IgA, IgD, IgE, IgG, and IgM) A class of serum proteins rich in antibodies. Often used, along with the more specific monoclonal antibodies, in diagnostic reagents in the health field.

Immunoglobulin A (IgA) The body's first line of defense against infectious diseases and is present in seromucous secretions such as saliva, tears, nasal fluids, sweat and secretions of the lung and genito-urinary and gastro-intestinal tracts.

Immunohistochemistry Pathologic examination technique involving tumor specific antibodies linked to a dye. These antibodies react with antigens located on the surface of tumor cells and allow for detection of even single cells within a microscopic slide.

Immunology Immunology is the study of the immune system and its reaction to pathogens, as well as its malfunctions, such as allergies and autoimmune diseases.

Immunoproteins All the proteins concerned with the immune system (antibodies, interferon, and cytokines).

Imperforate anus Caused by improper development of the baby's rectum and anus during pregnancy. The opening at the end of the rectum or anus is absent, so stool cannot leave the body normally.

Implantable cardioverter defibrillator (ICD) A device implanted in the abdomen or pectoral region which is used to treat potentially fatal fast heart rhythms by delivering electrical energy to the heart to restore the heart's normal rhythms.

Implantation Implantation into the Uterus Approximately 8 days after ovulation, if ou are pregnant, the blastocyst (as the baby is classified at this stage) begins to secrete a hormone that enables it to burrow into the lining of the uterus. Implantation [the burrowing] into the uterus usually happens in the upper one-third of the uterus and causes the placenta to begin to form.

Implanted Placed inside the body. The AICD system is an implanted system.

Imprinting A biochemical phenomenon that determines, for certain genes, which one of the pair of alleles, the mother's or the father's, will be active in that individual.

Impurity Any component present in the intermediate or API (Active Pharmaceutical Ingredient) that is not the desired entity. It may be either process or product related.

Impurity profile A description of the identified and unidentified impurities present in a typical batch of API (Active Pharmaceutical Ingredient) produced by a specific controlled production process. It includes the identity or some qualitative analytical designation (e.g. retention time), the range of each impurity observed, and type of each identified impurity. For each API there should be an impurity profile describing the identified and unidentified impurities present in a typical batch. The impurity profile is normally dependent upon the process or origin of the API.

In line An integral part of the flow path. In a fluid stream, something is said to be in-line if the entire fluid stream flows directly through or past it.

In process control Checks performed during production in order to monitor and if necessary to adjust the process and/or to ensure that the intermediate or API (Active Pharmaceutical Ingredient) conforms to its specification. (also called process control).

In situ In the natural or original position

In utero In utero-Within the uterus.

Inactivation Any process that destroys the ability of a specific microbiological agent or eukaryotic cell to self-replicate.

Inactive ingredient Any component other than an active ingredient.

Incidence The incidence of disease is defined as the number of new cases of disease occurring in a population during a defined time interval. The number is used to measure risk. High incidence may indicate an impending epidemic. Incidence is different from prevalence.

Incidence rate (IR) The number of new cases of a health problem or disease in a specified time that occurs in a population at risk of the disease in the same time period. The rate is expressed per 100, 1,000, 10,000 or 100,000.

Incidental release The discharge of a microbilogical agent or eukaryotic cell from a containment system that is expected when the system is appropriately designed and properly operated and maintained. Incidental releases are de minimis in nature.

Incision The cut or wound produced by cutting into the body in order to perform surgery; the cut becomes a scar after surgery.

Inclusion body Condensed particles of protein formed inside E. coli and other bacteria formed when the cells are forced to make large amounts of a product protein. The cells must be broken to harvest inclusion bodies.

Inclusions Particles of foreign material in a metallic matrix. The particles are usually compounds such as oxides, sulfides, or silicates, but may be any substance foreign to and essentially insoluble in the matrix.

Incomitant strabismus A condition also known as Noncomitant Strabismus. It occurs when the magnitude of deviation is not the same in the different positions of gaze or with either eye fixating. There is an abnormal restriction to movement or an over-action of one or more of the extraocular muscles. Generally, the magnitude must change by at least 5 PD to be incomitant (nonconcomitant).

Incompetent cervix Incompetent cervix– Cervix that dilates painlessly, without contractions.

Incomplete abortion Incomplete abortion-Miscarriage in which part, but not all, of the uterine contents are expelled.

Incontinence Inability to voluntarily control bowel or bladder function.

Incus The middle ossicle of the ear, that helps to conduct vibrations from the tympanic membrane to the oval window of the inner ear. Together, the incus and malleus look like an ice cream cone.

IND (investigational new drug) application A document filed with the FDA prior to clinical trial of a new drug. It gives a full description of the new drug, where and how is manufactured, all QC information, etc. The IND is followed by NDA (new drug application).

Indemnity Model A type of Long Term Care Insurance which pays a fixed level benefit when an individual becomes disabled and long-term care expenses are incurred. The payment may be larger or smaller than the actual cost of services and bears no direct relationship to such expenses.

Independent or Instrumental Activities of Daily Living (IADLs) Activities that include meal preparation, housework (e.g., cooking), managing finances (e.g., keeping a checkbook) or medications, telephone use, shopping, and transportation (e.g., how one moves up and down stairs, how one moves in and out of cars).

Indicator A variable that helps to measure changes directly or indirectly and permits one to assess the extent to which objectives and targets of a program are being attained. In medicine, indicators help to measure changes in the health situation of a population.

Indigestion Feeling of nausea, bloating, gas, and/or heartburn caused by poor digestion.

Indirect impact system An engineering system considered having no direct impact on product quality.

Indirect obstetric death Those deaths resulting from previously existing disease or disease that developed during pregnancy and which was not directly the result of obstetric conditions, but which was aggravated by the physiologic effects of pregnancy.

Individual Program Plan A written statement of the services to be provided, as developed by an interdisciplinary team, and based on a comprehensive functional assessment of an individual's active treatment needs.

Indurated Abnormally hard.

Indusium griseum A thin vestigial layer of gray matter located on the upper surface of the corpus callosum (supracallosal gyrus) continuous posteriorly with the fasciolar and dentate gyri. Imbedded within the indusium griseum are two longitudinal strands of white matter, the medial and lateral longitudinal striae which are rudimentary in man.

Inert Does not dissolve in water or react chemically with other substances.

Inevitable abortion Inevitable abortion– Pregnancy complicated with bleeding and cramping. Usually results in miscarriage.

Infarct A localized area of ischemic necrosis produced by the occlusion of the blood vessels - either arterial supply or venous drainage.

Infarction Death of a tissue or organ.

Infected Contaminated with extraneous biological agents and therefore capable of spreading infection.

Infectious Able to cause disease in a susceptible host.

Infectious agent A biological organism that can establish a process of infection.

Inferior (temporal) horn The portion of the lateral ventricle which stretches from the pars centralis, behind the thalamus, into the temporal lobe.

Inferior gluteal artery The artery which originates from the internal iliac and branches into the sciatic artery.

Inferior mesenteric artery Artery which originates from the abdominal aorta and branches into the left colic, sigmoid, and superior rectal arteries.

Inferior mesenteric vein The vein that parallels the inferior mesenteric artery and drains into the splenic vein.

Inferior or caudal Away from the head; lower (example, the foot is part of the inferior extremity).

Inferior orbital fissure Located in the inferolateral wall of the orbit, it allows for the passage of the infraorbital and zygomatic nerves and infraorbital vessels. It is surrounded by the greater wing of the sphenoid and the orbital process of the maxilla.

Inferior pubic ramus Portion of the pubic bone which projects posteroinferolaterally to join the ramus of the ischium.

Inferior vena cava The vein that begins at the junction of the two common iliac veins, at the level of the fifth lumbar vertebra, and empties into the right atrium. It drains blood from the lower extremities, and the pelvic and abdominal viscera.

Infiltration The entry of air from an adjoining room or from outdoors through wall and ceiling openings due to a difference in air pressure between the two areas.

Inflammatory bowel disease (IBD) Diseases that cause irritation and ulcers in the intestinal tract. Crohn's disease and ulcerative colitis are the most common inflammatory bowel diseases.

Informatics The study of the application of computer and statistical techniques to the management of information. In genome projects, informatics includes the development of methods to search databases quickly, to analyze DNA sequence information, and to predict protein sequence and structure from DNA sequence data.

Information management A method used to organize information to avoid information overload and to keep information in a format that is efficient to retrieve whenever needed. Filing systems, cognitive maps, manuals, and electronic databases are examples of devices that can prove useful in information management. A network of consultants is an additional way to ensure that necessary information will be readily available.

Informed Choice A decision-making process which involves the participation of the client as the primary decision maker and which is based upon a full exchange of information between the midwife and her client in a non-urgent, non-authoritarian, cooperative setting.

Informed Consent The person giving consent receives information necessary to make a health care decision, including information about the benefits, reasonable risks, alternatives, the right to refuse, and consequences of any treatment or service.

Infra (prefix) Beneath. e.g. infraorbital - beneath the eye.

Infraspinatus muscle Muscle responsible for the lateral rotation of the humerus. It originates from below the scapula spine (infraspinous fossa) and inserts onto the greater tubercle of the humerus.

Infratentorial Below the tentorium cerebelli and within the posterior cranial fossa.

Infundibulum Funnel-shaped evagination of the floor of the third ventricle from which the pituitary stalk arises.

Infusion The introduction of parenterals into a vein (intravenous).

Inguinal hernia Part of the small intestine that pushes through an opening in the abdominal muscle, causing a bulge underneath the skin in the groin area.

Inguinal lymph nodes Lymph nodes situated along the inguinal vessels.

Inion A craniometric landmark located at the apex of the external occipital protuberance.

Injection A preparation intended for parenteral administration and/or constituting or diluting a parenteral article prior to administration. The introduction of parenterals may be into the subcutaneous cellular tissue (subcutaneous or hypodermic), or the muscular tissue (Intramuscular).

Ink Jet Printer A type of printer that sprays ink, in very tiny droplets, from jet nozzles onto the paper. Ink jet printers can print in much higher resolutions than dot matrix printers, but not as high as laser printers.

Inner table of skull The inner layer of compact bone of the flat bones of the skull. The periosteal layer of the dura is attached to the inner table.

Innocuous Safe, not contaminated.

Inoculum Fermentation: an aliquot of a pure culture of microorganism added to the primary seed tank to initiate fermentation.

Inositol An active factor in the B-Complex vitamins which help convert food to energy. With Choline, Inositol is active in the metabolism of fats.

Input Data entered into the computer via some sort of input device such as the drive, lightpen, keyboard, microphone, mouse, modem, or scanner.

Insemination The placement of semen into a woman's uterus, cervix, or vagina.

Insertion Point A flashing vertical line showing where text will be inserted (cursor).

Install Loading and copying a program's files to a computer's disk drive and configuring it to run. Common when installing new software.

Institute for international medical education (IIME) A non-profit medical Institute established in 1999 by a grant from the China Medical Board of New York, which began its own operations in 1914 as a division of The Rockefeller Foundation. The IIME has been entrusted with the development of 'Global Minimum Essential (Core) Requirements' which include knowledge, clinical skills, professional ethical values and fundamental competencies to the practice of health care worldwide. These essential requirements represent only a portion of the educational experience, since each country and even each medical school has unique needs that the educational curriculum should address. Three committees composed of medical experts from around the globe supervise the work of IIME: the Core Committee, the Steering Committee and the Advisory Committee. The Institute is located just outside of New York City in suburban White Plains, New York.

Institutional LTC Institutional LTC is care provided in institutional settings such as services provided in residential homes, assisted living facilities, skilled nursing facilities, sub-acute care facilities.

Instrumental Activities of Daily Living Core life activities of independent living, including using the telephone, managing money, preparing meals, doing housework, and remembering to take medications.

Insula Cerebral cortical area within the depths of the lateral fissure (of Sylvius) beneath the frontal, temporal, and parietal opercula. It overlies the putamen and claustrum. Also known as the Island of Reil and somtimes consider ed the 5th "lobe".

Insulin An anabolic hormone that's supposed to take the sugar and traansport it into the muscle. Insulin also promotes increased amino acid entry into muscle and increases muscle protein synthesis. Too much insulin can cause sugar to bypass muscle, and be stored as bodyfat.

Integrated teaching A method of teaching that interrelates or unifies subjects frequently taught in separate academic courses or departments. In integrated teaching, subjects are presented together as a meaningful whole. Integration may be vertical or horizontal. Horizontal integration functions between parallel disciplines such as anatomy, histology, biochemistry or medicine, surgery and pharmacology. Vertical integration functions between disciplines traditionally taught in different phases of curriculum; it can occur throughout the curriculum with medical and basic sciences beginning together in the early years.

Intel Corporation A leading manufacturer of microprocessors, including the current standard, the Pentium I, II, and III Processors. Computers with Intel processors are usually identified by a "Intel Inside" logo.

Inter (prefix) Between. e.g. intercellular - between two cells.

Intercondylar eminences A projection on the proximal end of the tibia, set in between two tubercles.

Interdisciplinary Team A group of professionals from various disciplines who work together to provide services to the greatest benefit of the individual.

Interface The program or device that controls the way two pieces of equipment or programs work together. The term interface can also be used to describe the look and layout of a program on the screen for interaction with the user.

Interhemispheric fissure The cleft between the two cerebral hemispheres, containing CSF and the falx cerebri.

Intermediate Care Occasional nursing and rehabilitative care ordered by a doctor and performed or supervised by skilled medical personnel. A less-intensive type of care than Skilled Care, often involving a lot of Personal Care as well as occasional nursing care. Assistance needed for stable conditions that require daily, but not 24-hour, nursing supervision, ordered by a physician and supervised by registered nurses. Services that may be offered in an Intermediate Care Facility.

Intermediate Care Facility(ICF) A Nursing Home which provides less-extensive medical care than a Skilled Nursing Facility. ICFs have lower minimum staffing requirements than SNFs, and may not have a Registered Nurse on duty 24 hours a day.

Intermediate gray (zone) Zone of spinal cord gray matter that lies between the anterior and posterior horns corresponding to lamina VII of Rexed. This zone includes the nucleus dorsalis (of Clarke), intermediomedial, intermediolateral, and sacral autonomic nuclei.

Intermediolateral nucleus Cell column which occupies lateral part of lamina VII (of Rexed) in thoracic and upper lumbar segments (T1-L2) of the spinal cord only. It marks the location of neuronal cell bodies that give rise to preganglionic sym pathetic fibers.

Internal auditory meatus The channel that allows for the passaage of the facial, intermediate, and vestibulocochlear nerves, and the labrynthine artery to pass.

Internal capsule Concentration of protection fibers within the depths of each cerebral hemisphere between the thalamus, caudate and lenticular nuclei. It consists of an anterior limb, genu, and posterior (lenticulothalamic) limb. The corticipit al and corticofugal fibers contained within this confined region are on their way to and from widespread areas of the cerebral cortex.

Internal iliac artery Artery which is a continuation of the common iliac and branches into the iliolumbar, obturator, superior gluteal, inferior gluteal, umbilical, inferior vesicle, uterine, middle rectal, and internal pudendal arteries.

Internal iliac vein The vein originating from the parietal branches at the level of the greater sciatic notch, and extends to the brim of the pelvis where it joins the external iliac to form the common iliac vein.

Internal oblique muscle Muscles which originates at the inguinal ligamen, iliac crest, and lumbar aponeurosis, and inserts into the lower three or four costal cartilages, the linea alba, and the conjoined tendon to the pubis. It is responsible for flexion and rotation of the vertebral column and compression of the abdominal viscera.

Internal thoracic artery Artery which orginates from the subclavian, and branches into the mediastinal, thymic, bronchial, tracheal, sternal, perforating, medial mammary, lateral musculophrenic, and superior epigastric arteries.

Internal thoracic veins The two veins created from the junction of the venae comitantes of the internal thoracic arteries, and empties into the brachiocephalic vein.

Internet Originally a military project in the 1960's to connect the few relatively spread-out large computers more economically, the Internet is a network of computers connected to each other on a global scale,to share information. The Internet has expanded to become a common application, especially due to the appeal of the World Wide Web and E-Mail. Other features of the internet include newsgroups, mailing lists, chat, online audio and video files, coursework and games.

Internship A first postgraduate training year in which graduates practice medicine under supervision. In some countries this is a requirement for licensure. In many countries and for many specialties such as internal medicine, pediatrics and surgery, this is the first year of residency.. However, as there are some specialties that are too narrow to provide a broad medical practice experience, those residents may have to attend a transitional year in one of the above specialties or a rotating internship.

Interpeduncular fossa Depression along the midline of the ventral surface of the midbrain between the two cerebral peduncles.

InterStim Continence Control Therapy A therapy used in treating urge incontinence. A device, about the size of a pacemaker, that is implanted into the sacral nerves of the lower spine, where it delivers electrical impulses that help regulate bladder function.

Interstitial Between cells.

Interstitial laser A laser probe is placed within prostatic tissue. Laser energy is then used to destroy prostatic tissue which makes urination easier.

Interthalamic adhesion (massa intermedia) Midline nuclear mass found in about 80% of human brains which represents the fusion of the medial surfaces of the thalami across the third ventricle.

Intertrochanteric line The line that extends obliquely downward from the superior tubercle and then around the medial side of the femur, between the greater and lesser trochanter.

Interventricular septum The musculo-membreanous division that separates the left ventricle from the right ventricle of the heart.

Intervertebral disc space The space between the vertebrae, formed from a fibrous ring (the annulus) and a central "cushion" (nucleus pulposis).

Intestinal flora The normal bacteria, yeast, and fungi found in the intestines that aid in digestion.

Intestinal mucosa The lining of the intestines, through which nutrients and water are absorbed into the body.

Intestine Digestive organs found in the abdomen, also known as either the large or small bowel. The small intestine removes nutrients from food to be used for energy, while the large intestine absorbs water from the digested food and processes it into stool.

Intolerance Allergy to a food or other substance.

Intra (prefix) Within.

e.g. intracellular - within cells.

Intranet Similar to the Internet, an intranet is a smaller network of computers, usually within a single organization or building.

Intrinsic Sphincter Deficiency (ISD) Weakening of the urethra sphincter muscles. As a result of this weakening the sphincter does not function normally regardless of the position of the bladder neck or urethra. This condition is a common cause of stress urinary intinence.

Intussusception A disorder in which the intestine folds into itself in a telescope fashion, causing obstruction (blockage).

Invasive squamous-cell carcinoma Invasive squamous-cell carcinoma—Cancer of the cervix that extends beyond the cervix into surrounding tissues or deeper layers.

Inverse occlusion Covering the amblyopic eye.

Inzitol Inzitol is the trade name for Pinitol, a form ogff sugar than researchers are studying for use in insulin-deficient conditions, such as diabetes mellitus type 1. Taking Inzitol can show an increase in both glucose uptake and glycogen storange.

Ipriflavone One of many flavonoids, ipriflavone, formally known as 7-isopropoxyisoflavone, is synthesized from the soy isoflavone daidzein. It has anabolic effects that are especially pronounced in bone.

Ipsilateral Affecting or pertaining to the same side.

IRC Internet Relay Chat.

Iridology Diagnostic system based on the premise that every organ has a corresponding location within the iris of the eye, which can serve as an indicator of the organ's health or disease. Used by naturopaths and other practitioners, particularly when diagnosis achieved through standard methods in unclear.

Iris The colored part of the eye located between the lens and cornea; it regulates the entrance of light.

Iron deficiency anemia Iron-deficiency anemia—Anemia produced by lack of iron in the diet. Often seen in pregnancy.

Iron Mineral essential to oxygen transport in blood (via hemoglobin and myoglobin), enzyme production and immune support. A deficiency can cause the most common form of anemia. Teenagers need additional iron during their years of maximum growth; women need extra iron during the years they are menstruating and during pregnancy.

Irritable Bladder Involuntary contractions of muscles in the bladder, which can cause lack of control of urination.

Ischemia A local deficiency of blood due in part to functional constriction or actual mechanical obstruction of a blood vessel.

Ischial spine Process of bone projecting from the posterior border of the ischium, at the level of the lower border of the acetabulum, backward and medially.

Ischial tuberosity Elongated projection on the inferoposterior margin of the body of the ischial bone, that serves as the point of attachment for a number of muscles.

Ischiorectal fossa The space between the pelvic diaphragm and the skin below it. The fat in this region is almost a liquid at body temperature, allowing for changes in the size and shape of the rectum.

Ischium The inferior dorsal portion of the hip bone.

Isoflavones Phytonutrient antioxidants, including genisteine and diadzein, that act as estrogen receptor protectors (minimize PMS, menopause side effects) and lower cholesterol levels.

Isoimmunization Isoimmunization- Development of specific antibody directed at the red blood cells of another individual, such as a baby in utero. Often occurs when an Ph-negative woman carries an Ph-positive baby or is given Rh-positive blood.

Isoleucine One of the three branched chain amino acids. They are called BCAA's because they structurally branch off another chain of atoms instead of forming a line. Studies have shown that BCAA's help to stimulate protein synthesis and inhibit its breakdown, so BCAA's have powerful anabolic and anticatabolic effects on the body. They may also potentiate the release of some anabolic hormones, such as growth hormone. Regular ingestion of BCAA's help to keep the body in a state of postive nitrogen balance. In this state, your body much more readily builds muscle and burns fat. Studies have shown that athletes taking extra BCAA's have shown a loss of more bodyfat than those not taking BCAA's.

ISP Internet Service Provider. Also known as internet access providers, Internet service providers are local networks connected to the internet. When a user sets up an account with an ISP they are being connected to the ISP's local network which is then connected to the internet network, allowing the user access to the internet.

Itis (suffix) Inflammation. e.g. appendicitis - inflammation of the appendix.

IUGR Fetal-growth retardation (IUGR)— Inadequate growth of the fetus during the last stages of pregnancy.

IVP intra venous pyelogram An imaging study to look at the structure and function of the kidneys, ureters, and bladder. Also called an IVU - intravenous urogram. This test requires the injection of a *contrast agent*.

J

Jaundice Jaundice—Yellow staining of the skin, sclera (eyes) and deeper tissues of the body. Caused by excessive amounts of bilirubin. Treated with phototherapy.

Jejunum (jejunal loops) The portion of the small intestine located between the duodenum and the ileum (distal to the duodenum/proximal to the ileum).

Jin shin do Developed by a psychotherapist, it combines acupressure, Taoist yogic breathing and Reichian segmental theory (addresses how emotional tension affects the physical body) with the goal of releasing physical & emotional tension and armoring. Aims to promote a state in which the patient can address the emotional factors that underlie various physical conditions.

Joint capsule An membranous envelope consisting of a fibrous and synovial membrane that encloses the cavity of a synovial joint and attaches to the bone adjacent to the articular surfaces of the bones involved. A small amount of lubricating "synovial fluid" is contained within the capsule. (The fluid is not 10W-30.).

Joint Commission on Accreditation of Healthcare Agencies (JCAHO) An independent, not-for-profit organization that evaluates and accredits nearly 19,000 health care organizations and programs in the United States.

Joint space The area between the acticular cartilage surfaces making up a synovial joint. The synovial fluid lubricates the opposing articular cartilage. Normal cartilage is very smooth - like Teflon.

Justification To align text so that all the lines begin and/or end at the same place on a page. Justifications can be along the right side of the page, the left side, down the middle (center justification), or set to evenly distribute text across the page (full justification).

Juvenile Arthritis Juvenile rheumatoid arthritis (JRA) is arthritis that causes joint inflammation and stiffness for more than six weeks in children under 16. JRA can affect any joint and mobility may become limited. There are three types of JRA, one of them can affect the internal organs.

K

Karma Basic concept common to Hinduism, Buddhism, and Jainism. The doctrine holds that one's state in this life is the result of physical and mental actions in past incarnations and that present action can determine one's destiny in future incarnations. Karma is a natural, impersonal law of moral cause and effect.

Karyotype A photomicrograph of an individual's chromosomes arranged in a standard format showing the number, size, and shape of each chromosome type. It is used in low-resolution physical mapping to correlate gross chromosomal abnormalities with the characteristics of specific diseases.

Kegel Exercises Exercises is to strengthen the muscles of the pelvic floor, which leads to more control and prevents leakage.

Keratins Insoluble protective or structural proteins consisting of parallel polypeptide chains in a-helical or b-conformation.

Ketones Breakdown product of metabolism found in the blood, particularly in starvation or uncontrolled diabetes.

Ketose A simple monosaccharide having its carbonyl groups at other than a terminal position. Kilobase (kb) Unit of length for DNA fragments equal to 1000 nucleotides (kilo base pairs of DNA).

Keyboard An input device based on the standard QWERTY typewriter configuration. Computer keyboards typically have more keys and features than typewriters, but work in much the same way.

Kidney A pair of "bean shaped" organs in the upper posterior abdomen, behind the peritoneal cavity (retroperitoneal) that filter waste products from the blood. Water, sugar and other valuable materials are reabsorbed and conserved, while the "waste water" is drained by the ureters into the bladder.

Kidney stones Small mass or lesion found in the kidney or urinary tract. Can block the flow of urine.

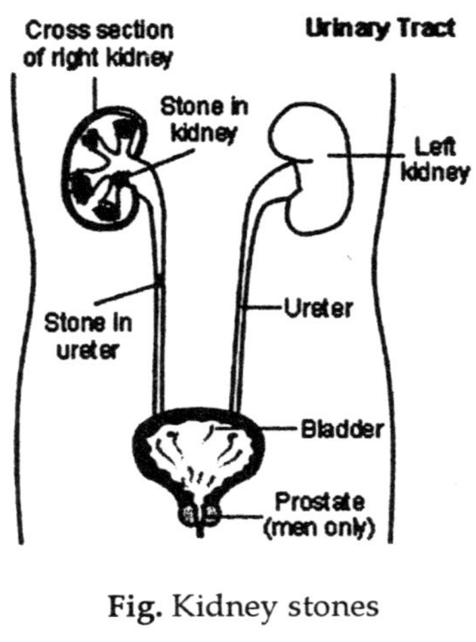

Fig. Kidney stones

Kilobyte A kilobyte or KB is approximately 1000 bytes. Hard drive manufacturers use an even number as a multiplier. In this case 1 KB would be 1,000 bytes.

Kinase An enzyme catalyzing phosphorylation of an acceptor molecule by adenosine triphosphate (ATP).

Kinesiology The study of muscles and their movement. Applied kinesiology is a system that uses muscle testing procedures, in conjunction with standard methods of diagnosis, to gain information about a patient's overall state of health. Practitioners analyze muscle function, posture, gait and other structural factors in addition to inquiring about lifestyle factors that may be contributing to a health-related problem.

Kinesthesia The sensation of bodily position, presence, or movement resulting chiefly from stimulation of sensory nerve ending in muscles, tendons, and joints.

Klinefelter Syndrome A genetic abnormality that is caused by an extra X chromosome in a male, and is typically identified as 47, XXY.

Knee The major joint of the leg, between the distal femur (condyles) and the proximal tibia (plateau).

Knee cap (patella) The roughly triangular sesamoid bone located in front of the knee, within the tendon of the quadriceps femoris muscle, a major extensor of the lower leg.

Knowledge The acquisition or awareness of facts, data, information, ideas or principles to which one has access through formal or individual study, research, observation, experience or intuition.

Kombucha A tea made from a fungus / yeast fermentation with high nutrient level used by people for immune protection, increase energy, and other postive effects. Sometimes called a Kombucha mushroom. It is two life forms, a yeast culture and bacteria living in symbiosis, from Manchuria.

Kynoselen Also called Kyno, it is a veterinary drug, not an anabolic steroid. It is used to treat abnormal muscle conditions in animals. Some bodybuilder use it to increase muscle hardness. Main ingredient in Kynoselen is AMP, a substance formed during the process of creating energy. Concerns for bodybuilders is that life threatening heart problems can arise with its use.

L

Laaoo Process of expelling a fetus from the uterus.

Labile Unstable or unsteady; not fixed; characterized by adaptability to alteration or modification, i.e., relatively easily changed, as in cleavage of a molecule or molecular rearrangement in a compound or complex chemical material.

Lacrimal glands The tear producing glands that are located in a bone depression (fossae) in the upper outer angle of the orbit. Tears serve several functions, including lubrication, moisturizing, and antisepsis for the eyeball. Tears have both a mucus layer, as well as a more liquid layer.

Lactase An enzyme in the small intestine needed to digest lactose, a sugar found in milk and milk products.

Lactase deficiency Lack of an enzyme made by the small intestine called lactase, which prevents the body from digesting lactose (a sugar found in milk and milk products) properly.

Lactoferrin It is a glycoprotein, which means its structure includes a carbohydrate attached to a simple protein. The single protein in lactoferrin contains 703 amino acids in a precise configuration. It appars to offer protectve benefits against a wide range of fungi and viruses.

Lactose Sugar in milk which many people, especially adults, have an intollerance to (indigestion) to to a lack of the enzyme lactasein their bodies.

Lactose tolerance test A test that checks the body's ability to digest lactose (a sugar found in milk and milk products). The child drinks a liquid with lactose in it, and then the amount of lactose in the bloodstream is measured with a blood sample.

Lag of accommodation A measure of the eye's ability to focus accurately on a given target. The dioptric difference between the eye's focusing response and the stimulus to focus.

LAL (limulus amoebocyte lysate) A material obtained by rupturing the cellular components of the blood of a horseshoe crab (Limulus Poliphemus). This material coagulates in the presence of LPS (lypopolysaccharides) and is a test used to quantitate bacterial endotoxins (pyrogens).

Lamina Any thin bone. The lamina of thé spine (arcus vertebrae) is a thin bone plate extending posteriorly from the pedicles and fusing to provide the dorsal portion of the neural arch (surrounding the spinal cord), forming the base for the spinous process.

Laminar airflow - clean work station A workstation in which the unidirectional airflow characteristics predominate throughout the entire airspace with a minimum of eddies (turbulence) to jeopardize critical surfaces.

Laminar flow Non-turbulent fluid flow is usually considered laminar if the Reynolds number is less than 2000 in a pipe. Depending upon many possible varying conditions, the flow may be laminar at a Reynolds number as low as 1,200 or as high as 40,000; however, such conditions are not experienced in normal practice. In the pharmaceutical industry, this term incorrectly refers to the air discharge of a clean air bench or wall.

LAN (local area network) Networks with computers geographically close together (that is, in the same building).

Langelier index A measure of the degree of saturation of calcium carbonate in water that is based on pH, alkalinity and hardness. If the Langelier Index is negative, the water is corrosive (pH value below 7 or acidic). If the Langelier Index is positive, calcium carbonate can precipitate out of solution to form scale (pH value above 7 or basic). The Langelier Index will vary for cold water and for warm water.

Laparoscope A tube with a camera lens attached that looks inside organs to check for abnormalities. Often used in surgery to look inside the body and avoid making large incisions.

Laparoscopic Lymph Node Dissection If a perineal prostatectomy is contemplated then prior to the operation the pelvic lymph nodes are sampled via three small incisions made in the abdomen, much like the procedure used to remove gallbladders.

Laparoscopic Refers to procedures performed with the laparoscope.

Laparoscopy A form of minimally invasive surgery in which viewing endoscopes and small-diameter surgical instruments are inserted into the abdominal cavity through multiple small incisions instead of through large abdominal incisions.

Large intestine (Also called the colon.) The last section of the digestive tract, from the cecum to the rectum; absorbs water from digested food and processes it into stool.

Larynx Head/Tomogram/hn033.html The cartilage support structures that connect the superior trachea, the pharynx inferior to the tongue, and the hyoid bone. It supports the sphincter at the entrance to the trachea (the glottis or true vocal cords) and is therfore also the organ responsible for voice.

Laser Printer A printer that uses a light beam to transfer images to paper. Laser printers print a full page at a time. A laser is used to 'paint' the dots of light onto a photographic drum or belt. The toner is applied to the drum or belt and then transferred onto the paper.

Last menstrual period (LMP) LMP Last menstrual period. Most caregivers date a pregnancy from the first day of your last menstrual period.

Latent heat The amount of heat needed to change a unit of substance, such as water, from a solid to a liquid without change in temperature or pressure.

Latent hyperopia Hyperopia (farsightedness) is compensated by accommodation and the tonicity (tension) of the ciliary muscle; identified by cycloplegic refraction. In mild cases of hyperopia (farsightedness), the eyes are able to compensate without corrective lenses; otherwise a plus lens (glasses or contacts) is prescribed. Vision therapy is not prescribed.

Lateral Away from the midline of the body (example, the little toe is located at the lateral side of the foot).

Lateral mass (C1) The lateral portions of the atlas bone (C1) that connect the arches (anterior/posterior), the articulating surfaces (superior/inferior), and the transverse processes for the first vertebral segment.

Lateral pterygoid plate A pair of projections (medial/lateral) from the greater wing of the sphenoid bone that forms the medial wall of the infratemporal fossa. The medial and lateral pterygoid muscles attach the mandible to the pterygoids.

Lateral semicircular canal Part of the vestibular system of the inner ear that provides sensation for balance and "inertial guidance". The lateral semicircular canal contains the ductus semicircularis lateralis.

Lateral ventricle The CSF filled cavities located in each cerebral hemisphere.

Lattisimus dorsi Muscle that originates from the spines of the thoracic and lumbar vertebrae, thoracolumbar fascia, iliac crest, lower ribs, and inferior angle of the scapula, and inserts into the humerus (along the crest of the intertubercular sulcus). It is responsible for the adduction, extension, and medial rotation of the humerus.

Lay In metallurgy, the direction of the predominant surface pattern ordinarily determined by the production method used.

Leach To dissolve by the action of a moving liquid. For example, high purity water leaches trace impurities from glass vessels.

Lead An insulated wire that carries the heart signal to the pulse generator and energy from the pulse generator to the heart. The leads are attached to the surface of the heart or passed into your heart through the veins.

Learner centered education A method of teaching in which the students' needs have priority. Learners are responsible for identifying knowledge gaps, actively participating in filling them, and keeping track of their learning gains. Teachers are expected to facilitate this process instead of supplying "spoon-fed" information. This approach increases the students' motivation to learn and prepares them for self-learning and continuous education. Learner-centered education is the opposite of teacher-centered education.

Learning disability (LD) A disorder that affects people's ability to either interpret what they see and hear or to link information from different parts of the brain. Learning disabilities can be divided into five broad categories: speech and language disorders, reading disorder, arithmetic disorder, writing disorder, and attention disorders. The term learning disability does not include children who have learning problems that are primarily the result of visual, hearing, or motor disorders.

Lecithin Dry powder source of phospholipids high in B-fatty acids.

Lecture An instruction or verbal discourse by a speaker before a large group of students. This teaching method has historically been quite prominent in education because it is an economic way to communicate information to large groups. However, increasing knowledge about the group's difficulties in maintaining concentration and absorbing extensive information while in a passive listening mode has brought the value of lectures under criticism. Audiovisual presentations, demonstration of patients and intermittent discussions can help activate learners.

Left atrium Chamber on the left side of the heart that recieves blood from the pulmonary veins, directing it to the left ventricle through the mitral valve.

Left colic artery Artery which originates from the inferior mesenteric, and supplies the descending colon.

Left common carotid artery The artery that originates directly from the aortic arch and splits into the left internal and external carotid arteries.

Left gastroepiploic artery Originating from the splenic artery it branches into the gastric and omental arteries.

Left mainstem bronchi Derived from the trachea, the left main bronchos that conducts air into the left lung.

Left marginal artery Artery which originates from the circumflex artery, and follows the left border of the heart, supplying the left ventricle.

Left pulmonary artery Artery originating from the main pulmonary trunk and branching into the arteries of the superior and inferior lobes of the left lung.

Left ventricle The major systemic pumping chamber of the heart that directs blood out through the aorta and into the systemic arteries.

Legacy systems Hardware and software applications in which a company has already invested considerable time and money. Legacy systems typically perform critical operations in companies for many years even though they may no longer use state-of-the-art technology. Replacing legacy systems can be disruptive and therefore requires careful planning and appropriate migration support from the manufacturer.

Leio (prefix) Smooth. e.g. leiomyoma - a benign tumor of smooth muscle cells.

Lens The transparent biconvex structure of the eye that is located between the posterior chamber and vitreous body. The lens is living tissue, but is almost "crystalline" in composition and is "crystal clear". It is one of the driest tissues in the body, and therefore has low signal intensity on MR.

Lensometer Also called Verometer, is a device used to measure the refractive power of eyeglasses and contact lenses.

Leptin This protein was been portrayed as the way to a cure for obesity. Leptin was first described as an apiodocyte - derived signaling factor, which, after interaction with its receptors, induced a complex response, including control of bodyweight and energy expenditure. It could be quite a fat burner. Research shows that people who used high doses of leptin for six months lost weight, most of it bodyfat.

Leptospira A genus of the family Treponemataceae, thin coiled organisms, flagellated at the extremities, one or both of which are bent back like a hook. Both pathogenic and innocent forms have been isolated.

Lesion An alteration or abnormality in a tissue or cell; a pathological change.

Lesser curvature (stomach) The medial/superior border of the stomach, site of attachment for the gastric mesentery.

Lesser trochanter (femur) A process on the medial surface of the posterior border of the neck of the femur.

Lesser wing of sphenoid The triangular plate of bone that extends from the anterior portion of the sphenoid bone and helps form the roof of the orbit and floor of the anterior cranial fossa.

Leuc, leuk (prefix) White.

e.g. leukocyte - a white blood cell.

e.g. leukopenia - reduction in the number of leukocytes in the blood.

Leucine One of the three branched chain amino acids. They are called BCAA's because they structurally branch off another chain of atoms instead of forming a line. Studies have shown that BCAA's help to stimulate protein

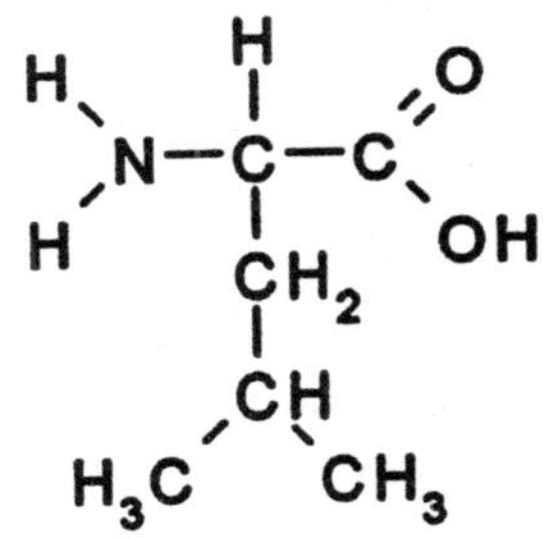

Fig. Leucine

synthesis and inhibit its breakdown, so BCAA's have powerful anabolic and anticatabolic effects on the body. They may also potentiate the release of some anabolic hormones, such as growth hormone. Regular ingestion of BCAA's help to keep the body in a state of postive nitrogen balance. In this state, your body much more readily builds muscle and burns fat. Studies have shown that athletes taking extra BCAA's have shown a loss of more bodyfat than those not taking BCAA's.

Leucine appears to be the most important BCAA for athletes, as it can affect various anabolic hormones, and have an effect on preventing protein degradation. HMB is a metabolite of Leucine. Some experts have suggested that if you do not have Leucine in your body, you will not have muscle growth.

Leukemia Cancer that begins in developing blood cells in the bone marrow.

Leukocyte A general name for white, nucleated blood cells found in the blood and lymphatic tissue.

Leukoencephalitis Inflammation of the white matter of the brain.

Leukorrhea Vaginal discharge characterized by a white or yellowish color. Primarily composed of mucus. Common during pregnancy.

Levator palpebrae muscle Muscle responsible for raising the upper eyelid. It originates at the upper border of the optic foramen/ orbital rim and inserts into the tarsal palate (cartilage) of the upper eyelid.

Level of Practice Four distinct stages that are characterized by a particular perspective, type of decision making and level of involvement with patients, families and colleagues.

Level of product protection The level of protection required for an area based on an assessment by the manufacturer of contamination risk.

LH (LH) Luteinizing Hormone A pituitary hormone that stimulates the gonads. In the man LH is necessary for spermatogenesis (Sertoli cell function) and for the production of testosterone (Leydig cell function). In the woman LH is necessary for the production of estrogen. When estrogen reaches a critical peak, the pituitary releases a surge of LH (the LH spike), which releases the egg from the follicle.

Liaison committee on medical education LCME A group organized under the sponsorship of the American medical association (AMA) and American Association of Medical Colleges (AAMC) to accredit educational programs leading to the MD degree in the US and Canada.

License Approval from a local or state health department to operate as a healthcare provider in that state. Facilities may be licensed as Skilled Nursing Facilities, Intermediate Care Facilities, Assisted Living Facilities, Home Health Agencies, or under a variety of other licensure types. Individuals may be licensed as physicians, nurses, certified nurse aides, therapists, or pharmacists. Provider types and licensure requirements vary greatly from state to state.

Licensed Practical Nurses Licensed practical nurses (LPNs), or licensed vocational nurses (LVNs) care for the sick, injured, convalescent and disabled under the direction of physicians and registered nurses. LPN training lasts about 1 year and is available in about 1,100 state-approved programs, mostly in vocational or technical schools. Most LPNs provide basic bedside care. LPNs in nursing homes provide routine care and help evaluate residents' needs. In doctors' offices and clinics, they also may make appointments, keep records, and perform other clerical duties. LPNs who work in private homes also may prepare meals and teach family members simple nursing tasks.

Licensure The process by which different governmental or non-governmental agencies, such as specialty boards or other bodies, grant permission to practice a profession to persons meeting predetermined qualifications to engage in a given occupation or use a particular title. In the case of physicians, licensure ensures that they have appropriate education and training and that they abide by recognized standards of professional conduct while serving their patients. This is typically done at a national or local level. In the United States licensure is a process by which physicians receive permission to practice medicine. Candidates for licensure first must complete the rigorous United States Medical Licensing Examination (USMLE), designed to assess a physician's ability to apply knowledge, concepts, and principles that are important in health and disease and that constitute the basis of safe and effective patient care. All applicants must submit proof of medical education and training and provide details about their work history. Results of the USMLE are reported to state medical boards for use in granting the initial license to practice medicine. Each medical licensing authority requires, as part of its licensing processes, successful completion of an examination or other certification demonstrating qualification for licensure.

Life Care A promise to provide care for the resident for the rest of his or her life, in exchange for a significant up-front payment. Once popular offerings of Continuing Care Retirement Communities, Life Care Contracts are less common now because of the significant risk to the issuer. However, older communities may still be obligated on contracts entered into in earlier years.

Life-long learning Continuous training over the course of a professional career. Because medical science changes so rapidly, it is vital that its practitioners are committed to and engage in life-long learning.

Lifestyle A general manner of living based on the interplay between living conditions in the broad sense and individual patterns of behavior as determined by socio-cultural factors and personal characteristics. The range of behavior patterns open to individuals may be limited or extended by social environmental factors. For this reason, lifestyles are usually considered in the context of both collective and individual experiences and general conditions of life. A change of lifestyle may include such activities as stopping cigarette smoking, changing the pattern of nutrition or engaging in regular physical exercise.

Ligand A molecule or ion that is bound to protein.

Ligase An enzyme used to catalyze the joining of single-stranded DNA segments.

Ligation Interruption with a suture or tie.

Light box A set of bright, full-spectrum light bulbs inside a box with a reflective background and diffusing screen; produces light that's 10 to 20 times stronger than ordinary indoor light. Used to treat winter depression, or SAD (seasonal affective disorder). Treatment typically involves spending 15 minutes to 3 hours in front of a light box every day in the fall, winter, and early spring. Research suggests that bright lights help regulate the body's internal clock, which controls hormone secretion and sleep patterns.

Light emitting diodes (LEDs) Tiny light sources (frequently used in digital watches and electronic equipment) that have been used in the field of phototherapy. Their power output is low enough to be safe for human exposure but strong enough to stimulate the biological responses involved in healing. Research indicates that LEDs may accelerate the healing of skin wounds and certain other conditions.

Lightening Change in the shape of the pregnant uterus a few weeks before labor. Often described as the baby "dropping."

Linea nigra Line of increased pigmentation running down the abdomen from the bellybutton to the pubic area during pregnancy.

Linkage The proximity of two or more markers (e.g., genes, RFLP markers) on a chromosome; the closer together the markers are, the lower the probability that they will be separated during DNA repair or replication processes (binary fission in prokaryotes, mitosis or meiosis in eukaryotes), and hence the greater the probability that they will be inherited together.

Linkage map A map of the relative positions of genetic loci on a chromosome, determined on the basis of how often the loci are inherited together. Distance is measured in centimorgans (cM).

Linoleic Acid An essential fatty acid (EFA) that your body cannot make itself. It is found in polyunsaturated oils such as safflower, sunflower, walnut oil, etc. This is considered a type of 'good' fat. You need approxiamately 2% of your daily calories as EFA's.

Linton Procedure A procedure involving ligation of venous perforators in the leg via an open longitudinal incision.

Lip(o) (prefix) Fat; lipid.

e.g. lipoma - a benign tumor of fat cells.

Lipids Hydrophobic biological compounds (fats and fatlike materials) that are insoluble in water, but soluble in nonpolar solvents such as benzene, chloroform, and ether. The major components in most lipids are fatty acids.

Lipoprotein A conjugated protein containing a lipid, prosthetic group.

Liposome An artificial phospholipid vesicle. Liposomes can be useful for the enclosure of macromolecules such as nucleic acids or, after loading with an appropriate drug. They may be used therapeutically to achieve slow release of the drug into circulation.

Lipotropic nutrients Substances that prevent or curtail the buildup of fat in the liver, such as B-fatty acids and methionine.

Lith (prefix) Stone. e.g. lithotomy - removal of a stone.

Lithotripsy A procedure done to break up stones in the urinary tract using ultrasonic shock waves, so that the fragments can be easily passed from the body.

Live at Level of practice that the clinician consistently practices at. There will always be times when a clinical situation can be described at another level (visiting) but it is not representative of practice. To live at a level is to be consistent with that level of practice. There are four levels of practice: Entry, Clinician, Advanced Clinician and Clinical Scholar.

Live birth The complete expulsion or extraction from its mother of a product of conception, irrespective of the duration of the pregnancy, which after such separation, breathes or shows other evidence of life, such as beating of the heart, pulsation of the umbilical cord, or definite movement of voluntary muscles, whether or not the umbilical cord has been cut or the placenta is attached. Each product of such a birth is considered liveborn.

Liver function tests Blood tests that indicate how well the liver is working.

Liver The liver is the largest solid organ in the body, just under the right upper quadrant of the abdoment, just under the diaphragm. It's primary role is in support of digestion, where it processes nutrients absorbed by the intestinal mucosa. The venous drainage from the intestines enters the liver through the portal veins. The liver also has a separate arterial supply, and the hepatic veins empty directly into the inferior vena cava. The liver also secretes bile, and "filters" the gastrointestinal blood. The liver has 'reticuloendothelial cells' that can trap microsopic particles from the blood. The liver may be imaged by US, CT, MR and functional Nuclear Medicine studies.

Load To transfer programs or data from secondary to primary storage. For example, when a program is started, the information contained in its files are copied from the hard drive to the RAM.

Local Anesthesia Provides pain control at the site of a surgical procedure by injection of the site with a medication. No sedation or relaxation is induced.

Localize Determination of the original position (locus) of a gene or other marker on a chromosome.

Locus The position on a chromosome of a gene or other chromosome marker; also, the DNA at that position. The use of locus is sometimes restricted to mean regions of DNA that are expressed.

Long Term Care(LTC) Widely-used terminology to describe care provided for people who need assistance or care on a long term basis, as opposed to the short term of a hospital stay or acute illness. An umbrella term for Skilled Care, Intermediate Care, Personal Care, Home Care, Adult Day Care, Respite Care, and other types of non-acute care. Long term care is often provided for people with chronic illnesses, physical or mental disabilities, or problems with activities of daily living, all of which generally lead to the need for life-long assistance once they occur.

Long Term Care Facility Terminology used to refer to licensed care facilities other than nursing homes. They might include an Assisted Living Facility, an Alzheimer's facility, a Christian Science setting, a Hospice facility, a Personal Care Home, a Residential Care Facility, an Adult Foster Home, a Domiciliary Care Facility, or an Adult Congregate Care Facility. Terminology and licensing requirements vary widely by region.

Long Term Care Insurance Insurance which provides a benefit for nursing home stays or other long term care services. Benefits and qualifying services vary considerably from policy to policy, however all policies cover at least some stays in a licensed nursing home. Some, but not all, policies cover other non-acute services, such as stays in assisted living facilities or home care services. Premiums may be tax-deductible and benefits may be exempt from income tax for qualified plans.

Long range restriction mapping Restriction enzymes are proteins that cut DNA at precise locations. Restriction maps depict the positions on chromosomes of restriction enzyme cutting sites. These are used as biochemical "signposts", or markers of specific areas along the chromosomes. The map will detail the positions on the DNA molecule that are cut by particular restriction enzymes.

Longus capitus muscle Muscle responsible for flexing the head. It originates at the transverse processes of the third to the sixth cervical vertebrae, and inserts into the basal portion of the occipital bone.

Longus colli muscle The long muscles of the neck, responsible for flexion and support of the cervical vertebrae.

Low birth weight Less than 2,500 g (up to and including 2,499 g).

Low Level Care In low level care residents can live independently, but get help with meals and laundry, and personal care like dressing and bathing.

Lower Esophageal Sphincter The last few centimeters of esophagus which are intro-abdominal and form a functional mechanism to prevent the reflux of material from the stomach into the esophagus yet relaxes in a coordinated fashion to permit passage of a food bolus into the stomach.

Lower flammability level (LFL) The minimum concentration of vapor in air at which propagation of flame will occur in the presence of an ignition source. LFL is sometimes referred to as LEL or Lower Explosive Limit.

Lower GI series A study that looks at the rectum, the large intestine, and the lower part of the small intestine. A fluid called barium that shows up well on x-rays is given into the rectum as an enema. X-rays of the abdomen shows strictures (narrowed areas), obstructions (blockages), and other problems.

LP needle Lumbar puncture needle.

LPS (lipopolysaccharide) Molecule found in the outer cell walls of some bacteria that trigger the immune response resulting in fever. Also referred to as pyrogens or as endotoxins, though, strictly speaking, they are not endotoxins but predominant components of endotoxins produced by gram-negative bacteria. Common cause of pyrogenic reactions in parenteral products.

Lumbar Relating to the lower back.

Lumbar artery A segmental artery which originates from the abdominal aorta and branches into dorsal and spinal branches.

Lumbar spine Portion of the vertebral column located between the thorax and the pelvis.

Lupus Lupus is an autoimmune disease, caused by the body's immune system mistakenly attacking its own tissues and organs. Lupus is a chronic inflammatory condition that can affect one or more organs, including the skin, blood, joints, heart, lungs and kidneys. There are four different types of lupus.

Luteal Phase The Luteal Phase (in relation to conception) is the time period beginning with the day after ovulation and running through the remainder of your menstrual cycle (it ends the day before your next period). Typically, the duration of the luteal phase phase lasts between 10 and 16 days - and is generally consistent from cycle to cycle, averaging for most women at 14 days.

Lutein A carotenoid phytonutrient with antioxidant properties especially important to eye protection.

Luteinizing Hormone Luteinizing Hormone (LH) A pituitary hormone that stimulates the gonads. In the man LH is necessary for spermatogenesis (Sertoli cell function) and for the production of testosterone (Leydig cell function). In the woman LH is necessary for the production of estrogen. When estrogen reaches a critical peak, the pituitary releases a surge of LH (the LH spike), which releases the egg from the follicle.

Luteinizing Hormone Surge (LH Surge) The spiking release of luteinizing hormone (LH) that causes release of a mature egg from the follicle. Ovulation test kits detect the sudden increase of LH, signaling that ovulation is about to occur (usually within 24-36 hours).

Lycopene Most powerful of the carotenoid antioxidants; shown to be beneficial in prostate protection and treatment.

Lymph nodes Regions of lymphoid tissue organized into lymphoid organs located along the lymphatic vessels. They are the main source of production of circulating lymphocytes and "filter" lymph to remove noxious agents.

Lymphangiectasia Dilation of the lymphatic vessels; may be congenital or acquired.

Lymphatic vessels Vessels through which lymph is transported throughout the body.

Lymphatics The vast network of vascular channels that drain all tissues, process the drained fluid through lymph nodes and ultimately return the fluid to the blood.

Lymphedema A pattern of tissue swelling related to obstruction of lymphatic flow.

Lymphocintogram A nuclear medicine study in which an area of the body is injected with a radioactive isotope and an x-ray image of the lymphatic flow pattern is obtained.

Lymphocyte A type of white blood cell accounting for 20-25% of the white cells in humans. They are mostly non-phagocytic and actively mobile and are continuously made in the bone marrow. They are the immediate precursors of all antibody-forming cells.

Lymphoma A neoplastic disorder of lymphocytes.

Lyophilization Also known as freeze drying, it is a means of stabilizing wet substances by freezing them, then evaporating the resulting ice, to leave a substantially dry, porous residue which has the same size and shape of the original frozen mass.

Lyophilizer A freeze dryer.

Lysate A product of lysis, which is the disintegration or dissolution of the cell walls.

Lysine As essential, basic amino acid obtained from many proteins by hydrolysis.

Lysis The dissolution or destruction of red blood cells, bacteria, or other antigens by a specific lysin (antibody), or by the action of detergents, thus allowing the cell contents to escape.

Lysosome A membrane-surrounded organelle in the cytoplasm of eukaryotic cells; it contains many hydrolytic enzymes.

M

Ma Huang A herb that yields the stimulant Ephedra.

Mab Monoclonal Antibody).

Machine lines/process lines Surface topography created from machining or honing/polishing lines will normally run parallel but bisecting (perpendicular) lines may occur when the honing stone mandrel is removed from the work piece.

Machine welding Welding with equipment that performs the welding operation under the constant observation and control of a welding operator. The equipment may or may not perform the loading and unloading of the works.

Macintosh A highly successful line of personal computers designed by Apple Computers. Called a "Mac" for short, Macintosh computers, with their operating system called "System", practically pioneered the graphical user interface. Using a system of a desktop work area and icons to represent files, Macs were a long-time favorite for people wanting ease-of-use and a visual interface.

Macro A mini-program which will execute a series of commands in series, saving the user having to repeat typing or data input. Macros are typically created to perform frequently used tasks.

Macromolecules Molecules whose molecular weights are greater than about 5,000 Daltons.

Macroparticle Particle with an equivalent diameter greater than 5 μm. ISO/FDIS 14644-1.

Macrophage A phagocytic cell of the immune system found in blood and connective tissue and involved in removing debris after injury.

Macrorestriction map Map depicting the order of and distance between sites at which restriction enzymes cleave chromosomes.

Macroreticular resin An ion exchange resin with a reticular porous matrix that makes it effective for removing colloids and bacteria from process streams, as well as dissolved anions. It is especially useful for preventing colloidal and organic fouling of mixed-bed resins and premature clogging of final filters.

Macula The most sensitive part of the retina that is about the size of a pinhead and is where our most detailed vision occurs.

Macular degeneration A deterioration of the central portion of the retina known as the macula.

Magnesium Mineral necessary for energy metabolism, protein and fat synthesis, neuromuscular transmission, amonia scavenging and binding of calcium to teeth, etc. Aids in bone growth, and is necessary for proper functioning of nerves and muscles.

Magnetic resonance imaging (MRI) A radiologic imaging procedure that uses a magnetic field and radiofrequency waves to produce an image.

Magnetic therapy Magnetic field therapy or bio-magnetic therapy involves the use of magnets, magnetic devices or magnetic fields to treat a variety of physical and emotional conditions, including circulatory problems, certain forms of arthritis, chronic pain, sleep disorders, and stress.

Main pulmonary artery Artery originating from the conus arteriosus of the right ventricle, and dividing into the right and left pulmonary arteries under the arch of the aorta. Carries deoxygenated blood to the lungs.

Maintainability Ease with which maintenance can be performed.

Makeup air External air introduced to the air handling system for ventilation and pressurization.

Malabsorption syndrome Problems with how the small intestine absorbs nutrients from the foods we eat.

Malacia (suffix) Softening.

e.g. osteomalacia - softening of the bone.

Malignant GTN Malignant GTN-Cancerous change of gestational trophoblastic disease.

Malingering A voluntary or intentional reduction in visual acuity or other examination data.

Malleolus Rounded bone process located at either side of the ankle joint. The medial malleolus is part of the distal tibia, the lateral malleolus is the distal fibula.

Malleus The largest auditory ossicle (small bone), which attaches to the tympanic membrane (ear drum) and connects to the incus. Through mechanical linkages, the sound vibrations are amplified and transmitted to the oval window of the cochlea.

Malnutrition A situation caused by eating a poorly balanced diet, or by not eating enough food to meet the body's needs.

Malposition Faulty or abnormal position of a part of the body.

Maltitol This is a sugar alcohol that is used as a sweetener. It has half the caloric value of sucrose because it is not completely absorbed by the body.

Maltodextrin A long chain of glucose molecules (carbohydrates) that provides sustained energy without sharply increasing insulin levels. Essentially a chain of molecules of the simple sugar glucose linked together. There are an average of seven glucose molecules linked together to form a maltodextrin molecule.

Mammary Duct Ectasia An inflammatory breast condition caused by ductal obstruction but which may produce symptoms which may be confused with carcinoma, notably a mass and nipple retraction.

Mammillary bodies Two small protuberances located on the ventral surface of the cerebrum. They are created by the underlying medial, intermediate and lateral mammillary nuclei and mark the most posterior border of the ventral hypothalamus. The medial mamillary nucleus receives the postcommissural fornix and giv es rise to the mammilothalamic and mammillotegmental tracts.

Mammogram Mammogram—X-ray study of the breasts to identify normal and abnormal breasttissue.

Managed Care Programs where a health plan manages the care needs of its enrollees and a pool of money to pay for those needs. The health plan is paid on a capitated (or per capita) basis for the people in its program, and then provides services directly, or contracts for them using third parties.

Contracts with other providers may include capitated payments, or may be fee-for-service payments.

Managed competition Health care market regulations which use competition as the means to promote efficiency of the health care system. Within the framework of government intervention, managed competition helps to achieve policy objectives including price control, cost containment, quality control, control of pattern of service provision, greater accountability of local managers, closure of surplus facilities, control of powerful professional groups and greater equity in service access.

Mandible The lower jaw bone.

Mandibular condyles Posterior superior process of the mandibular ramus that articulates with the mandibular fossa of the temporal bone. (You can feel this while chewing, by putting your finger in your external ear canal.

Manganese Needed for normal tendon and bone structure.

Manipulation Application of manual force for healing. Term describes the techniques used in osteopathy, chiropractic, massage, and other bodywork therapies. Manipulation may involve various forms of massage, muscle pressure, and joint realignment or adjustment.

Mantra In Hinduism and Buddhism, mystic word used in ritual and meditation. It is believed to have power to bring into being the reality it represents. Use of such mantras usually requires initiation by a guru, or spiritual teacher.

Manual welding Welding in which the entire operation is performed and controlled completely by hand.

Manubrium The cranial part of the sternum that articulates with the first two pairs of ribs and the clavicles.

Manufacture All operations of receipt of materials, production, packaging, repackaging, labelling, relabelling, quality control, release, storage and distribution of APIs and the related controls.

Manufacturer The party responsible for the quality of the drug product.

Manufacturing process (biotechnology) The basic processes for rDNA fermentation and purification normally include the following steps:

1. Inoculum Preparation: The aim is to develop for the production stage fermentation a pure inoculum in sufficient volume and in the fast-growing (logari-thmic) phases so that a high population density is obtained. This is accomplished through a seed fermentation train.

2. The Medium: This is designed to provide the microorganism with all the nutrients it requires. Provision is usually made to add nutrients during fermentation.

3. Oxygen Supply: An adequate supply of oxygen is required. As oxygen is only slightly soluble in water, a number of methods are used to make oxygen more readily available to the microorganisms in the broth, including sparging, mechanical agitators, and dispersion baffles in the fermenter tank.

4. Temperature Control: Heat is generated both by the metabolism of nutrients and by the power dissipated in stirring and has to be removed by controlled cooling. Tank jackets or internal coils are used to control temperature.

5. Antifoam Agents: Microbiological systems that are vigorously stirred and aerated usually produce foam. Excessive foam cannot be tolerated and so provisions have to be made for adding antifoam agents.

6. Harvesting: This is the removal of the cells from the broth. This can be accomplished by cross-flow filtration or centrifugation.

7. Cell Lysis: With E. coli fermentations, the product protein is contained within the cell in the form of an inclusion body. High-pressure homogenizers are often used to chop up the E. coli bacteria into fine fragments, liberating the inclusion bodies for further processing.

8. Purification: This is the separation of the desired product from the other constituents in the harvested broth. Various processes including refolding, ultrafiltration/diafiltration, centrifugation, and chromatographic columns are employed to purify the product. Mapping

Marker An identifiable physical location on a chromosome (e.g., restriction enzyme cutting site, gene) whose inheritance can be monitored. Markers can be expressed regions of DNA (genes) or some segment of DNA with no known coding function but whose pattern of inheritance can be determined.

Mask of pregnancy Mask of pregnancy—Increased pigmentation over the area of the face under each eye. Commonly has the appearance of a butterfly.

Massage therapy This is a general term for a range of therapeutic approaches with roots in both Eastern and Western cultures. Involves the practice of kneading or otherwise manipulating a person's muscles and soft tissue.

Masseter muscle One of the muscles of mastication (chewing). Muscle raises the mandible and closes the jaw.

Mastoid air cells The air spaces within the mastoid process of the temporal bone. The communicate with the pharynx via the eustachian tube.

Mastoid process Process projecting inferoanteriorly from the petrous portion of the temporal bone, anterior to the ear.

Material A general term used to denote raw materials (starting materials, reagents, process aids, solvents) intermediates, APIs (Active Pharmaceutical Ingredients) and packaging and labelling materials.

Material containment The method to incorporate suitable measures into design procedures and operational practices for the containment of materials that can harm personnel and the workplace environment, and minimize potential for cross contamination and housekeeping concerns in the fine chemical, bulk pharmaceutical and pharmaceutical industries. Solids and/or liquids are normally most hazardous in the form of powders and have been divided into the following three categories:

1. Biologically Hazardous additives are compounds that when contacting a living cell, will alter, endanger, or damage the cell in some shape or form. These should be treated as requiring total containment.

2. Chemically Hazardous additives are compounds that when coming into contact with an oxidant, will cause harm to its surroundings due to reaction and/or oxidation. These products usually require containment and/or blanketing with an inert gas.

3. General Intermediates are compounds that are neither biologically nor chemically hazardous additives but they will cause a housekeeping problem. They usually require dusting prevention.

Maternal death The death of a women while pregnant or within 42 days of termination of pregnancy, irrespective of the duration and the site of the pregnancy, from any cause related to or aggravated by the pregnancy or its management, but not from accidental or incidental causes. Maternal death is subdivided into two groups

Maternal mortality rate The number of maternal deaths per 100,000 women of reproductive age (15-49).

Maternal mortality ratio The number of maternal deaths per 100,000 live births during the same time period.

Maxilla The upper jaw bone that contributes to the formation of the orbit, nasal cavity, and the palate.

Maxillary antrum The large paranasal sinus under the cheekbones, also called the maxillary sinus.

Maxillary artery Originates from the external carotid artery and gives these branches: pterygoid rami, deep auricular, anterior tympanic, inferior alveolar, middle meningeal, masseteric, deep temporal, buccal, posterior superior alveolar, infraorbital, descending palatine, spheno-palatine, and artery of the pterygoid canal ("Vidian artery").

Maxillary sinus One of the paransal sinuses, located on either side of the body of the maxillary bone.

Maximize Button In Windows, a button in the upper right corner of a Window that, when clicked, enlarges the window to its maximum size. When the window is already at its maximum size,the maximize button switches to the restore button, which returns the window to its previous size.

Maximum Cr/Fe ratio The maximum ratio of chromium to iron and the depth at which it occurs are the most direct measures of the chromium enrichment in a material oxide layer. Typical ratios are about 1.5 or greater for well-electropolished 316L stainless steel. The depth at which the maximum Cr/Fe ratio is found varies but is usually about one-half the oxide thickness.

Maximum depth of enrichment In stainless steel the chromium enrichment layer comprises all depths at which the chromium concentration is greater than the iron concentration. For well electropolished 316L stainless steel, the maximum depth of this layer is typically 20 to 25 angstroms (Å). Chromium Enrichment Layer Thickness).

Maximum working pressure The pressure at which the system is capable of operating for a sustained period.

Maximum Working Temperature The maximum temperature at which the system may operate for a sustained period. The maximum working temperature should relate to the maximum working pressure and the fluids involved.

McDonald cerclage Surgical procedure performed on an incompetent cervix. A drawstring-type suture holds the cervical opening closed during pregnancy.

Mean kinetic temperature (MKT) The single calculated temperature at which the degradation of an article would be equivalent to the actual degradation that results from actual temperature fluctuations during the storage period. It is not a simple arithmetical mean. The MKT is calculated from average storage temperatures recorded over a one-year period, with a minimum of 12 equally spaced storage temperatures being recorded.

Meatus M. (Internal Acoustic): A short passage on the posterior surface of the petrous temporal bone that transmits the facial and vestibulocochlear nerves and the labyrinthine artery.

Mechanical completion The point in a project at which all equipment and materials have been installed, but not commissioned (started-up).

Meckel's diverticulum A problem that occurs as a baby is developing during pregnancy, in which a small pouch (or sac) forms in the ileum.

Meconium First intestinal discharge of the newborn; green or yellow in color. It consists of epithelial or surface cells, mucus and bile. Discharge may occur before or during labor or soon after birth.

Media (plural of medium) Substances used to provide sterile nutrients to the fermentation or cell growth process supporting the growth of the live microorganisms. Media may be liquid (broth) or solid, and generally include sucrose or glucose as a carbon source, various minerals, a nitrogen source, and selected growth factors.

Media prep The act of preparing nutrient media for cell culture or fermentation.

Medial Toward the midline of the body (example, the middle toe is located at the medial side of the foot).

Medial articular facet (tibial plateau) The articulating surface of the proximal tibia, forming a joint with the medial and lateral condyles of the distal femur.

Medial geniculate boby (nucleus) Nuclear mass that is part of the ventrocaudal thalamus (metathalamus). It is the auditory relay nucleus which receives afferents from the inferior colliculus via the brachium of the inferior colliculus and giv es rise to the auditory radiation.

Medial meniscus A semicircular disk of fibrocartilage between the medial condyle and medial tibial plateau, attached to the medial margin of the superior articulating surface of the tibia.

Torn Meniscus.

Medial pterygoid plate On of a pair of projections from the greater wing of the sphenoid bone that help form the lateral wall of the nasal cavity.

Median Lying in the midline.

Median eminence (of the tuber cinereum) Midline part of the tuber cinereum that forms the floor of the thid ventricle

Median plane Sagittal plane through the midline of the body; divides the body or any of its parts into right and left halves.

Mediastinum That area in the middle of the chest containing the heart, great vessels, esophagus and other structures.

MedicalInformatics Medical informatics is a scientific field that deals with the storage, retrieval and optimal use of information and data. Rapid development is due to advances in computing, communication technology and an increasing awareness that the knowledge base of medicine is essentially unmanageable by traditional paper-based methods.

Medical devices Any health care product that does not achieve its principal intended purposes by chemical action in or on the body or by being metabolized. The term "devices" also includes components, parts, or accessories of medical devices, diagnostic aids such as reagents, antibiotic sensitivity disks, and test kits for in vitro diagnosis of diseases and other conditions. There are three classes of medical devices:

1. Class I, General Controls (registration of manufacturers, recordkeeping and labeling requirements, compliance with GMPs).
2. Class II, Special Controls (including performance standards, posmarket surveillance, and patient registries).
3. Class III, Premarket Approval (implanted and life supporting or life sustaining devices).

Medical Doctor (MD) A physician licensed by state law to practice medicine.

Medical education The process of teaching, learning and training of students with an ongoing integration of knowledge, experience, skills, qualities, responsibility and values which qualify an individual to practice medicine. It is divided into undergraduate, postgraduate and continuing medical education, but increasingly there is a focus on the "lifelong" nature of medical education.

Undergraduate education or basic medical education refers to the period beginning when a student enters medical school and ends with the final examination for basic medical qualification. This period of education comprises a pre-clinical and a clinical period. It can result in granting a license to practice, which may be provisional and subject to conditions as to supervision; or permitting the start of postgraduate education. In the United States, however, undergraduate education refers to pre-medical college education, which results in a Bachelor's degree and is the training most students receive before entering medical school.

Postgraduate education, graduate medical education or specialty training is used to designate the more or less continuous period of post-basic training which, when it occurs, normally directly follows undergraduate training and is designed to lead to competence in a chosen branch of medical practice.

Medical Nutrition Therapy A diet ordered by a physician as part of treatment for a disease or clinical condition, or to eliminate, decrease or increase specific nutrients in the diet. (May also be called Therapeutic Diet).

MedicalEducator A professional who focuses on the educational process necessary to transform students into physicians. Some medical educators are physicians, but an increasing number have backgrounds in education, behavioral or other health sciences.

Medicalschool A higher education or university level institution offering a prescribed course of medicine. The following are examples of the names that such institutions may bear and which vary from one country to another or even within countries: Medical College; College of Surgeons; Medical Institute; Institute of Medicine and Pharmacy; Institute of Medicine and Surgery; Faculty of Medicine; Faculty of Medical Sciences; Faculty of Medicine and Surgery; Academy of Medicine or Medical Academy; University Center for Health Sciences; Medical University; Faculty of Medicine and Pharmacy.

Medicare The national health insurance program for people age 65 or older in the United States. Medicare pays for acute medical care services under either Part A Hospital Insurance (HI) or Part B Supplementary Medical Insurance (SMI). Medicare is not a needs-based program, but provides coverage for acute care services to most people age 65 or over. Most chronic care services, including many nursing home stays, are not covered under the Medicare program.

Medication Error Medications not given as intended by prescriber, as required by the drug manufacturer, or according to acceptable professional standards.

Medicinal product Any substance or combination of substances presented for treating or preventing disease in human beings or animals. Any substance or combination of substances that may be administered to human beings or animals with a view to making a medical diagnosis or to restoring, correcting or modifying physiological functions in human beings or in animals is likewise considered a medicinal product.

Medicine, Holistic/Wholistic Wholistic medicine is a broadly descriptive term for a healing philosophy that views a patient as a whole person, not as just a disease or a collection of symptoms. In the course of treatment, wholistic medical practitioners may address emotional and spiritual dimensions as well as the nutritional, environmental and lifestyle factors that may contribute to an illness. Many wholistic practitioners combine conventional forms of treatment with natural or alternative treatments.

Medigap Private insurance which covers some of the gaps in Medicare coverage, such as the deductibles and coinsurance.

Medilla oblongata The tapering posterior most division (myelencephalon) of the hindbrain or rhombencephalon. It is interposed between the pons and the spinal cord.

Meditation Discipline in which the mind is focused on a single point of reference. Employed since ancient times in various forms by all religions, the practice gained greater notice in the recent times, as interest in Zen Buddhism rose. Meditation is now used by many nonreligious adherents as a method of stress reduction; known to lower levels of cortisol, a hormone released in response to stress. Enhances recuperation and improves the body's resistance to disease.

Medium (filter) The material from which a filter is constructed.

Medium Chain Triglycerides (MCT) MCT's are technically fats, but they have very unique properties. The difference between them and other fats lies in their molecular structure. MCT's are shorter than other fats, which allows them to be burned rather quickly by the body for energy. MCT's enter the mitochondria, the powerhouse of a cell, without assistance, and do not require the usual transport mechanism.

MCT's are an attractive supplement because of their calorie density. They have 9 calories per gram, like fats, but lack the disposition to be stored as fat. All fats are not created equal. Research shows that animals maintain a lower bodyfat when they use MCT's in place of traditional fats.

They can help you increase lean muscle tissue, decrease excess bodyfat and fuel precompetition workouts.

Medulla (Oblongata) The cone of nerve tissue anterior to the cerebellum and connecting the pons with the cervical spinal cord. It contains nerves responsible for respiration, circulation and special senses.

Medullary cavity Within a long bone, the portion of the diaphysis containing marrow.

Mega (prefix) Great.

e.g. megakaryocyte - the giant cell of the bone marrow that has a greatly lobulated nucleus and gives rise to blood platelets.

Megabase (Mb) Unit of length for DNA fragments equal to 1 million nucleotides and roughly equal to 1Centimorgan (cM).

Megabyte or MB A unit of data measurement equal to approximately one million bytes. Hard drive manufacturers use an even number as a multiplier. In this case 1 MB would be 1,000,000 bytes.

Megaly (suffix) Great, large.

e.g. splenomegaly - enlargement of the spleen.

Megohm cm/B A measure of ionic purity in water.

Meiosis The process of two consecutive cell divisions in the diploid progenitors of sex cells. Meiosis results in four rather than two daughter cells, each with a haploid set of chromosomes.

Melan (prefix) Black.

e.g. melanin - black pigment of the hair, skin, ciliary body, choroid, retina, and certain nerve cells.

Melanoma A cancer that begins in skin cells called melanocytes and spreads to internal organs.

Melatonin Hormone produced by the pineal gland in the brain and released mainly at night in the absence of light on the retina. Regulates the onset and timing of sleep and seasonal changes in the body such as winter weight gain. Levels of melatonin decline with age. Melatonin is being investigated as a sleep promoter and to prevent or reduce jet lag. Synthetic melatonin and melatonin derived from bovine pineal glands are available as over-the-counter dietary supplements. Melatonin occurs naturally in some foods but in fairly small amounts. Reported side effects include reduced fertility, inhibition of male sexual drive, hypothermia, damage to the retina. Some physicians and scientists advise against taking melatonin as a long-term supplement.

Membrane A barrier, usually thin, that only permits the passage of particles of a certain size or special nature. Filtration membranes are thin polymer films that are permeable to water and other fluids:

1. Microporous membrane filters have measurable pore structures that physically remove particles or microorganisms larger than pore size.

2. Ultrafiltration membranes (sometimes called molecular sieves) also remove molecules larger than a specified molecular weight.

3. Reverse osmosis membranes are permeable to water molecules and very little else, rejecting even dissolved ions and endotoxins in water.

Membraneous urethra The portion of the urethra located between the pars prostatica ("prostatic urethra") and pars spongiosa ("penile urethra") in the male.

Mengingioma A hard, firm, or rubbery, slowly growing extraaxial neoplasm, hypervascular, and arising from the arachnoid. They are usually attached to the dura. Meningiomas may cause erosion and thinning of the skull, as well as hyperostosis (bone thickening).

Meningioma.

Meninges The three membranes covering the brain and spinal cord - the dura mater, arachnoid, and pia mater.

Meningiomas Benign brain tumors of arachnoid origin.

Meningo (prefix) Membrane; meninges.

e.g. meningoencephalitis - inflammation of the brain and its meninges.

Meningomyelocele Meningomyelocele-Congenital defect of the central nervous system of the baby. Membranes and the spinal cord protrude through an opening or defect in the vertebral column.

Meniscus Thin cartilaginous discs, found in the knee between the femur and the tibia, in the jaw between the mandibular condyle and fossa, that reduce friction. The menisci can be damaged by trauma or chronic stress.

Torn Meniscus.

Menopause The period that marks the permanent cessation of menstrual activity, usually occurring between the ages of 40 and 58.

Menstrual age Menstrual age .

Menstruation Menstruation-Regular or Periodic discharge of a bloody fluid from the uterus.

Mental Illness (MI) Individuals with organic or non-organic psychiatric diagnoses. Nursing homes are not normally allowed to admit and care for individuals with non-organic psychiatric diagnoses between the ages of 22 64 if they wish to receive reimbursement.

Mental Retardation (MR) Individuals with significant limitations in intellectual functioning and adaptive behavior characterized by impaired learning ability and impaired practical, social, and vocational skills. The application of the term mental retardation reflects the need for personalized supports that consider limitations in context of the individual's cultural community, linguistic diversity, and age peer group. (Adopted from the AAMR definition.)

Menu A list of operations or tasks available to a user in a given program, usually organized in some logical fashion. Users access a function or command by selecting it from the menu.

Meristem The growing point or area of rapidly dividing cells at the tip of a stem, root, or branch.

Mesencephalon The middle of the three primary brain vesicles in the embryonic brain. The adult derivative of which is the midbrain which is located between the diencephalon and the pons.

Mesentery Attachment of an organ to the body by a broad double layer of connective tissue in which blood vessels, nerves, lymphatics and other structures are contained.

Mesodermal germ layer Mesodermal germ layer—Tissue of the embryo that forms connective tissue, muscles, kidneys, ureters and other organs.

Mesophile An organism that grows best in the temperature range of 20°C to 50°C (68°F to 122°F).

Mesothelium The layer of flat cells lining the body cavity of the embryo; in the adult, it forms the simple squamous epithelium that covers the true serous membranes of the body. Mesothelium is derived from mesoderm.

Messenger RNA (mRNA) RNA that serves as a template for protein synthesis.

Metabolism The sum of the physical and chemical changes in living cells by which energy is provided for vital processes and growth in cell mass.

Metabolite Any of the various organic compounds produced by metabolism.

Metadata Electronic records that include processing parameters and audit trail logs. Metadata allows reviewers to replay the original result, or reconstruct a final report from raw data. In chromatography, metadata include integration parameters and calibration tables. An example of metadata can be in long division "1,000 ÷ 5" would be the raw data, the work you had to show on your paper in fourth grade math class would be the metadata, and "200" would be your result.

Metaphase The stage of cell division when chromosomes are aligned at the cell center prior to separation. A "metaphase spread" refers to the view of a cell's chromosomes in the metaphase stage on a slide.

Metaphysis Portion of a long bone, usually funnel-shaped between the shaft (diaphysis) and the epiphyseal (growth) plate. This is a region of growth and remodelling during development.

Metaplasia Change in the structure of a tissue into another type that is not normal for that tissue.

Metastases The plural of metastasis.

Metastasis In cancer, it is the appearance of neoplasms in parts of the body remote from the seat of the primary tumor. It also applies to the transportation of bacteria from one part of the body to another through the blood streams (hematogenous metastasis) or through lymph channels (lymphogenous metastasis).

Metastatic A tumor that has transfered from one organ (or part) to another not directly connected to it.

Metastatic lesion The transfer of any pathologic process from one body part to another. Metastasis is usually distinguished from "local extension". Metastasis can be carried by blood-flow ("hematogenous metastasis"), by lymphatic fluid, through the CSF dissemination, by the bronchi (lepidic spread), along the urinary tract, etc.

Metastasis.

Metatarsal phalangeal joint The point of junction between the metatarsals and phalanges of the foot.

Metatarsals The five long tubular bones of the foot between the tarsus and the phalanges.

Metathalamus A ventrocaudal subdivision of the thalamus which consists of the medial and lateral geniculate bodies.

Metencephalon The rostral subdivision of the hindbrain or rhombencephalon in the embryonic brain. It is situated between the midbrain (mesencephalon) and the medulla oblongata (myelencephalon). The adult derivative is the pons and cerebellum.

Methionine A sulfur bearing essential amino acid important in hair, nail and muscle production, liver maintenance (lipotropic effects), and production of creatine and other aminos.

Methods validation Establishing, through documented evidence, a high degree of assurance that an analytical method will consistently yield results that accurately reflect the quality characteristics of the product tested.

Methoxyflavone Also called 5-methyl-7-methoxyisoflavone. A synthetic isoflavone that is highly anabolic, yet free of any androgenic effects. It halts the muscle wasting, and increases lean tissue growth. It increases calcium phosphorous, potassium and nutrogen retition to a significant degree.

Methyl cellulose A common viscosity-increasing agent used in ophthalmics preparations. It is inversely soluble with temperature.

Mho Unit of measurement for conductance; the reciprocal of ohm (resistance).

Micro (prefix) Small.

e.g. microhepatia - a small liver.

Microbe A microscopic one-celled organism, animal or vegetable, a microorganism.

Microbiology The study of microscopic life such as bacteria and viruses.

Microcephaly Microcephaly- Abnormally small development of the head in the developing fetus.

Microcomputer The smallest and least expensive class of computers. Also called a personal computer.

Microencapsulated Surrounded by a thin, protective layer of biodegradable substance referred to as microsphere.

Microglia Small supporting cells of the central nervous system (neuroglia) derived from the mesoderm (blood histiocytes) and having a phagocytic function.

Microhmo A measure of conductance equal to one millionth of a mho.

Microinch A unit of length equal to one millionth of an inch (0.000001 inches).

Micrometastasis Refers to metastatic deposits of tumor that may consist of only a few cells.

Micron or micrometer A unit of length equal to one millionth of a meter (μm) or thousandth of a millimeter (25μm are approximately 0.001 inch.). Bacteria range in size from 0.5μm to 20μm.

Microorganism A microbe - A microscopic plant or animal, such as a bacterium, protozoan, yeast, virus, or algae.

Microphthalmia Microphthalmia-Abnormally small eyeballs.

Microsoft Corporation An incredibly successful supplier of computer software founded in 1975 by Bill Gates and his partner Paul Allen. Microsoft has grown to become the world leader in the software industry by supplying software to the world's largest computer base (IBM-compatibles). A large portion of Microsoft's success is due to its popular Windows operating environment.

Microsoft Internet Explorer Microsoft's World Wide Web browser.

Microsoft Windows 98 Windows 98 is the fifth version of Windows from Microsoft. However, unlike its predecessors, which were merely operating environments that ran on top of DOS, Windows 98 is its own stand-alone operating system. Integrating some of the most popular aspects of its rival, Macintosh's System, as well as the best elements of earlier Windows versions, Windows 98 is extremely easy to use and very powerful. Windows 98 is so named because it was released in 1998. Windows 2000 is now in early launch mode.

Microsoft Windows Windows was introduced as a graphical operating environment that simplified DOS commands and tasks by converting programs and commands to icons that were "clicked" (selected with a mouse or other pointing device) to initiate.

Windows also introduced the feature multi-tasking to the IBM-based computer.

Microstrabimus Also called microtropia, monofixation syndrome, and small angle strabismus. A small angle deviation (inward or outward, commonly inward) that is less than five degrees with some amount of stereopsis (depth perception) and anomalous retinal correspondence (ARC). Possible mild amblyopia, eccentric fixation, and/or anisometropia may also be present. It frequently results from the treatment of a larger-angle deviation (esotropia or exotropia) by optical correction, vision therapy, pharmacological agents, and/or extraocular muscle surgery. Treatment for microstrabimus consists mostly of correcting significant refractive errors and any coexisting amblyopia. The use of vision therapy and prisms to establish bifoveal fusion has been successful in selected cases.

Microwave (Targis) A catheter is placed within the bladder and positioned within the prostate, then the antenna emits microwaves. This procedure increases the passageway allowing for easier urination.

Midbrain (Mesencephalon)The portion of the brain developed from the middle of the three primary vesicles in the embryo. In cross-section, the midbrain resembles "Mickey Mouse": the ears are the cerebral peduncles.

Middle colic artery Artery which originates from the superior mesenteric artery, and supplies the transverse colon.

Middle ear bone complex The small bones (malleus("hammer"), incus ("anvil") and stapes ("stirrup"))that conduct sound from the tympanic membrane ("ear drum") to the oval window of the inner ear.

Middle sacral artery The continuation of the abdominal aorta, that branches into the lowest lumbar artery.

Midwifery Midwives provide education and support during pregnancy, assist the mother during labor and delivery and provide follow-up care. Practitioners of childbirth support include childbirth educators, childbirth assistants and women labor coaches who also provide post-partum home care.

Milk Thistle A herbal formula. Popular with bodybuilders because certain steroids are known to negatively impact the liver. Silymarin (the active ingredient of milk thistle) has been found to play a role in human regeneration of liver cells after damaged from alcohol, or liver disease, as a means for promoting would healing, and as a strong antoixidant. It also has been known to decrease elevated liver enzymes induced by certain type of drugs.

Milliequivalent To simplify the calculation of ion exchange resin capacity, total dissolved ion concentrations are usually converted into equivalent concentrations of calcium carbonate, the most common source of dissolved ions in water. Resin capacity is normally given in ppm as CaCO3, or in grains per gallon as CaCO3 (7,000 grains = 1 pound). However, it may also be given as milliequivalents per liter (meq/L). Since calcium carbonate has a molecular weight of 100 and an equivalent weight of 50 (because calcium has a valence of two) ppm as CaCO3 can be converted to meq/L by dividing by 50. Thus, 1 ppm of CaCO3 = 0.02 meg/L.

Mineral (Chelated) A chelated mineral is generally attached to a protein transporter molecule with the intent of improved transport across the gut to the blood stream. Although some of the minerals are well absorbed in this manner it does not necessarily always indicative of the best form for absorption.

Mineral Inorganic substances necessary for good health as an ingrediant or a catalyst.

Minienvironment The actual localized control space limited by a defined enclosure that separates or isolates the inside from the outside environment, such that the transfer of potential contamination from one side to the other is minimized or completely eliminated, depending on the design. Minienvironments are not always isolators.

Minimally invasive surgery (MIS) Procedural techniques which limit the size of the abdominal incisions by using small incisions to gain access to the surgical site.

Minimize Button In a Windows environments, the button is in the upper right corner of the window. When clicked it reduces the window to an icon (in Windows 3.x) or a taskbar button (Windows 95 and 98) in order to display the desktop.

Minimum Data Set A resident assessment which must be done for every resident in a nursing home. The MDS must be completed within a certain period of time from admission to the facility, and must be reviewed on a scheduled basis or whenever there is a significant change in the resident's condition. In the MDS, the resident's needs are scored in a variety of areas, and the results of those scores trigger treatment protocols which should be addressed in the care plan. The MDS data are transmitted electronically to a designated state agency.

Minimumessentialrequirements This specifies the knowledge, skills and attitudes related to the sciences basic to medicine, clinical practice, professional behavior and ethical values. The graduate of undergraduate medical education should possess these to ensure that he or she is prepared to begin further graduate medical education (specialty training) or to start practicing medicine under supervision.

Mini Tower A configuration of PCs similar to a tower case (taller than it is wide), but typically houses fewer drives and expansion cards than its larger counterpart.

Minus (-) lens Concave lens, stimulates focusing and diverges light. The lens is thinner in the center than the edges. It is used in glasses or contact lenses for people who are nearsighted (myopia).

Misappropriation The deliberate misplacement, exploitation, or wrongful, temporary, or permanent use of a resident's (patient's) belongings or money without the resident's consent.

Missed abortion Failed pregnancy without bleeding or cramping. Often diagnosed by ultrasound weeks or months after a pregnancy fails.

Mitosis The process of nuclear division in cells that produces daughter cells that are genetically identical to each other and to the parent cell.

Mittelschmerz Pain that coincides with release of an egg from the ovary.

Monilial vulvovaginitis Monilial vulvovaginitis-Infection caused by yeast or monilia. Usually affects the vagina and vulva.

Mixed airflow room Room which is supplied of air by conventional "turbulent" means, such as a diffuser or terminal HEPA filter but also includes an unidirectional flow zone (such as a hood over a critical area). Total air changes of the room are greatly enhanced by the operation of the hood.

Mixed Incontinence Having both stress and urge incontinence.

Mixed bed ion exchange Mixing both anion and cation resins in the same deionizer results in higher efficiency, but lower capacity, than separate-bed deionizers.

MMX A recent technology created by Intel Corporation to enhance their Pentium processor's handling of multimedia applications.

Modem Acronym for modulator/demodulator, a device that translates digital impulses from a computer into analog signals for telephone transmission, and analog signals from the telephone into digital pulses the computer can understand. Provides communication capabilities between computer equipment over common telephone facilities.

Modifiedessayquestion(MEQ) A measurement instrument which allows for assessment of clinical reasoning skills, understanding and knowledge of clinical and basic science and application of basic science to clinical problems. MEQ's constitute a series of questions which must be answered in the sequence asked, with no review and no possibility of correcting previous answers. Questions must be answered within the allocated time which may vary from 40 to 90 minutes. In general, a brief patient clinical scenario (presentation) is followed by a few questions exploring diagnostic hypotheses and mechanisms underlying the clinical presentation. Subsequent questions may focus on applied basic science, interpretation of diagnostic information, management issues, disease complications, ethical issues or prognosis, for example. The initial scenario is either repeated or reformulated as the reporting process progresses, and as further information is provided, the assessed area narrows. Thus the medical problem is progressively defined with questions being directed to increasingly specific areas. A well-written MEQ assesses the approach of students to a problem, their reasoning skills and understanding of concepts, rather than recall of factual knowledge.

Moiety A part or portion of a molecule, generally complex, having a characteristic chemical or pharmacological property.

Moist air A binary mixture of dry air and water vapor. Each component behaves as if the other is not present and each occupies the complete volume of the mixture.

Molds Filamentous fungi that have a mycelial structure.

Mole One gram molecular weight of a compound.

Molecular genetics Deals with the study of the nature and biochemistry of genetic material. Includes the technologies of genetic engineering.

Molecular weight The weight of a molecule that may be calculated as the sum of the atomic weights of its constituent atoms. Atomic weight is the weight of an element in relation to some element taken as the standard, usually oxygen (16) or carbon (12).

Molecule A group of atoms arranged to interact in a particular way; one molecule of any substance is the smallest physical unit of that particular substance.

Monitor A screen which allows the user to watch and interact with the computer. A monitor is different from a television because it does not have a tuner for pulling in TV signals, is of a much higher resolution than TVs are.

Monoclonal antibody (Mab or MoAb) Antibodies derived from a single source or clone of cells that recognize only one type of antigen. They are produced from hybridomas formed by the hybridization of two cells: a single antibody-producing cell and a cell that can be grown indefinitely in culture. Monoclonal antibodies have found markets in diagnostic kits and show potential for use in drugs and industrial purification processes.

Monocular vision Only one eye having useful vision.

Monomer The basic subunit from which, by repetition of a single reaction, polymers are made. For example, amino acids (monomers) condense to yield polypeptides or proteins (polymers).

Monosaccharides The building blocks of carbohydrates, hence known as "simple sugar". They are classified by the number of carbon atoms in the molecule, pentoses have five and hexoses six.

Monounsaturated Fats An essential fatty acid (EFA) that seems to reduce the risk of cardiovascular disease. This is considered a type of 'good' fat. Olive oil, and canola oil have this in them. You need approxiamately 2% of your daily calories as EFA's.

Monozygotic twins Monozygotic twins-Twins conceived from one egg.

Moratorium A limit on the number of healthcare facilities or services which can be built in a state or a geographic area, by restricting permission for a Certificate of Need (CON) needed to start new facilities or services. The stipulated reason for establishing moratoriums is usually to control healthcare costs by preventing overbuilding and excess capacity in the system.

Morning sickness Morning sickness-Nausea and vomiting, with ill health, found primarily during the first trimester of pregnancy.

Morphologic diagnosis The interpretation of the abnormalities in terms of severity, time, lesion and anatomic site. For example: severe, chronic, glomerulonephritis.

Moruaa Moruaa-Cells resulting from the early division of the fertilized egg at the beginning of pregnancy.

Mosaicism A single embryo that has two or more cell types of different chromosomal makeup. Such abnormalities can arise from defects in embryonic development or can emerge artificially when fetal cells are grown in a laboratory prior to analysis.

Mother liquor The residual liquid that remains after the crystallization or isolation processes. A mother liquor may contain unrecovered products (i.e., unreacted starting materials, intermediates, levels of the API and/or impurities). It may be used for further processing.

Motherboard The main circuit board in a computer. The motherboard houses a variety of microchips, sockets, and plugs, and plays an integral part in connecting all of a computer's parts together.

Motility The movement of food through the digestive tract, aided by contractions of muscles in the stomach and intestines known as peristalsis.

Mouse A common pointing device that senses its movement across a flat surface and transmits that information to the computer, typically to control the position of a cursor or pointer. A mouse is usually equipped with 1-3 buttons that also send signals to the computer.

MSDS (material safety data sheet) Document describing the chemical and physical properties of a substance as related to its safe handling and storage. The substance manufacturer originates it.

Mucosa Innermost tissue layer lining the gastro-intestinal tract.

Mucosal fold A fold of mucous membrane protruding into the lumen (cavity).

Mucosal Referring to the lining of most hollow organs.

Mucous Describes drainage or secretions that are made of mucus.

Mucus A thick, jelly-like substance made by the intestines and other organs of the body (such as the nose), that helps coat and protect the lining of the organ. Mucus also helps stool pass through the large intestine and rectum more easily.

Multicellular Referring to organisms composed of more than one cell - often billions of them, arranged in various organs, tissues, and systems.

Multimedia A combination of various types of media, including sound, animation, video and graphics. Due to the generally large size of "multimedia" files, a CD-ROM is usually necessary to store files. As well, appropriate sound and video cards and speakers are also necessary.

Multiplechoicequestions(MCQ) An assessment tool that requires examinees to identify the one correct answer to a question. It consists of a stem that directly or indirectly poses a question and a set of distracters from which the answer is selected. In its simplest form, it comprises a stem statement followed by related statements which an examinee marks as either true or false. Another type asks examinees to select a correct or best answer from a number of options. In the 'extended matching' type test, a short vignette about a patient is presented and the examinee is asked to select the best response from approximately 15-20 choices. Such extended matching questions, a relatively new form of MCQ, reduce the potential for guessing to marginal terms. The test reliability is achieved by formulating a large number of well-constructed questions; this requires considerable skill. The great strength of the multiple-choice format is its ease and reliability of scoring. Checking answers is mechanical and requires neither interpretation nor special knowledge. Most commonly administered multiple-choice exams are scored by machine and provide statistical information about the exam, such as item difficulty and item-test correlations. For these reasons, multiple-choice questions are popular among instructors offering the advantage of allowing different kinds of questions, at various levels of difficulty. The computerized version of MCQ can cover a large area of knowledge in a short space of time. And poor questions which fail to discriminate between candidates of different ability can be easily identified. Using a greater number of questions is beneficial, as a larger set of questions provides better coverage of course material, and students' test scores are more reliable. The correct answers are pre-specified and hence marking in some respects is objective. A large number of examinees can be tested with relatively few resources. The major disadvantage to multiple-choice questions is that they are time-consuming to construct. However, once constructed, multiple-choice questions can be used again, in either original or modified form. Since these tests primarily measure knowledge only, they are now often being replaced with more performance-basedassessmentmethods.

Multiplexing A sequencing approach that uses several pooled samples simultaneously, greatly increasing sequencing speed.

Multitasking The ability of an operating system to run more than one program simultaneously, allowing the user to easily switch and share information between applications.

Multi-use Equipment used to process more than one product.

Murine Relating to a member of the rodent family Muridae, including rats and mice; such as murine monoclonal antibodies derived from mice.

Mutagen An agent that induces cellular DNA to undergo mutation (e.g. X-rays, mustard gas radiation).

Mutagenesis The induction of mutation in the genetic material of an organism; researchers may use physical or chemical means to cause mutations that improve the production of capabilities of organisms.

Mutant The altered cell resulting from mutation of the original wild type or any subsequent alteration.

Mutation An abrupt change of genotype involving either the structure or number of complete chromosomes or, more commonly, a change in the structure of a single gene so that its function is altered or lost. Certain chemicals called mutagens can induce it.

Mutations Change in the character of a gene. Passed from one cell division to another.

My Computer An icon present on the Windows 95 and 98 desktop that enables users to view drives, folders, and files.

My, myo (prefix) Muscle.

e.g. leiomyosarcoma - a malignant tumor of smooth muscle cells.

Mycelium The mat or complex group of protoplasmic units, or the entangled mass of tubelike or filamentous structures, i.e., hyphae, that represents the "body" of plant forms classified as Eumycetes (including Phycomycetes, Ascomycetes, Deuteromycetes (Fungi Imperfectii), and Basidiomycetes).

Mycobacterium A genus of the family Mycobacteriaceae containing slender, aerobic, usually acid fast, Gram positive, rod-shaped organisms of various forms, club shaped, swollen, but seldom branched or with filaments; it includes many species which were formerly and are still called bacilli, such as the pathogens of tuberculosis and leprosy.

Mycoplasma The smallest, free-living organism with a size range from 1.25μm to 0.5μm. Pleomorphic (many shapes) because of a lack of a cell wall. Cannot be quantitatively removed by 0.2μm filtration.

Myelencephalon The caudal subdivision of the hindbrain or rhombencephalon which develops into the medulla oblongata in the adult.

Myelin The lipid substance forming a sheath around the axons of certain nerve fibers.

Myelogram A roentgenogram of the spinal cord taken after contrast material has been injected (through an LP needle) into the subarachnoid space of the spinal canal.

Myeloma A malignant human plasma cell that can synthesize excessive amounts of whole antibody or single immunoglobulin chains.

Mylohyoid muscle Muscle which originates at the mylohyoid line of the mandible, and inserts into the body of the hyoid bone and median raphe. It elevates the hyoid bone and supports the floor of the mouth.

Myocardial infarction (MI) Also called a heart attack. This occurs when an artery that feeds the heart becomes blocked. As a result, blood does not get to some parts of the heart and some of the heart tissue dies. Symptoms may include nausea, shortness of breath and pain in the chest, arm or neck.

Myocardial ischemia Oxygen deprivation of the heart muscle caused by a blockage in the blood vessels serving a particular region of the heart.

Myofascial release Trauma, posture, or inflammation can create a binding down of fascia resulting in excessive pressure on nerves, muscles, blood vessels, osseous structures and/or organs. This hands-on technique seeks to free the body from the grip of tight fascia, or connective tissue, thus restoring normal alignment and function and reducing pain. Therapists apply mild, sustained hand-pressure in order to gently stretch and soften fascia. Treatment is used to treat neck and back pain, headaches, recurring sports injuries, and scoliosis, and other conditions.

Myopia Nearsightedness, an individual will have difficulty seeing clearly at distance. Light entering the eye focuses in front of the retina when the eye is at rest and is corrected with a minus lens. A condition known as high myopia occurs when myopia is greater than 6 diopters. Typically, vision therapy is not prescribed for myopia.

Myx (prefix) Mucus. e.g. myxedema - mucinous edema (swelling).

N

N-Acetyl Cysteine A stable form of the essential amino acid L-cysteine. Cysteine is a precursor for glutathione, an important antioxidant in the body. Cysteine also serves as a major sulfur source for many body components.

NADH (Nicotinamide Adenine Dinucleotide) Also known as coenzyme 1, is the coenzymatic form of vitamin B3. NADH is involved in the production of energy in every cell. It supports healthly neurotransmitter functions.

Nasal septum The vertical (sagittal) midline partition separating the left and right nasal cavities.

Nasal turbinates Curved plates of cartilage and bone, located on the lateral walls of the nasal cavities. Covered by mucous membrane and vascular tissue, they serve to warm and humidfy the air for respiration.

Naso-gastric tube Aplastic tube inserted through the nose used to provide drainage of gastric contents.

Nasopharynx The portion of the pharynx located above the horizontal level of the soft palate.

National formulary (NF) A compendium of purity and testing criteria for chemicals, usually used in combination with the USP.

Nausea A feeling of needing to vomit (throw-up).

Navicular A "boat shaped" bone of the hand and foot. Also called the "scaphoid". Note: In the hand, this bone is prone to develop aseptic necrosis after a fracture.

FX Scaphoid (Carpal Navicular)

FX Scaphoid (Carpal Navicular)

FX Tarsal Navicular.

Near acuity The eye's ability to distinguish an object's shape and details at a near distance such as 16 inches (40 cm).

Near point of convergence (NPC) The closest point at which the two eyes can maintain a single united image.

Near point of convergence test Measures the patient's ability to point the eyes at an approaching object and to keep them fixed on the object as it reaches the patient's nose. Normal range is 0 to 4 inches away from the nose.

Necr (prefix) Death.

e.g. necrosis - the morphologic changes indicative of cell death, indicated by characteristic nuclear and cytoplasmic changes.

Necropsy Examination of a body after death.

Necrosis The pathological death of one or more cells, or of a portion of tissue or organ, resulting from irreversible damage to the nucleus.

Necrotizing enterocolitis A situation that may affect underweight or premature infants, and occurs when part of the intestine is damaged or destroyed by a bacterial infection.

Necrotizing Fasciitis A fulminant infection involving the connective tissue layer under the skin and subcutaneous fat. May result in "Gas Gangrene" leading to a high degree of morbidity and mortality.

Necrotizing pancreatitis A most severe form of pancreatitis in which there is significant death of pancreatic tissue associated with high morbidity and mortality.

Negative relative accommodation (NRA) A measure of the maximum ability to relax accommodation while maintaining clear, single binocular vision.

Neglect Failure to provide goods and services to prevent resident (patient) harm.

NEMA (national electrical manufacturers association) Enclosures As a way of standardizing enclosure performance, NEMA uses a rating system to identify the enclosure's ability to resist external environmental influences. Resistance to everything from dripping liquid to hose-down to total submersion is defined by this rating system.

Neocerebellum The most recently evolvèd part of the cerebellum and comprising its largest expanse. It includes mainly the lateral or hemispherical part of the cerebellum situated between the primary and posterolateral fissures (posterior lobe).

Neonatal mortality rate Number of deaths in the neonatal period during a given time period per 1,000 live births during the same time period.

Neonatal period Commences at birth and ends 28 completed days after birth. Neonatal deaths (deaths among live births during the first 28 completed days of life) may be subdivided into early neonatal deaths, occurring during the first seven days of life, and late neonatal deaths, occurring after the seventh day but before 28 completed days of life.

Neopallium The most recently evolved part of the cerebral cortex. It consists of six layers and forms most of the cerebral cortex in man. Also known as neocortex or isocortex.

Neoplasia Tumor formation.

Neoplasm Any new growth of cells or tissues but the term is customarily used with rather specific reference to a focus (or a relatively large mass or region) of intermittently or constantly progressive, comparatively unlimited, or uncontrolled new growth that manifests varying degrees of autonomy.

Neostriatum Phylogenetically, the most recently evolved component of the corpus striatum. It is equivalent to the caudate nucleus and the putamen. Sometimes abbreviated to Striatum.

Nephelometer Any apparatus used to measure the size and concentration of particles in a liquid by analysis of light transmitted through or reflected by the liquid.

Nephelometry The semiquantitative estimation of the concentration of particles in a suspension (e.g. bacterial cells in an antigenic preparation), by means of comparing it with the standard suspensions in a nephelometer.

Nephr (prefix) Kidney.

e.g. nephrectomy - surgical removal of the kidney.

Nephrectomy Removal of an entire kidney.

Nephrotoxin A cytotoxin that is specific for cells of the kidney.

Nerve root The portion of a nerve adjacent to the CNS centers of the brain and spinal cord that they innervate.

Netscape Corporation A pioneer in the design of World Wide Web browser technologies.

Netscape Navigator Netscape Corporation's popular World Wide Web browser.

Network Two or more computers connected together to share files and resources.

Network chiropractic Uses Network Spinal Analysis, a method characterized by the sequential application of a number of gentle, specific chiropractic adjusting techniques. Care progresses through a series of levels that parallel spinal and quality-of-life changes.

Network Computer Also called NC. A computer designed specifically for use on the internet or some other type of network. NCs typically have no drives of their own and rely heavily on a remote internet server to download and run applications.

Neural foramen The passage for a nerve. For the spine, the spinal nerves and vessels, pass through the intervertebral neural foramen, formed by the inferior notch of the pedicle above, and a superior notch of the pedicle below.

Neural therapy A form of therapy based on the idea that illness is the result of disruptions in biological energy and that the disruptions are caused by changes in the electric activity of the autonomic nervous system (which controls involuntary functions like breathing).

Neural tube defects Neural-tube defects- Abnormalities in the development of the spinal cord and brain in a fetus.

Neuroglia The non-neuronal supporting cells of the central nervous system which includes the macroglia (astrocytes and oligodendrocytes) and the microglia.

Neurohypophysis Division of the hypophysis cerebri (pituitary) consisting of the median eminence, infundibular stem and the infundibular process (neural lobe).

Neuropil The feltwork of unmyelinated neuronal processes (axonal and dendritic) within the gray matter of the central nervous system.

Neurotopic injection Treatment involves dozens of injections of small amounts (0.5 cc or less) of sterile saline solution (0.9 percent salt) into the muscles at both sides of the spine near the places where the nerves enter into the back muscles. According to this theory, salt injection helps the nerves function better, leading to improved circulation, control of pain, and healing of numerous disorders. Statistics on successful treatment of back and neck pain, sciatica, disk problems, headaches, arthritis, prostate and thyroid problems, asthma, and allergies have been presented at more than 15 international medical congresses. Technique is being evaluated in double-blind studies at the National College of Naturopathic Medicine in Oregon.

New drug application (NDA) The New Drug Application contains most of the information included in the IND. Only after FDA approval of the NDA, can distribution and marketing of a new drug begin.

Newsgroup A popular feature of the Internet. Sort of an electronic bulletin board, newsgroups are organized by subjects, and members can post messages for other members to read, as well as reply to any posted messages.

NHSA (normal human serum albumin) A blood plasma fraction usually prepared by Cohn cold ethanol precipitation. Dispensed as a 5% to 25% protein solution.

Niacin (Vitamn B-3) A vitamin Important in carbohydrate metabolism, formation of testosterone and other hormones, formation of red blood cells and maintaining the integrity of all cells. Helps body utilize protein, fats, and carbohydrates. Necessary for a healthy nervous system and digestive system. It also lowers elevated blood cholesterol levels when taken in large amounts of more than 1,000 milligrams a day.

Nissen fundoplication An operation that helps treat gastroesophageal reflux disease (GERD). The fundus (top of the stomach) is pulled around the esophagus and sewn. This helps prevent food from moving back from the stomach into the esophagus by creating a muscular band at the top of the stomach, which becomes tighter as the stomach fills up.

Nitrogenous base A nitrogencontaining molecule that has the chemical properties of a base.

Nominal (rating of filter) An arbitrary micrometer value indicated by filter manufacturers. Based upon removal of some percentage of particles of a given size or larger, but rarely well defined and consequently not reproducible.

Nominal A numerical identification of dimension, capacity, rating, or other characteristics used as a designation, not as an exact measurement.

Nominal outside diameter A numerical identification of outside diameter to which tolerances apply.

Nominal pore size Based on retention efficiency, a filter should retain 99.9% of particles larger than its nominal rated pore size.

Nominal wall thickness A numerical identification of wall thickness to which tolerances apply.

Non Ambulatory Inability to walk independently, usually bedridden or hospitalized.

Non Coiled Umbilical Cord During an ultrasound, your baby umbilical cord might be noted as being "straight". 5% of umbilical cords start out uncoiled, but 30% of those become coiled by the time the baby is born. If you baby's umbilical cord remains severely non-coiled it could indicate that there will be problems with the baby/ pregnancy.

Noncarbonate hardness Hardness in water caused by chlorides, sulfates, and nitrates of calcium and magnesium.

Non-GMP technology Facility design requirement resulting from decisions to address issues outside the realm of GMPs or manufacturer preferences. Often these do affect GMP related design features.

Nonsteroidal anti-inflammatory drugs (NSAID) A class of drugs used to treat inflammatory symptoms in the body caused by arthritis, rheumatism and other similar conditions.

Nonunidirectional airflow Air distribution where the first air entering the controlled space mixes with the internal air by means of induction. The airflow that does not meet the definition of unidirectional airflow; previously referred to as "turbulent" or "non-laminar" airflow.

Norandrostenedione Naturally occuring prohormone that works in a manner similar to Androstenedione, however, results can be much better, and side effects less.

Norepinephrine A hormone produced by your adrenal glands. Important for many bodily activities, including brain function.

Normal retinal correspondence (NRC) The foveas of the two eyes are corresponding neural points in the visual cortex and binocular vision can occur.

Normal saline A very common LVP that has a physiologic (0.9gm%) concentration of sodium chloride.

Northern blot A recombinant DNA technique used for the detection of specific RNA transcripts.

Nosocomial Infection in the Long Term Care Facility An infection that develops after admission to the LTCF. Infections that are incubating at the time of admission, or develop within 48 to 72 hours of admission, usually are community-acquired, or hospital associated if the person was transferred from the hospital.

Nosode A homeopathic remedy made from diseased tissue or bodily secretions rather than from a plant or animal. Taken like a homeopathic immunization to build up an immune response against a specific disease. Nosodes are often named for the disease present in the material they were made from - for example, the flu nosode and the infectious mononucleosis nosode.

Not exposed or closed Drug substance is protected from exposure to the environment during processing.

Not for Profit Status of ownership and/or operation characterised by government by community-based boards of trustees who are all volunteers. Board members donate their time and talents to ensure that a not-for-profit organisation's approach to caring for older people responds to local needs. Not-for-profit homes and services turn any surplus profit back into improving or expanding services for their clients or residents. Many not-for-profit organisations are often associated with religious denominations or ethnic groups.

NPDWR water Potable water meeting EPA National Primary Drinking Water Regulations.

Nubain Bodybuilding steroid. Real name is Nalbuphine Hydrochloride. A lot of bodybuilders get addicted to Nubain, as it helps them relax or sleep better. It makes them feel like they can really relax, especially during the times when you are stressed before a contest preperation. You inject it.

Nuclear medicine Radioactive materials with specific biological properties can be used to produce images, diagnose illness, and in some cases can be used to treat diseases.

Nuclease An enzyme that breaks down nucleic acids. Exonucleases cleave the nucleotides only at the ends of polynucleotide chains (e.g. phosphodiesterase). Endonucleases attack certain linkates wherever they occur in the polynucleotide chain

Nucleic acid A large molecule composed of nucleotide subunits.

Nucleic acid hybridization Matching of either DNA or RNA (depending on the organism) from an unknown organism with DNA or RNA from a known organism. This method is used in tropical disease research for identifying species and strains of organisms.

Nucleoid The compact body that contains the genome in a bacterium.

Nucleolus A discrete region of the nucleus created by the transcription of rRNA genes. The nucleolus disappears during mitosis, or cell division.

Nucleotide The structural unit of nucleic acids. A subunit of DNA or RNA consisting of purine bases (adenine, guanine), pyrimidine bases (thymine, or cytosine in DNA; uracil, or cytosine in RNA), a phosphate molecule, and a sugar molecule (deoxyribose in DNA and ribose in RNA). Thousands of nucleotides are linked to form a DNA or RNA molecule.

Nucleus The cellular organelle present in eukaryotes cells and separated from the cytoplasm by a nuclear membrane. It contains the genetic material and is essential for the continued life of the cell.

Num Lock A key on the keyboard that toggles the Number Pad between arrow keys and number keys.

Number Pad An extra set of numeric keys on the right side of the keyboard, used in the same manner as a calculator's 10-key pad. The number pad can also double as a set of arrow keys if the Num Lock toggle switch is set to off.

NUN The Network UserName (NUN) identifies the facility (or corporation) from which you have logged on to the ePIP website. Each facility (or corporation) receives one NUN that is used by all of its members.

Nurse A registered nurse (RN) or a registered practical nurse (RPN). Only registered members of the College of Nurses can call themselves a nurse, or practise as a nurse.

Nurse Aide Competency State training and capability requirements needed for employment of nurse aides in nursing homes.

Nurse Aide Registry A listing of nurse aides who have met State training and competency requirements needed for employment in nursing homes.

Nurse Aide, Nursing Assistant (NA) An unlicensed caregiver, under professional nurse supervision, who provides nursing and personal care.

Nurse midwife Nurse who has received extra training in the care of pregnant patients and the delivery of babies.

Nurse Practitioner A registered nurse who meets additional state requirements to meet this designation. In some states, nurse practitioners may act as physician extenders to conduct certain activities such as ordering tests and medications.

Nursing Home A state-licensed healthcare facility that is staffed with nurses around the clock and a physician on call, and which has approved procedures for maintaining medical records and administering medications. Rooms are often shared, and communal dining is common. Nursing homes may be freestanding Skilled Nursing Facilities, Skilled Nursing Units in hospitals, or Intermediate Care Facilities.

Nursing theory Nursing theory is the term given to the body of knowledge that is used to support nursing practice. In their professional education nurses will study a range of interconnected subjects which can be applied to the practice setting. This knowledge may be derived from experiential learning, from formal sources such as nursing research or from non-nursing sources. To speak of nursing theory is often difficult. Nursing is many things to many people. Most universally agreed upon is that Nursing is a science involving people, environment and process fueled by a vision of transcendence in the context of healthcare. It is interesting to note that 90% of all Nursing theories have been generated in the last 20 years. Many schools encourage students to formulate theories of Nursing as part of their curriculum.

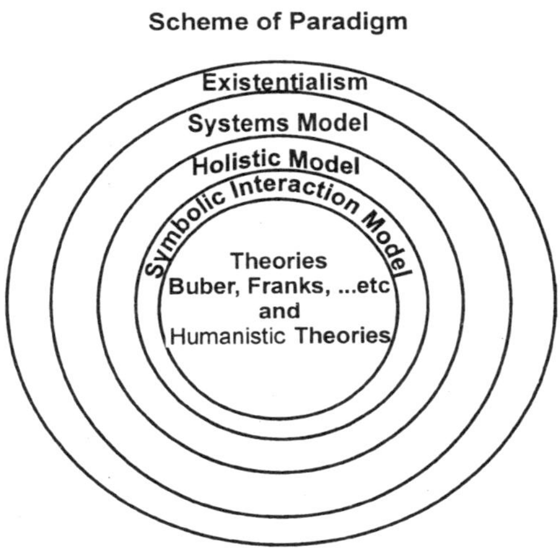

Fig. Nursing theory

Nystagmus Rhythmic oscillations or tremors of the eyes which occur independent of the normal eye movements. Generally nystagmus is not curable, but it is manageable. Treatments include prescri-ption glasses or contact lenses, prisms, and vision therapy.

O

Obex The apex of the caudal midline boundary of the fourth ventricle.

Object database management system (ODBMS) A database management system specifically designed to manage and store complex objects and their complex relationships; that is, such items are stored as objects rather than as tables or fields. They support modeling and creation of data as objects, allowing for greater flexibility in tracking parent method sets and subcomponents. Such systems may be better than relational database management systems at meeting the data integrity requirements.

Objective In medical education, it is what the learner will be able to know or do after taking part in educational activities. Objectives should result from assessment of the needs ofthepatientorpopulation.

Objective structured clinical examination (OSCE) A method introduced in 1972 as a more standardized way of assessing clinical competencies. It provides a standardized means to assess physical examination and history-taking skills, communication skills with patients and family members, breadth and depth of knowledge, ability to summarize and document findings, and ability to make a differential diagnosis or plan treatment. The examiners carefully plan the tested areas and objectives of the test are identified and recorded. The clinical competency to be tested is broken down into its various components such as taking a history, auscultation of the heart, interpretation of an ECG, or making a conclusion on a basis of findings. Candidates rotate through a series of "stations", usually 12-20, and in a specified time perform a standardized task.

The format of individual OSCE varies significantly. Clinical models and standardized patients or simulated patients can be used to allow large numbers of students to be tested on the same clinical problem without causing fatigue or stress to real patients. Direct or indirect observations as well as checklists and rating scales measure the performance against predetermined standards resulting in a more objective examination than with traditional methods. This provides a more valid and more reliable examination permitting the move away from testing factual knowledge to testing a wide range of skills. The variables of the examiner and the patient are, to a large extent, removed. OSCE is particularly suited to situations where a pass/fail decision has to be taken and where a decision has to be made as to whether a student has reached a prescribed standard. It is cost-effective when many candidates are examined at once, as it is difficult to create and administer and requires resources and expertise. With succeeding examinations, less time is required and both time and effort can be reduced if a bank of objective test items and checklists is maintained.

Use of OSCE for formative assessment has great potential and value as the learners can gain insights into the elements making up clinical competencies as well as feedback on personal strengths and weaknesses. However, in the OSCE, the student's knowledge and skills are tested in compartmentalized fashion and he/she is not tested on the ability to look at a patient as a whole being. Still, OSCE may be combined with other forms of assessment, such as the clerking of cases in the wards. The previously used term for this assessment method was Multiple Station Exercises/ Exam (MSE).

Oblique orbital line The radiographic shadow of the greater wing of the sphenoid bone, projected through the orbit.

Oblique view A view or perspective that is rotated off axis from the three cardinal imaging planes:Sagittal - Coronal – Axial.

Obstetrician Obstetrician-Physician who specializes in the care of pregnant women and the delivery of babies.

Obstruction A blockage in the digestive tract that prevents the forward movement of foods and liquids as they are digested.

Obtundation A state of decreased awareness, near coma.

Obturator externus muscle Muscle which originates at the pubis, ischium, and the superficial surface of the obturator membrane, and inserts into the trochanteric fossa of the femur. It contributes to the lateral (external) rotation of the thigh.

Obturator foramen The opening between the os pubis and the ischium.

Obturator internus muscle Muscle which originates at the pelvic surface of the hip bone, the margin of the obturator foramen, the ramus of ischium, the inferior ramus of pubis, and the internal surface of the obturator membrane, and inserts into the greater trochanter of the femur. It contributes to lateral rotation of the thigh.

Obturator Relating to the obturator foramen of the pelvis.

Occipital artery Originates from the external carotid and branches into the auricular, meningeal, mastoid, descending occipital, and sternocleidomastoid rami arteries.

Occipital bone The bone situated at the inferior and posterior portion of the cranium, articulates with the two parietal bones (at the lambdoid suture) and the temporal bones as well as the sphenoid bone and the atlas (C1).

Occipital lobe That part of the cerebral hemisphere delimited from the parietal lobe on the medial surface by the parieto-occipital fissure and on the lateral surface by an arbitrary line extending from the parieto-ccipital sulcus to the preoccipital notch. The primary visual cortex resides on the medial surface of this small lobe.

Occipital lobe The cerebral lobe from the posterior pole to the parietooccipital fissure medially and continuous with the parietal lobe laterally. The occipital lobe is immediately above the tentorium, and is supplied by the posterior cerebral artery.

Occlusion To block out light. An eye can be completely or partially blocked. This procedure is used to promote the use of one eye or both eyes. This therapy procedure may be used for people with amblyopia, strabismus, or closed head trauma. It may also be used in a vision therapy program for someone with amblyopia, eye focusing (accommodation) disorder, or poor eye tracking (oculomotor) skill. An eye patch, black contact, or another device may be used to block out light from an eye.

Occult blood Blood in the stool that is not visible to the naked eye.

Occupancy The purpose for which a building or part thereof is used or intended to be used.

Occupational Therapist (OT) A person licensed, certified, or registered under State statutes to perform as an occupational therapist. Generally these individuals are certified by the American Occupational Therapy Association (AOTA).

Ocular motility Pertaining to binocular alignment and eye muscle movement.

Ocular motor (OM) General eye movement ability, which include pursuits (to visually track and/or follow moving objects) and saccades (to direct and coordinate eye movement as the eye quickly and voluntarily shift from one target to another).

Ocular motor dysfunction Poor eye movement skills. Vision therapy is an effective treatment option.

Oculomotor skills The ability to quickly and accurately move our eyes. These are sensory motor skills that allow us to move our eyes so we can fixate on objects (fixation), move our eyes smoothly from point to point as in reading (saccades), and to track a moving object (pursuits).

Oculus dexter (OD) Rght eye.

Oculus sinister (OS) Lft eye.

Oculus uterque (OU) Bth eyes.

Odontoid process (DENS) (C1) The "tooth-like" projection from the superior surface of the axis, which ascends to articulate with the atlas, allowing the head to rotate on the cervical spine.

Office Suite A collection of powerful programs for business and other uses. Suites make it easy for users to create and share information in databases, spreadsheets, and word processors, as well as other applications. Microsoft Office is a leading office suite, as are Corel's WordPerfect Suite and Lotus SmartSuite.

Official Sources The institutions that provide the information used to evaluate your application for registration. They include schools, employers, nurse registration boards and language testing services. Occasionally, official sources may send incorrect or incomplete information. In some cases, no information exists. You and the assessment team work together to obtain the documents and information required for the evaluation.

Off-line Describes the state of a computer when it is turned off. Also refers to work that is done on your local computer, rather than on a network.

Oid (suffix) Like, resembling.

e.g. leukemoid - like leukemia.

Oil (Canola) Canola Oil is a good choice for bodybuilders seeking an oil low in saturated far. It has a fat profile of eight grams monounsaturated, four grams polysa-turated, and only one gram of saturated fat per tablespoon. Monounsa-turated fat contains Omega-3 fatty acids. At high temperatures, canola oil releases free radicals and loses its Omega-3 benefits.

OLE Object Linking and Embedding. A feature of Windows and other graphical user interfaces that allows the user to share information and documents created in one program with another. For instance, you can easily insert a spreadsheet created in Microsoft Excel into a report created in Microsoft Word using OLE.

Olecranon process The bony projection of the distal ulna at the elbow, which helps form the trochlear notch. On extension of the arm, the olecranon "hides" in the olecranon fossa of the distal humerus.

Olestra A fake fat substitute. This will save you calories, but may also deplete your body of nutrients. If you use this product, or products containing this, make sure you good your 2% dose of essential fatty acids (EFA).

Olfactory trigone The point at which the olfactory tracts as they pass toward the anterior perforated substance divide into medial, lateral and intermediate stria.

Oligo (prefix) Few; scanty.

e.g. oligochromemia - deficiency of hemoglobin in the blood.

Oligodendroglia Neuroglial cells of ectodermal origin (from bipotential O-2A progenitor cells) introduced by Del Rio Hortega and forming part of the non-neuronal interstitium the central nervous system. Interfascicular oligos are common to white matter whereas perineuronal forms are found in gray matter. These cells make myelin and can be identified by their content of carbonic anhydrase, surface galactocerebroside, myelin, and MBP.

Oligohydramnios Oligohydramnios-Lack or deficiency of amniotic fluid. A complication of pregnancy defined as the volume of the amniotic fluid (AF) being less than 300 ml during the third trimester of pregnancy. This condition is associated with a high probability of postmaturity, fetal growth retardation, congenital anomalies, and perinatal mortality. The volume of the AF may be determined by a variety of methods including ultrasound and dye-dilution tests.

Olive A smooth ovale eminence located on the ventrolateral surface of the rostral medulla oblongata. It marks the location of the underlying inferior olivary nucleus.

Ologous (suffix) Relating to.

e.g. homologous - of similar structure.

Oma (suffix) Tumor.

e.g. osteoma - tumor of bone.

Ombudsman A Long Term Care Ombudsman is an advocate for residents of nursing homes, board and care homes, and assisted living facilities. Ombudsmen provide information about how to find a facility and what to do to get quality care. They are trained to resolve problems. If you want, the ombudsman can assist you with complaints. However, unless you give the ombudsman permission to share your concerns, these matters are kept confidential. Every state is required to have an Ombudsman Program that addresses complaints and advocates for improvements in the long term care system.

Omega-3 Fatty Acids An essential fatty acid (EFA) that seems to reduce the risk of cardiovascular disease. This is considered a type of 'good' fat. Sources include fish, salmon, mackerel, sardines. You need approxiamately 2% of your daily calories as EFA's.

Omphalocele Omphalocele-Presence of congenital outpouching of the umbilicus containing internal organs in the fetus or newborn infant.

Oncogene A gene that when expressed as a protein can lead cells to become cancerous, usually by removing the normal constraints on growth.

Online Describes the state of a computer when it is turned on and connected to the Internet via an ISP.

Opacified Made to be opaque to X-ray irradiation, due to the introduction of contrast material - as in a barium study (Upper GI, Barium Enema), arteriogram, myelogram, etc.

Opathy (suffix) Disease.

e.g. nephropathy - any disease of the kidney.

Open Exposed to the environment, not closed.

Open Nephrolithotomy is the most invasive procedure for removing kidney stones. Because it is so traumatic, most kidneys can withstand no more than two such operations. Deep anesthesia is required, after which the surgeon makes a large (10-20 centimeter) incision in the patient's back or abdomen, depending upon where the stone is located. Either the ureter or the kidney isopened and the stone extracted. Most patients require prolonged hospitalization afterward, and recovery may take up to two months.

Open system A system that fails to meet one or more of the requirements that set the criteria for a closed system.

Operating Environment Also called a shell. A software program designed to simplify an operating system. Earlier versions of Microsoft Windows were operating environments for MS-DOS, and several computer manufacturers are now providing their own "companions" to Windows 95, which are also operating environments.

Operating parameter Any information entered into an automated system that is used for automated equipment operation. Or, a parameter indicative of the operating condition of a system.

Operating range The validated acceptance criteria within which a control parameter must remain, wherein acceptable product is being manufactured.

Operating system (OS) The most important program run on a computer because it manages all the other programs. Operating systems perform basic tasks, such as recognizing input from the keyboard, sending output to the display screen, keeping track of files and directories on the disk, and controlling peripheral devices such as disk drives and printers. For large systems, the OS has even greater responsibilities and powers. It regulates traffic, making sure that different programs and users running at the same time do not interfere with each other. The operating system also is responsible for security, ensuring that unauthorized users do not access a system. Microsoft Windows NT, LINUX, and UNIX are operating systems.

Operating variables All factors of operation, including control parameters that may potentially affect process state of control and/or fitness for use of the product.

Operation Room condition when normal process operations are undertaken.

Operational cleanroom ISO 14644-1 defines "operational" occupancy state as "condition where the installation is functioning in the specified manner, with the specified number of personnel present and working in the manner agreed upon".

Operculum Adjoining parts of the frontal, parietal and temporal lobes which overhang and conceal the insula from view.

Ophthalmic artery Originates from the internal carotid and branches into the lacrimal, supraorbital, central artery of the retina, ciliary, posterior and anterior ethmoid, palpebral, supratrochlear, and dorsal nasal arteries.

Ophthalmics Pertaining to products for the eyes. GMP requirements for the preparation of ophthalmics are essentially identical to those for parenterals.

Ophthalmologist A physician (doctor of medicine (M.D.) or doctor of osteopathy (D.O.) who specializes in the comprehensive care of the eyes and visual system in the prevention of eye disease and injury. The ophthalmologist has completed four or more years of college premedical education, four or more years of medical school, one year of internship, and three or more years of specialized medical and surgical training and experience in eye care. The ophthalmologist is a physician who is qualified by lengthy medical education, training and experience to diagnose, treat and manage all eye and visual system problems, and is licensed by a state regulatory board to practice medicine and surgery. The ophthalmologist is the medically trained specialist who can deliver total eye care: primary, secondary and tertiary care services (i.e., vision services, contact lenses, eye examinations, medical eye care and surgical eye care), and diagnose general diseases of the body. An ophthalmologist is not trained to provide vision therapy.

Ophthalmoscope A device used to illuminate the inside of the eye and enlarge the image for examining the retina, optic nerve entrance, arteries, and veins.

Optic chiasm A Landmark for the rostral-most border of the hypothalamus on the ventral surface of the brain. It is the point of convergence of the optic nerves and where optic nerve fibers from the nasal halves of each retina cross the midline on their way to the contralateral thalamus and visual cortex.

Optic nerve The second cranial nerve, responsible for the special sensation of sight. This is not really a "nerve", but is actually a post-synaptic white-matter tract that connects the retinal ganglion cells to the occipital (visual) cortex, via the chiasm, lateral geniculate body, and the optic radiations.

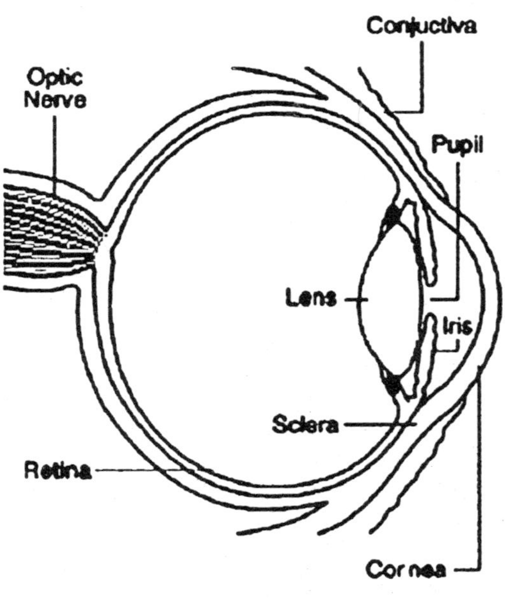

Fig. Optic nerve

Optical Character Recognition Also called OCR; A method of recognizing text that has been photographically scanned into a computer. OCR analyzes the shapes of scanned characters and determines which letters in the ASCII character set they resemble most and creates a text file with this information.

Optician Is a professional in the field of designing, finishing, fitting and dispensing of eyeglasses and contact lenses, based on an eye doctor's prescription. The optician may also dispense colored and specialty lenses for particular needs as well as low-vision aids and artificial eyes.

Optometric vision therapy (VT) As defined by the American Optometric Association: Optometric vision therapy is a treatment plan used to correct or improve specific dysfunctions of the vision system. It includes, but is not limited to, the treatment of strabismus (turned eye), other dysfunctions of binocularity (eye teaming), amblyopia (lazy eye), accommodation (eye focusing), ocular motor function (general eye movement ability), and visual-perception-motor abilities.

Optometric vision therapy is based upon a medically necessary plan of treatment which is designed to improve specific vision dysfunctions determined by standardized diagnostic criteria. Treatment plans encompass lenses, prisms, occlusion (eye patching), and other appropriate materials, modalities, and equipment. (Vision therapy can also be called visual or vision training, orthoptics, eye training, or eye exercises.).

Please note that the definition above describes Optometric Vision Therapy, which has been clinically shown to improve certain eye disorders, which are described above. However Optometric Vision Therapy is NOT the same as the Bates Method, vision therapy using Bates, integrated vision therapy, or natural eye exercises. These holistic programs use some form of eye exercises associated with relaxation techniques, which claim to improve nearsightedness, farsightedness, astigmatism, decreasing vision with age, and other disorders. There is virtually no statistical studies/results indicating the success of these methods.

Optometrist A health care professional who is state licensed to provide primary eye care service. These services include comprehensive eye health and vision examinations; diagnosis and treatment of eye disease and vision disorders; the detection of general health problems; the prescribing of glasses, contact lenses, low vision rehabilitation, vision therapy, and medications; the performing of certain surgical procedures; and the counseling of patients regarding their surgical alternatives and vision needs as related to their occupations, avocations and lifestyle. The optometrist has completed pre-professional undergraduate education in a college or university and four years of professional education at a college of optometry, leading to the doctor of optometry (O.D.) degree. Some optometrists complete a residency.

OQ (operational qualification) Documented verification that aspects of a facility system that can affect product quality perform as intended throughout anticipated operating ranges.

Oral Relating to the mouth.

Oral cavity Cavity of the mouth including the inside of the cheek, palate, oral mucosa, teeth, tongue, and glands that open into the cavity itself.

Oral product A pharmaceutical product meant to be introduced through the mouth in the form of a tablet, capsule, or suspension.

Oral solid dosage drug Formulated in a solid or powder form for patient to ingest orally.

Orbital welding Automatic or machine welding of tubes or pipe in-place with the electrode rotating (or orbiting) around the work. Orbital welding can be done with the addition of filler material or as a fusion process without the addition of filler.

Orchiectomy The surgical removal of one or both of the testicles.

Orchitis Inflammation of a testicle.

Organ based teaching In this approach, medical competence is gained by focusing on one organ system at a time. It is an approach that integrates different disciplines (subjects) such as biochemistry, physiology and anatomy, and has ultimately led to the more common problem-based approach, which is currently more commonly used.

Organelles Membrane-surrounded structures found in eukaryotic cells; they contain enzymes and other components required for specialized cell function.

Organic Organic matter is a broad category that includes both natural and man-made molecules containing carbon and hydrogen. All living matter in water is made up of organic molecules. The most common are by-products of vegetative decay such as tannins, lignins, and humic acid.

Organic amblyopia Gradual or sudden loss of central vision (partial loss) affecting visual acuity with no treatment options.

Types of organic (irreversible) amblyopia:

nutritional amblyopia- vision loss caused by low levels of vitamin B12 due to poor nutrition and poor absorption associated with drinking alcohol.

tobacco-alcohol amblyopia- clinical evidence exists that a nutritional deficiency is the underlying cause of this vision loss; however, many still believe that the toxic effects of alcohol and/or tobacco are contributing factors.

toxic amblyopia- caused by exposure to toxins such as ethambutol, methyl alcohol (moonshine), ethylene glycol (antifreeze), cyanide, lead, and carbon monoxide.

Organic peroxide An organic compound that contains the bivalent -0-0- structure and which may be considered to be a structural derivative of hydrogen peroxide where on or both of the hydrogen atoms have been replaced by an organic radical. Organic peroxides can present an explosion hazard (detonation or deflagration) or they can be shock sensitive. They can also decompose into various unstable compounds over an extended period.

Organism A single, autonomous living thing. Bacteria and yeasts are organisms; mammalian and insect cells used in culture are not.

Origin Point or region where DNA replication is begun. Often abbreviated Ori.

Ornithine A non-essential, non-structural amino acid made from Arginine shown to influence growth hormone release: most anabolic when combined with alpha-ketoglutarate (OKG).

Oropharynx The portion of the pharynx below the soft palate and above the upper edge of the epiglottis.

Orphan drug The FDA grants Orphan Drug status to one company for a drug that is believed to substantially increase the life expectancy of the treated patient for a particular disease. This excludes other companies from receiving an FDA license to produce a similar drug for a finite period (usually 7 years), thereby allowing the company producing the drug to recuperate their R&D expenses.

Orrhea (suffix) Flow; discharge.

e.g. leukorrhea - white discharge.

Orthomolecular medicine A form of nutrient therapy that uses combinations of vitamins, minerals, and amino acids normally found in the body to maintain good health and to treat specific conditions, such as asthma, heart disease, depression, and schizophrenia. "Orthomolecular" means an approach based on a correct (ortho) balance of substances present in the body.

Orthophoria (ortho) The absence of either esophoria or exophoria. The eyes do not have a tendency to want to turn more inward than necessary or want to turn more outward than necessary when pointed on an object.

Orthoptics The science of correcting defects in binocular vision. The technique of eye exercises to correct strabismus (esotropia or exotropia), convergence insufficiency (exophoria), or convergence excess (esophoria), amblyopia, and ocular motility disorders. Orthoptics was pioneered by French ophthalmologist Javal in the mid to late 1800's. Today ophthalmologists use specialty-trained healthcare professionals called orthoptists to evaluate patients and treat them with orthoptics. In America, the non-surgical technique of orthoptics is less commonly used by ophthalmologists compared to other countries. Orthoptics is a limited form of optometric vision therapy.

ORYX A project of the Joint Commission on the Accreditation of Healthcare Organizations (JCAHO) to use performance measurement data to support its survey and accreditation activities. All JCAHO accredited hospitals, long term care organizations and home health agencies must participate in the program by using an acceptable performance measurement system. CHSRA is a JCAHO accepted performance system for long term care organizations.

Oscopy (suffix) View. e.g. endoscopy - to view the inside, specifically: the intestine.

Osis (suffix) A process, especially a morbid one. e.g. diverticulosis - involvement with diverticula.

Osmosis The diffusion of a solvent through a semipermeable membrane from a solution of higher concentration to one of lower concentration until there are equal concentrations of fluid on both sides of the membrane.

Osmotic pressure Pressure generated by the osmotic flow of water through a membrane into a (aqueous) phase containing a solute in a higher concentration.

Osteo (prefix) Bone. e.g. osteomyelitis - inflammation of bone.

Osteoarthritis Osteoarthritis (OA) is a joint disease that affects the cartilage. It is the most common type of arthritis, especially among older people. Also called degenerative joint disease.

Osteoid Resembling bone.

Ostia The opening of a tubular organ or between two cavities.

Ostomy An operation that is done when there is damage to a section of intestine. It creates an opening in the wall of the abdomen, and brings a portion of intestine through the opening so stool can leave the body.

Otomy (suffix) Cut. e.g. cholecystotomy - incision into the gallbladder.

Out of hospital birth A birth conducted by a midwife where other specialized medical care (obstetrical, paediatric, surgical and/or anaesthetic skills) is not provided on site. Such sites may include homes, birth centres, nursing stations and some hospitals.

Out of Pocket The amount of a medical bill that is not covered by Insurance, or other third-party payors. These costs include Deductibles and Coinsurance, as well as uncovered Costs. Some insurance policies put a cap, or a maximum, on the total amount of Deductibles and Coinsurance that the patient must pay in a year, but uncovered costs still must be paid.

Out of specification An examination, measurement, or test result that does not comply with preestablished criteria.

Outcome All possible demonstrable results that stem from casual factors or activities. In medical education, outcome refers to a new skill, knowledge or stimulus to improve the quality of patient care. Setting outcomes can be very useful for developing a framework of various results expected from various educational activities. Outcomes may be related to the educational process (process outcomes), to the product of undergraduate medical education (learning outcomes), or to the professional role of the physician (performance outcomes).

Outcome and Assessment Information Set (OASIS) A group of data elements that represent core items of a comprehensive assessment for an adult home care resident (patient) and used for measuring patient outcomes in quality improvement.

Outcome based education This approach emphasizes educational outcomes rather than the educational process and focuses on the product of medical education such as what kind of doctors will be produced, and with what professional knowledge, skills, abilities, values and attitudes. Educational outcomes must be clearly specified as they determine the curriculum content, the teaching methods, the courses offered, the assessment process and the educational environment. The scope and definition of competence and the levels of its attainment is defined in terms of student development within the natural progression in medical school. Consequently, the assessment system will ensure that the expected variation of levels of attainment is defined and assessed.

An example of such a framework is the 12-outcomes paradigm of Dundee- a model presented in the form of three-circles which describes the following:

What the doctor is able to do: clinical skills; practical procedures; patient investigations; patient management; health promotion; disease prevention and communication.

How the doctor approaches his practice: appropriate understanding of basic, social and clinical sciences and underlying principles; with appropriate attitudes and ethical understanding and legal responsibilities and with the appropriate decision-making skills and clinical reasoning and judgment.

The doctor as a professional: understanding of the doctor's role within the health system and the understanding of personal development.

In addition, some medical schools have already incorporated advanced levels of progression in the early phases of their curriculum such as problem-based learning programs, early clinical exposure, and self-directed learning programs.

Outer table of skull The outer layer of compact bone, part of the flat bones of the skull.

Outliers Providers that fall so far outside of acceptable levels that investigation is warranted. "Outlier" implies an extreme condition. In terms of CHSRA QI reports, an outlier would be above the threshold of the 90th percentile.

Output In the health field, this indicates the immediate result of professional or institutional health care activities, usually expressed as units of service such as patient hospital days, outpatient visits or laboratory tests performed.

Over the wire (OTW) catheters Balloon catheters which are delivered over a separate guidewire to position the balloon across the lesion.

Overactive bladder A condition characterized by involuntary bladder muscle contractions during the bladder filling phase which the patient cannot suppress.

Overflow UI Leakage of small amounts of urine from a bladder that is always full.

Oxidation (on metals) The formation of an oxide layer on a metal surface. When oxidation occurs because of welding, it is visible as discoloration. The discoloration or heat tint produced by oxidation has been associated with the onset of corrosion in stainless steel piping systems.

Oxide layer In welding, an area usually located in the heat-affected zone (HAZ) of the weldment where an oxidation reaction has taken place.

Oxide thickness The depth at which the oxide signal has fallen to half the maximum peak height. Typical values for well electro-polished 316L stainless steel range from 20 to 50 angstroms (Å).

Oxidizer A material other than a blasting agent or explosive, that readily yields oxygen or other oxidizing gas, or that readily reacts to promote or initiate combustion of combustible materials. Oxidizers are subdivided as follows:

1. Class 4 - An oxidizer that can undergo an explosive reaction due to contamination or exposure to thermal or physical shock. In addition, the oxidizer will enhance the burning rate and may cause spontaneous ignition of combustible materials.

2. Class 3 - An oxidizer that will cause a severe increase in the burning rate of combustible materials with which it comes in contact or that will undergo vigorous, self-sustained decomposition due to contamination or exposure to heat.

3. Class 2 - An oxidizer that will cause a moderate increase in the burning rate or that may cause spontaneous ignition of combustible materials with which it comes in contact.

4. Class 1 - An oxidizer whose primary hazard is that it slightly increases the burning rate but does not cause spontaneous ignition when it comes in contact with combustible materials.

Oxygenated Carrying oxygen within. Blood that is carrying oxygen from the lungs to all the body tissue is oxygenated.

Ozone Formed by an electric discharge or by the slow combustion of phosphorus, ozone is a modified and condensed form of oxygen, in which three atoms of oxygen are combined to form the molecule, O3. Because it is a powerful oxidizing agent it is used in deionized water systems to kill bacteria and to reduce by oxidation the amount of Total Organic Carbon (TOC) in the water. Air containing a perceptible amount of ozone has an odor suggesting chlorine or sulfurous acid gas.

P

Paba (Para Aminobenzoic Acid) Important for the formation of red blood cells. Aids in the conversion of protein into energy. Necessary for healthy skin, and hair pigmentation.

Pacemaker lead An electrically insulated conductor that carries signals between the pulse generator (pacemaker) and the heart. Some leads enter the heart through a vein, and other leads attach to the outer surface of the heart.

Pacemaker system A two-part electrical system that includes a pulse generator (pacemaker) and one or two leads. It helps pace the heart when the natural rate is too slow to pump enough blood to the body.

Packaged equipment An assembly of individual pieces or stages of equipment, complete with inter-connecting piping and connections for external piping. The assembly may be mounted on a skid or other structure prior to delivery.

Packaging All operations, including filling and labeling, which a bulk product has to undergo in order to become a finished product.

Packaging material Any material intended to protect an intermediate or API (Active Pharmaceutical Ingredient) during storage and transport.

Paleocerebellum Phyolgenetically old part of the cerebellum represented by the anterior lobe in man. It is concerned with regulation of muscle tone.

Paleopallium (or paleocortex) Remnants of phylogenetically old 3 layered cortex found in the rhinencephalon or olfactory areas in man.

Paleostriatum Oldest component of the corpus striatum, the globus pallidus.

Palliative Care Management and support provided for the reduction or abatement of pain, for other physical symptoms and for psychosocial and spiritual needs of individuals with terminal illness and includes physician services, skilled nursing care, medical services, social services, services of volunteers and bereavement services, but does not mean treatment provided to cure a medical condition or disease or to artificially prolong life.

Pallidal Pertaining to the globus pallidus or paleostriatum.

Pallium Cerebral cortex.

Pancreas The pancreas is a combined 'endocrine' and 'exocrine' solid organ. The endocrine function includes the secretion of insulin that regulate the blood sugar levels. Pancreatic exocrine secretions are basic (pH

> 7.0) and are secreted into the duodenum to neutralize the acid from the gastric contents. The exocrine secretions also include digestive enzymes.

Pancreatic duct The main excretory duct of the pancreas that flows into the common bile duct. Pancreatic secretions are basic and neutralize the acid from the gastric contents.

Pancreaticoduodenal branches The branches of the SMA (superior mesenteric artery) that supply the pancreas and duodenum.

Pandemic disease An epidemic over an especially wide geographic area.

Panniculitits A rare, multifactorial inflammatory condition involving subcutaneous fat.

Panniculus A layer of membrane.

Pantothenic Acid (Vitamin B-5) A vitamin which supports carbohydrate, protein and fat metabolism; hemoglobin synthesis. Helps release energy from protein, carbohydrates, and fat. Needed to support a variety of body functions, including the maintenance of a healthy digestive system.

Papillary Having small nipple-shaped projections.

Papilloma Refers to a small benign tumor on a stalk, may occur in many locations including; within the duct in the breast, on the mucous membranes of the nose and mouth, larynx or esophagus and around the anus or genitals. The causes and implications are different in these different locations.

Papillotomy The creation of a small incision in the entrance of the bile duct into the duodenum such as to enlarge this entrance and permit easier passage of stones and debris.

Papules A small circumscribed, solid, elevated lesion of the skin.

PAR (proven acceptable range) A range for a critical parameter that has been determined to be achievable and appropriate for the process or processes with which it is associated. It is established by knowledge gained through relevant documentation and actual testing. A process should perform consistently and as intended when all critical parameters are held within the established PARs.

Para (prefix) Beside.

e.g. para-aortic - beside the aorta.

e.g. parauterine - beside the uterus.

Paraaortic lymph nodes The abdominal lymphnodes that are adjacent to the aorta.

Paracenrical block Paracenrical block—local anesthetic for cervical dilatation.

Parahippocampal gyrus A convolution located on the medial surface of the temporal lobe bounded by the collateral and hippocampal sulci and continuous posteriorly with the lingual gyrus. It is separated from the occipitotemporal (fusiform) gyrus laterally by the collateral and rhinal sulci.

Parailiac lymph nodes The lymphnodes that are adjacent to the iliac arteries.

Parallel Port A port through which many units of data can move simultaneously, usually over several different wires. Printers are typically connected to the computer via a parallel port.

Parasympathetic Craniosacral division of the autonomic nervous system that functions to conserve energy, build up reserves and restore the resting state of the body.

Paraterminal gyrus Vertical cortical convolution located just rostral to the lamina terminalis and anterior commissure. It is sometimes also referred to as the subcallosal gyrus. The paraterminal gyrus along with the subcallosal area comprise the septal area.

Paratracheal stripe The soft-tissue line produced by air inside the trachea and air in the lung outlining the wall of the trachea. Seen on the frontal (PA or AP) chest film, it is thin (usually 2-3 mm, always < 5mm).

Paratransit Types of passenger transportation that are more flexible than conventional Fixed-Route transit but more structured than the use of private automobiles. Paratransit includes Demand-Response transportation services, subscription bus services, shared-ride taxis, car pooling and vanpooling, jitney services, and so on. Most often refers to wheelchair-accessible, demand-response van service.

Parenchyma The essential or functional elements of an organ.

Parenteral drug (LVP, SVP) A parenteral drug is defined as one intended for injection through the skin or other external boundary tissue, rather than through the alimentary canal, so that active substances they contain are administered, using gravity or force, directly into a blood vessel, organ, tissue, or lesion. They are infused when administered intravenously (IV), or injected when administered intramuscularly (IM), or subcutaneously into the human body. A large volume parenteral (LVP) is a unit dose container of greater than 100ml that is terminally sterilized by heat. Small volume parenteral (SVP) is a "catch-all" for all non-LVP parenterals products except biologicals.

Parenteral nutrition A means of providing protein, fats, carbohydrates, fluid, and vitamins to the body through a special solution given through a vein into the bloodstream.

Paresis A paralysis that when occurring in ocular muscles causes double vision when looking in some directions.

Parietal lobe Bounded by the central fissure, lateral fissure, parieto-occipital sulcus and an imaginary line extending from the superior margin of the parieto-occipital sulcus to the pre-occipital notch. This lobe includes the primary somesthetic area association cortex concerned with understanding and interpreting multi-sensory (auditory, visual, somatic) input.

Particle concentration Number of individual particles per unit volume of air.

Particle size The apparent maximum linear dimension of a particle in the plane of observation as seen with a microscope or the equivalent diameter of a particle detected by automatic instrumentation. The equivalent diameter is the diameter of a reference sphere having known properties and producing the same response in the sensing instrument as the particle being measured.

Particle Solid or liquid object which for purposes of classification of air cleanliness, falls within a cumulative distribution that is based upon a threshold (lower limit) size in the range from 0,1 μm to 5 μm.

Particulate Usually a solid particle large enough to be removed by filtration. Nonfilterable solids are usually referred to as colloids.

Passivation A final chemical treatment/ cleaning process that removes exogenous iron or iron compounds from the surface of stainless steel piping and equipment by the use of a mild oxidant, such as a nitric acid solution, or by "in-situ electropolishing. The purpose of passivation is to restore and/or enhance the spontaneous formation of the chemically inert surface or protective passive film.

Passive immunity Temporary immunity produced by administration of gamma globulin.

Passive layer A passive oxidized film that forms naturally on a stainless steel surface when exposed to air or similar oxidizing environment thus protecting the underlying base metal from corrosion. Welding disturbs the passive layer by reducing the chromium and increasing the iron, thus altering the chromium/iron ratio (measure of corrosion resistance). Upon completion and approval of the weld, the weld surface and adjacent boundary area must be brought back to a passive state. Additionally, normal operating conditions in typical Water For Injection, reverse osmosis, deionized water, clean steam, Clean In Place, and process piping often lead to formation of the most prevalent form of self catalyzing corrosion called "rouge" (French for red), which is a colloidal form of rust containing iron oxide, chromium and nickel in various forms. This problem is further accentuated by high temperature. The rouge layer acts as a passive layer until it becomes so thick that it "sloughs off" into the process or water stream.

Passivity The state in which a stainless steel exhibits a very low corrosion rate. Also known as passivity, is the loss (or minimizing) of chemical reactivity exhibited by certain metals and alloys under special environmental conditions.

Paste A command on the Edit menu that inserts data copied to the clipboard into a document.

Pasteurization The heating of milk, wines, fruit juices, etc., for about thirty minutes at 68°C (154.4°F) whereby the living bacteria are destroyed, but the flavor or bouquet is preserved; the spores are unaffected, but are kept from developing by immediately cooling the liquid to 10°C (50°F) or lower.

Patella The roughly triangular sesamoid bone located in front of the knee, within the tendon of the quadriceps femoris muscle, a major extensor of the lower leg.

Patent Open, exposed or unobstructed.

e.g. patent ductus arteriosus - an abnormal persistence after birth of an open lumen in the ductus arteriosus, between the pulmonary artery and the aorta.

Path The location of a file in the directory tree.

Pathogen Any microbiological or eukaryotic cell containing sufficient genetic information, which upon expression of such information is capable of producing disease in healthy people, plants, or animals.

Pathogenesis The sequence of events that leads to a disease or morbid process. It may be, for example, hormonal, chemical, infectious, genetic or traumatic in nature.

Pathogenic Causing or capable of causing disease.

Pathogenic organisms Organisms capable of causing disease, either directly (by infecting) or indirectly (by producing a toxin that causes illness).

Pathology The science and study of disease, especially the causes and development of abnormal conditions both gross and microscopic.

Pathophysiology The relationship between pathology and function.

Patient Terminology used by hospitals, physicians, and home health agencies to identify their customers. Long term care facilities prefer the term resident.

Patient Days A measurement of the utilization of institutional care programs, such as nursing homes and assisted living facilities. Patient days are calculated by multiplying each person cared for by the number of days they were cared for in the month, and combining the totals. Licensed patient days would be the total of each licensed bed times the number of days in the month. Actual patient days would be the total of each resident cared for times the number of days of care each received.

Patient management problem (PMP) A written method that attempts to assess clinical problem-solving abilities. To improve its validity, recent improvements include an attempt to focus testing on the key features within a clinical case, which represents the diagnostic or problem-solving challenge. The main advantage of this innovation is that many more 'clinical cases' can be administered to candidates in a given period of time than with conventional PMP.

Computer-Based Patient Management Problem (e-PMP) is a related method that has been used for some years, which more recently has been enriched with the ability to link computers to various audiovisual inputs such as videodiscs and optical holograms produced by lasers extending realism of the simulations and conceivably providing enhanced educational opportunities. The cost of developing, establishing and maintaining the required facility may constitute a significant constraining factor for broader use.

Patient surveys Questionnaire used to assess patient satisfaction with different aspects of their health care. The questions address general aspects of the physician's care such as the amount of time spent with the patient, overall quality of care, physician competency (skills and knowledge), courtesy, and interest or empathy. Specific patient care competencies can be assessed including interpersonal and communication skills, professional behavior, listening skills, provision of information about examination findings etc. Each rating may generate a single score overall or separate scores for different clinical care activities or settings. Most patient satisfaction surveys are completed at the time of service and require less than 10 minutes. Improvements to this tool may include utilizing more effective survey design and using computers to collect and summarize survey data.

Payor Mix The composition of payors for the residents or patients of a healthcare organization. A favorable payor mix includes a high percentage of payors with attractive reimbursement rates.

Payor The source of payment for a healthcare product or service. Payors include, insurance, private pay or self pay, and other miscellaneous entities.

PC Acronym for Personal Computer. Is also a line of microcomputers manufactured by IBM Corporation. Often used to refer to any PC-Compatible computer.

PC-Compatible A computer that can run the same programs as an IBM PC.

PCD, immotile cilia syndrome (ICS) and kartagener's syndrome (KS) Refer to the same condition, with the exception that in KS the heart is located on the right side of the body. [Immotile Cilia Syndrome]

PE (polyethylene) A thermoplastic material that varies from type to type according to the particular molecular structure of each type, i.e. its crystallinity, molecular weight, and molecular weight distribution. These variations are possible through changes in polymerization conditions used during manufacturing. Low-density polyethylene (LDPE) has a melt point of 221°F (105°C), specific gravity of 0.91 to 0.925 g/cc, increased toughness, stress cracking resistance, clarity, flexibility, and elongation. It also has reduced creep and mold shrinkage. Polyethylene of higher density such as HDPE has better permeation barrier properties, hardness, abrasion resistance, chemical resistance, and surface gloss. It is important to note that photo or light oxidation will occur when natural PE is exposed to UV radiation, usually from the sun.

Pectin A soluble fiber found in the skins of fruits (apples and peaches) and vegetables. One study found that eating Pectin will make you feel full longer. Researchers speculate that Pectin may slow digestin and keep food in your stomach longer.

Pectoral The area near the breast or upper chest.

Pectoralis major Muscle which contributes to the adduction, flexion, and medial rotation of the arm. It originates at the clavicle, sternum, six upper ribs, and the aponeurosis of obliquus externus abdominus, and inserts into the crest of intertubercular groove of the humerus. The major muscle of the upper chest wall.

Pectoralis minor Muscle which originates at the third, fourth and fifth ribs, and inserts into the coracoid process of the scapula. It contributes to drawing the shoulder forward and downward.

Pediatric gastroenterologist A physician who treats infants and children with diseases of the digestive system.

Pediatrician Pediatrician-Physician who specializes in the care of babies and children.

Pedicle The short tubular bone process of the vertebral arch that forms the connection between the lamina and vertebral body (centrum).

Peduncle Generic term usually denoting a stalk-like bundle of connecting nerve fibers.

P. Cerebral: The robust bundles of fibers located bilaterally in the ventral midbrain .

P. Cerebellar: Large bundles of fibers that connect the cerebellum with the midbrain (superior cerebellar peduncle or brachium conjunctivum), pons (middle cerebellar peduncle or brachium pontis) and medulla oblongata (inferior cerebellar peduncle or restiform body).

Pedunculated Elevated, as on a stem (peduncle).

Peer Groups The other providers in a group that are used for comparison purposes.

Peer review or peer evaluation Method for evaluating professional attitudes and behavior, used by trainees to assess each other and also used by supervisors, nurses and patients to assess trainees. Typical measurement tools for this form of testing are checklists and questionnaires.

Pelvic diaphragm The floor of the pelvis formed by the coccygei and levatores ani muscles and their fascia. The pelvic diaphgram is fenestrated (holes) for the anus and vagina.

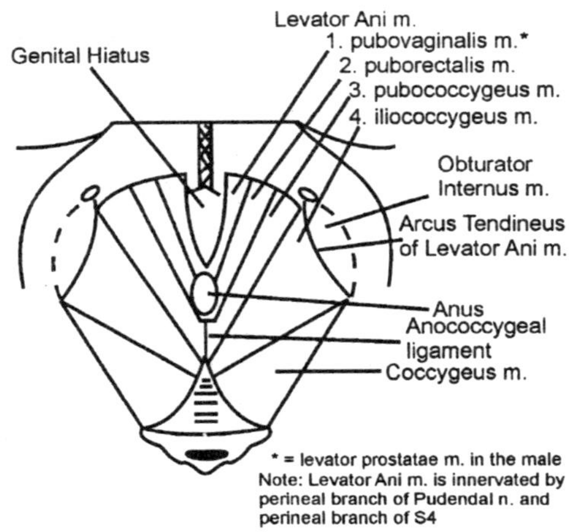

Fig. Pelvic diaphragm

Pelvic muscle exercises Pelvic muscle exercises are intended to improve your pelvic muscle tone and prevent leakage for sufferers of Stress Urinary Incontinence. Also called Kegel exercises.

Pelvimetry Pelvimetry-Evaluation of the size of the birth canal or pelvis. Performed by X-ray.

Pelvis A group of bones that join the lower extremity to the spine: sacrum, ilium, ischium, pubis.

Penalization To prevent sight out of the good eye and force the weaker, amblyopic eye, to function. A filter, eye patch, or eye drops such as atropin or miotics are used on the good eye.

Penetrance A term indicating the likelihood that a given gene will actually result in disease.

Penia (suffix) Poverty. e.g. thrombocytopenia - decrease in blood platelets.

Penicillin An antibiotic containing a ß-lactam ring that inhibits an enzyme responsible for making peptide cross-links in the bacterial cell wall. It is obtained from cultures of the molds Penicillium Notatum or Penicillium Chrysogenum.

Penicillium The genus of mold causing a zone of inhibition in an agar plate of bacteria. It is the organism, which produces natural penicillin.

Penis The male sexual organ, suspended from the pubic symphysis, supporting the urethra.

Pentium Name given to Intel's successor to the 486 processor (the "pent-" in Pentium refers to the fact that this chip is, in essence, a 586 processor). Pentium technology is currently the standard, with processor speeds ranging from 120 mHz to 600 mHz

Peptic Related to the stomach and the upper part of the small intestine (duodenum).

Peptic ulcer A sore in the lining of the esophagus, stomach, or duodenum (beginning of the small intestine); often caused by a bacteria called Helicobacter pylori.

Peptide A secondary protein derivative defined as "a definitely characterized combination of two or more amino acids, the carboxyl (COOH) group of one being united with the amino (NH2) group of the other, with the elimination of a molecule of water". They form a peptide bond.

Peptide hormones A diverse class of hormones that are synthesized and excreted at various sites within the body. Examples include: insulin, relaxin, glucagons, growth hormone, vasopressin, ACTH (Adrenocorticotropic Hormone), endorphins, and encephalins.

Per Capita A measurement based on the number of persons cared for. Per capita reimbursement rates may be paid on a per member, per month (PMPM) basis, under "capitation," as compared to per diem rates or fee-for-service payments.

Per Diem A measurement based on the days a person is cared for. Per diem reimbursement pays a set amount for each day the person is under care. Contrast per diem reimbursement rates to per capita reimbursement rates where payment is a flat amount per person cared for, whether or not they received services, and to fee schedule reimbursement where standard amounts are charges based on the units of service provided.

Per Member Per Month A monthly fee paid to a provider or plan for each member under care, also called capitation.

Per Patient Day A measurement of revenue and expenses on a per diem basis, calculating the revenue and cost per patient day. Revenue and expenses are divided by patient days to calculate PPD revenue and costs, to calculate an average of the daily revenue and expense of caring for a resident. PPDs may be calculated on a facility-wide basis, by unit, or by level of care.

Percent recovery In reverse osmosis or ultrafiltration, the ratio of pure water output to feedwater input.

Percent rejection In reverse osmosis or ultrafiltration, the ratio of impurities removed to total impurities in the incoming feedwater. For example, RO membranes typically remove (reject) 90% of the dissolved inorganic contaminants in water.

Percentile Rank For the CHSRA QIs, a means of ranking providers based on how they compare with each other on each separate QI. The higher a provider's percentile ranking, the more apt the provider is to have a care concern.

Perceptual skills Includes the identification, discrimination, spatial awareness, and visual-sensory integration. These are visual cognitive skills used to processes visual information to the brain to be organized and interpreted.

Percutaneous Nephrolithotomy (PCN) Percutaneous means "though the skin." In PCN, the surgeon or urologist makes a 1-centimeter incision under local anesthesia in the patient's back, through which an instrument called a nephroscope is passed directly into the kidney and, if necessary, the ureter. Smaller stones may be manually extracted. Large ones may need to be broken up with ultrasonic, electrohydraulic or laser-tipped probes before they can be extracted. A tube may be inserted into the kidney for drainage.

Percutaneous Through the skin.

Percutaneous transluminal coronary angioplasty (PTCA) Percutaneous (through the skin) transluminal (through the blood vessel) coronary (of the heart) angioplasty (plastic repair of the blood vessels) is a minimally invasive procedure which uses balloon dilation catheters to enlarge and treat blocked coronary arteries.

Perforation A hole in the wall of an organ.

Performance based assessment An evaluation that demands trainees be engaged in specified clinical activities. This permits evaluation of an ability to perform clinical tasks and not merely the recitation of medical knowledge. Typical measurement tools for this form of testing are checklists, observation logs, and anecdotal reports.

Performance Denotes what an individual actually does in a real life situation. In medicine, it denotes what a student or doctor actually does in an encounter with a patient when applying learned knowledge and skills, mediated by clinical judgment and the use of interpersonal communication skills. From this standpoint, competence implies professional maturity and ease in making difficult decisions. And, although these elements are inherent in good practice, it is not easy to demonstrate them. Assessment of clinical performance is of the greatest importance but is often difficult to measure.

Perfusion A feature available on balloon catheters where holes in the catheter shaft on either side of the balloon allow uninterrupted blood flow to the heart muscle during inflation.

Peri (prefix) Around.

e.g. peribronchial - around the bronchus.

Periamygdaloid area Small region of the anterior parahippocampal gyrus (near the uncus) dorsal and rostral to the amygdaloid nuclear complex.

Pericardium The fibroserous sac enclosing the heart and the roots of the great vessels of the heart. It is composed of a fibrous external layer and a serous inner layer.

Perikaryon The cytoplasmic component of a nerve cell body excluding the nucleus and processes. The term is often used synonymously with neuron and soma.

Perimetry The measurement of a visual field function (the total area that can be seen while looking straight ahead) using targets of different sizes and brightness (light levels). The visual field is measured in degrees. In a normal eye the peripheral field of vision is about 180 degrees. An instrument called a perimeter is used for mapping all areas of a person's eyesight, including peripheral (side) vision. Visual field testing can help detect certain patterns of visual loss, indicating specific types of eye diseases or vision conditions. It is the single best test for diagnosing glaucoma.

Perinatal mortality rate Number of deaths in the perinatal period during a specified period of time per 1,000 total births (live births plus fetal deaths) during the same period of time.

Perinatal period Commences at 22 completed weeks (154 days) of gestation (when birth weight is normally 500 g) and ends seven completed days after birth.

Perinatologist Perinatologist-Physician who specializes in the care of high-risk pregnancies.

Peripheral nervous system The cranial nerves (12 pair), spinal nerves (31 pair), nerve plexuses, and the spinal and autonomic ganglia associated with them.

Peripheral vision The ability to see or be aware of what is surrounding us, our side vision.

Peristalsis Wave-like movements of food forward through the digestive tract.

Peristaltic pump A type of positive displacement pump that operates by pulsations of flow caused by passing rollers over flexible tubing. Operating pressure limited by tubing tolerance.

Peritoneal cavity The thin space between the parietal and the visceral peritoneum, normally containing a small amount of serous fluid.

Peritoneum The lining of the inside of the abdomen.

Peritonitis An infection inside the abdominal cavity.

Periurethral bulking injections A surgical procedure in which injected implants are used to "bulk up" the area around the neck of the bladder allowing it to resist increases in abdominal pressure which can push down on the bladder and cause leakage.

Permeability The ability of a body to pass a fluid under pressure.

Permeate In reverse osmosis, the water that diffuses through the membrane, thereby becoming purified water.

Permissible exposure limit (PEL) The maximum permitted eight-hour time-weighted average concentration of an airborne contaminant. For Permissible Exposure Limits .

Permissions or privileges Security codes that define or restrict which users can read, write, and execute the associated files, directories, or programs. Some departments need to look only at data, some need to input data or run programs, and others may not need to look at the data at all.

Peroneal artery (Fibular Artery)Originates from the posterior tibial artery and branches into the superficial epigastric, superficial circumflex iliac, external pudendal, deep femoral, and descending geniculate arteries.

Peroxisome Very small membrane-bound particles responsible for photorespiration in plants. Similar to lysosome in structure, but not in function.

Perpendicular plate of ethmoid The thin bony plate that projects off the inferior surface of the cribriform plate of the ethmoid bone that helps form the nasal septum.

Person with midwifery skills A person who has successfully completed the prescribed course in midwifery and is able to give the necessary supervision, care and advice to women during pregnancy, labour and the postpartum period. This person is also able to conduct deliveries alone, to provide lifesaving obstetric care, and to care for the newborn and the infant.

Personal Care Personal Care refers to assistance with activities of daily living. It is usually provided by home health aides (some aides are non-licensed), transportation and shopping aides, certified nursing assistants or therapy aides. It may be provided by home health agencies, adult foster care or adult day care, as well as in residential and assisted living facilities.

Personal Computer Another name for a microcomputer designed for use by a single user.

Personal development plan (PDP) A list of educational needs, development goals and actions and processes, compiled by learners and used in systematic management and periodic reviews of learning. It is an integral part of reflective practice and self-directed learning for professionals. It can be equally valuable in teacher-directed medical training for maintaining learner-centered approaches and shared objectives. PDP can be used to manage learning needs systematically, to set development and performance improvement goals, organize learning activities and review outcomes.

Some educational organizations accept completed plans for accredited professional development and health managers link them with appraisals.

Pes hippocampi The enlarged anterior foot-like part of the hippocampus located in the floor of the inferior horn of the lateral ventricle.

Pet therapy A therapeutic approach based on the idea that expressing affection for a pet helps people feel happier, maintain a positive outlook, and therefore improve their health. According to several studies, having a pet can reduce stress, lower blood pressure, and ward off loneliness and depression. Many nursing homes and some prisons have developed pet therapy programs, with excellent results.

Petechia A pinpoint, non-raised, purplish-red spot caused by intradermal or subcutaneous hemorrhage. Plural is petechiae. These are tell-tale symptoms of Ebola and Lassa Fevers.

Petit mal seizure Petit mal seizure—Attack of a brief nature with possible short impairment of consciousness. Often associated with blinking or flickering of the eyelids and a mild twitching of the mouth.

Petrolatum White petrolatum is a purified mixture of semi-solid hydrocarbons obtained from petroleum. It is a common base or carrier for ointments. It can be sterile filtered at elevated temperatures.

Petrous pyramid A pyramid of dense bone within the temporal bone, located at the base of the cranium, and housing the hearing and vestibular sensory structures.

Petrous ridge The lateral division between the middle and posterior cranial fossae, oriented at about 45 degrees between sagittal and coronal in the axial plane.

Peyer's patches Ovoid, elevated patches of closely packed lymphoid follicles in the mucosa and submucosa of the small intestine. Also called aggregated lymphoid follicles.

PH The pH value of an aqueous solution is a number describing its acidity or alkalinity. A pH is the negative logarithm (base 10) of the concentration of hydrogen ions (equivalent per liter). The pH value of a neutral solution is 7. An acidic solution has a pH less than 7, while a basic solution has a pH greater than 7, up to 14.

Phage (suffix) Eat; devour.

e.g. macrophage - a cell which devours (phagocytoses).

Phago (prefix) Eat; devour.

e.g. phagocyte - any cell that ingests foreign material, other cells or microorganisms.

Phagocyte A cell that engulfs foreign particles from its surroundings by a process called phagocytosis. The cell releases hydrolytic enzymes from intracellular bodies called lysosomes that partially digest the foreign particle, after which it is further degraded in the phagocyte cytoplasm.

Phalanges The small tubular bones of the fingers and toes.

Pharmaceutical A medicinal drug, or relating to or engaged in pharmacy or the manufacture and sale of pharmaceuticals. A pharmaceutical product is generally one that is made up using available chemical compounds.

Pharmaceutical area A general manufacturing area classification designated by the need for a change of clothing (e.g., Packing Hall).

Pharyngeal recess A lateral extension in the wall of the nasopharynx that is situated cranial and dorsal to the pharyngeal orifice of the auditory (Eustachian) tube.

Phaseolus Vulgaris An ingredient which has been shown to effectively prevent the body from absorbing up to 35 grams of unwanted starch per meal. It is found in white kidney beans.

Phasic Fast, jump movement.

Phenol An organic acid often used as a disinfectant. Proper strength for a bacteriocidal preparation is 5%. Sometimes dispersed as an aerosol "fog" in manufacturing rooms.

Phenylalanine An amino acid, one of the main ingredients to enhance brain function. It has also been used to relieve stress.

Pheochromocytoma (pheo=dusky) (chromo =color) (cyt=cell) (oma=tumor) A small tumor of chromaffin cells, usually of the adrenal medulla, but occasionally of the chromaffin tissue of sympathetic paraganglia. Functional tumors secrete catecholamines.

Phleb (prefix) Vein.

e.g. phlebitis - inflammation of the vein.

Phlegm (obsolete word, no longer used) Thick, gluey, stringy mucus secreted in the respiratory passages as a result of inflammation, iritation or infection of the airways, and discharged through the mouth. (often synonymous with mucus)

Phosphatidyl glycerol Phosphatidyl glycerol-lipoprotein present when fetal lungs are mature.

Phosphatidylserine (PS) A phospholid. An ingredient which may block cortisol (a hormone which breaks down muscle cells into fuel). Alsom reported to increase levels of glucose, the brain's energy source.

Phospholipids Phospholipids-Fat-containing phosphorous. The most important are lecithins and sphingomyelin, which are important in the maturation of fetal lungs before birth.

Phosphorus Mineral that is structural component of all cells (including muscle); necessary for energy metabolism, protein synthesis, and growth / mainteneance of al tissues.

Photo oxidation The mechanism by which ultraviolet light reduces Total Organic Carbon (TOC) to Carbon Dioxide. If halogenated organics are present, both CO2 and mineral acids can be formed.

Photoautotrophs Facultative autotrophs that obtain their energy from light.

Photoluminescent The property of emitting light as the result of absorption of visible or invisible light, which continues for a length of time after excitation.

Photophobia Unusual sensitivity to light.

Phototherapy Phototherapy-Treatment for jaundice in a newborn infant.

Phycomycetes Algalike fungi that do not posses chlorophyll and cannot photosynthesize. Aquatic and terrestrial molds belong to this category.

Physical barrier Any equipment, facilities, or devices (e.g., fermentors, factories, filters, thermal oxidizers) that are designed to achieve containment.

Physical hazard A classification of a chemical for which there is scientifically valid evidence that it is a combustible liquid, compressed gas, cryogenic, explosive, flammable gas, flammable liquid, flammable solid, organic peroxide, oxidizer, pyrophoric, unstable, (reactive), or water-reactive material.

Physical manipulation A process other than a chemical reaction that may change the purity of the physical properties of the material, including but not limited to, crystallization, recrystallization, gel filtration, chromatography, milling, drying, or blending.

Physical map A map of the locations of identifiable landmarks on DNA (e.g., restriction enzyme cutting sites, genes), regardless of inheritance. Distance is measured in base pairs. For the human genome, the lowest-resolution physical map is the banding patterns on the 24 different chromosomes; the highest resolution map would be the complete nucleotide sequence of the chromosomes.

Physical Restraint Devices that prevent or restrict resident (patient) movement. A device or manual method that works to treat a medical symptom(s) but is attached to or adjacent to the individual's body so that freedom of movement or normal access to one's body is restricted.

Physical Therapist A person licensed, certified, or registered by State statute to perform as a physical therapist. Generally these individuals are certified by the American Physical Therapy Association (APTA).

Physician A professional, qualified by education and authorized by law to practice medicine. The essence of being a professional is an ability to find solutions to difficult problems for which there are no easily discovered answers and to effectively handle medical situations where no two patients are identical even if they have the same condition. This differentiates the professional, who must deal with complex problems that tend not to have unambiguous, clear-cut solutions, from the technician.

Physician Assistant (PA) A person licensed or certified by State statute to perform as a Physician Assistant.

Physician Extender A Physician Assistant or Nurse Practitioner acting under the general supervision and direction of a physician.

Physiologic anemia Physiologic anemia of pregnancy—Anemia during pregnancy caused by an increase in the amount of plasma (fluid) in the blood compared to the number of cells in the blood.

Physiological diplopia A normal diplopia (double vision) that occurs when an individual is not pointing his/her eyes on a certain object.

Physis (growth plate) The portion of long bones concerned with growth in length.

Pia mater The innermost of the three meninges investing the brain and spinal cord. It is a delicate vascular connective tissue membrane that is closely adherent to the neural surface. Together with the arachnoid comprises the leptomeninges.

Pickle An acid or other chemical solution used as a bath to remove scale and oxides fro the surface of metals before plating or finishing.

Pineal gland A small cone-shaped component of the epithalamus attached in the midline by a stalk to the dorsocaudal 3rd ventricle. Also known as the epiphysis cerebri. This endocrine organ secretes serotonin and melatonin in sync with light cycles. Prior to puberty the pineal exerts an inhibitory influence of the reproductive system. After the age of 16 the gland becomes infiltrated with calcareous material which renders it a useful landmark for determining the presence of space-occupying intracranial masses in radiographs.

Pink puffer Term describing the COPD or emphysematic patient whose symptoms are breathlessness, hyperinflation, mild hypoxemia and a low PCO_2.

Pinna The projecting part of the ear; also known as the auricle.

Pipe A pressure-tight cylinder used to convey a fluid or to transmit a fluid pressure ordinarily designated "pipe" in applicable material specifications. Materials designated "tube" or "tubing" in the specifications are treated as pipe when intended for pressure service. Types of pipe, according to the method of manufacture, are: 1. Electric resistance-welded pipe (ERW)

2. Furnace butt welded pipe, continuous welded

3. Electric-fusion welded pipe

4. Double submerged-arc welded pipe

5. Seamless pipe

6. Spiral welded pipe.

Pipe size Pipe size is determined by diameter and schedule. For bioprocessing equipment, pipe does not include tube.

Piriform sinus Fossa in the wall of the laryngeal pharynx that is lateral to the arytenoid cartilage and medial to the thyroid cartilage.

Pit A small surface void resulting from a localized loss of base metal by corrosion or etching, or by the removal of surface inclusions during electropolishing or passivation. A pit may or may not be detectable during liquid penetrant inspection.

Pitch To cause to be set at a particular angle or slope. Degree of slope or elevation.

Pituitary An endocrine organ located at the base of the skull in the sella turcica ("turkish saddle"), and connected to the hypothalamus by a thin stalk.

Pituitary Adenoma

Pituitary Adenoma.

Pixel Abbreviation for Picture Element, a pixel is the smallest element on a display screen. Images on a computer screen are made up of hundreds to thousands of pixels, and the screen's resolution is determined by the size, number, and closeness of these pixels.

Placebo An inert or innocuous substance used in controlled experiments testing the efficacy of another substance.

Placenta Organ inside the uterus that is attached to the baby by the umbilical cord. Essential during pregnancy for growth and development of the embryo and fetus. Also called afterbirth.

Placenta accreta Placenta that attaches to muscle of uterus.

Placenta increta Placenta that grows into muscle of uterus.

Placenta percreta Placenta that penetrates muscle of uterus.

Placenta previa Low attachment of the placenta, covering or very close to the cervix. If the placenta is covering the cervix, a cesarean section may need to be performed.

Placental abruption Premature separation of the placenta from the uterus. There may be a partial separation or complete separation of the placenta in a placental abruption.

Placentamegaly Abnormally large growth of the placenta during pregnancy.

Plan of Correction (POC) A provider's plan for how and when it will correct State violations.

Plankton Those microorganisms that are passively floating or drifting in a body of water.

Plano lens A lens that has no prescription. No variance between the curvature of the front and back lens surfaces. It is a flat lens.

Plaque A clear zone in a bacterial culture grown on an agar plate caused by localized destruction of bacterial cells by a bacteriophage. Applying the fluid to a culture and counting the number of plaques formed can estimate the concentration of infective virus in a fluid.

Plasia (suffix) To form.

e.g. hyperplasia - an increase in the number of cells in a tissue or organ, usually as a physiologic response to a stimulus.

Plasma The liquid portion of blood in which the cellular elements are suspended. As a fresh liquid obtained by centrifugation, plasma is a clear, amber-colored solution containing eight to nine percent solids; of these, 85 percent are proteins while the other components are the lipids, which include the neutral fats, fatty acids, lecithin, and cholesterol. Also present are sodium, chloride and bicarbonate, potassium, calcium and magnesium. A most essential function of plasma is the maintenance of blood pressure and the exchange with tissue of nutrients for waste. Contains fibrinogen.

Plasma cell A cell derived from a B-lymphocyte and solely responsible for the production of antibodies. Each plasma cell forms only one type of antibody and is characterized by an eccentric nucleus, a prominent Golgi zone, bulky basophilic cytoplasm (due to an extensive endoplasmic reticulum) and large numbers of mitochondria.

Plasma membrane The physical barrier that surrounds the cytoplasm of all cells. It is composed of lipid, protein, and carbohydrate and is semi-permeable.

Plasma proteins The proteins found in plasma, usually divided into albumin, globulin and fibrinogen fractions.

Plasma Protein Fraction (PPF)

Plasmid Self-replicating, extrachromosomal circular DNA molecules, distinct from the normal bacterial genome and nonessential for the cell survival under nonselective conditions. Some plasmids are capable of integrating into the host genome. A number of artificially constructed plasmids are used as cloning vectors.

Plastics High molecular weight polymers or copolymers. The wide range in physical properties of polymeric materials allows for utilization as elastomers, fibers, adhesives, rigid castings, composites, and laminates. ASTM D883 defines a plastic as a material that contains as an essential ingredient, one or more organic polymeric substances of large molecular weight, is solid in its finished state, and, at some stage in its manufacture into finished articles, can be shaped by flow. Plastics, or more appropriately polymers, are composed primarily of carbon, hydrogen, oxygen, silicon, chlorine, fluorine, and nitrogen, in various combinations and permutations. Plastics are grouped into two categories: 1. Thermoplastics: can be melted, cooled and remelted without destroying the physical or mechanical characteristics of the polymer. This property permits components to be molded or extruded. Thermoplastic polymers include: Chlorinated Vinyls, Fluorinated plastics, Ketone, Nitrile, Nylon, Polyamide-imide, Polyolefin, Polycarbonate, and Acrylonitrile butadiene styrene (ABS). 2. Thermosets: begin as a liquid or powder that through chemical reaction with a second reactant or through catalyzed polymerization result in anew product with characteristics different from either starting material. Thermoset resins include: Epoxy, Phenolic, Polyurethane, Silicone, Urea and Melamine, Polyester, Vinyl ester, Furan, Bisphenol A fumarate.

Platelets (also called thrombocytes) Platelets are tiny blood particles that help the clotting process by sticking to the lining of blood vessels. Platelets are made in the bone marrow and survive in the circulatory system for an average of about 10 days before being removed from the body by the spleen.

Platform A generic term used to refer to a computer's operating system.

PLC (programmable logic controller) An automated system with analog capability as well as binary (discrete). PLCs must be equipped with a digital interface to a "front end" computer for data collection and for programmer interface.

PLC controlled automated system Any automated system using a Programmable Logic Controller as its primary controller. Plumbing Code

Plena The plural of plenum.

Plenum An enclosure in which air or other gas is at a pressure greater than that outside the enclosure.

Pleomorphic Of varying shape and size.

Pleoptics A method of eye exercises created to stimulate and train an amblyopic eye. The goal is to have eyesight which is produced by the fovea.

Plethysmography or body box An airtight chamber with clear doors where you sit to have your lung volumes measured. Breathing is accomplished through a mouthpiece.

Pleura Either of a pair of two-walled sacs of serous membrane that covers and protect the lung.

Pleural cavity The space between the two layers of pleura; the chest cavity

Pleural space The fluid-filled "space" between the two pleural walls (visceral and parietal pleura).

Pleurisy Inflammation of the pleura with or without diffusion of an exudate into the pleural cavity

Pleuropneumonia A specific infectious disease in cattle characterized by inflammation of the lung and pleura, generally called contagious pleuropneumonia. It is due to a virus.

Plotter A printing device that draws images on paper using ink pens or pencils. A plotter draws images as a series of point-to-point lines.

Plug 'n Play Also called PnP, Plug n' Play refers to technology that allows you to simply install a new peripheral device on your computer, then start the computer and the operating system will automatically identify the device and load the necessary drivers. PnP was a reaction to the widespread difficulty of having to manually configure each add-on device and driver.

Plus (+) lens Convex lens (thicker in the middle) relaxes focusing and converges light. It is typically used in glasses or contact lenses for people who are farsighted (hyperopic). Although it may also be prescribed for other visual conditions as well.

Pnea (suffix) Breath.

e.g. dyspnea - labored or difficult breathing.

Pneumonitis Pneumonitis-Inflammation of the lungs.

Pneumothorax (PTX) Presence of air in the pleural cavity, caused by by rupture of the plural membrane or by trauma through the chest wall; often referred to as a collapsed lung. Compare to Spontaneous Pneumothorax

Poison Any substance which when taken into the body in a single dose of 1.0 gm. or less, is injurious to health or dangerous to life.

Polarity therapy Based on a theory of energy flow in the body developed by Randolph Stone, a doctor of naturopathy, osteopathy, and chiropractic. Asserts that balancing the flow of energy in the body is the foundation of health. Specific points along the currents are said to hold positive or negative energies. Practitioners use gentle touch and guidance in diet, exercise and self-awareness to help clients balance their energy flow, thus supporting a return to health.

Polaroid lens A lens used in sunglasses and sometimes 3D glasses which consists of two glass or plastic surfaces with a plastic lamination between the two surfaces, and designed to reduce reflected glare. In optometric vision therapy, these lens are used with 3D pictures such as vectograms and stereograms, which are also polarized.

Polished water High purity water after it has undergone a second treatment step. Ultrapure water usually undergoes two or more treatment steps. More economical pretreatment processes (e. g., reverse osmosis) are used to remove all but a very small fraction of the impurities. Highly efficient polishing processes (e. g., mixed-bed deionization) are used to remove the impurities that remain.

Polyalphaolefin (PAO) A synthetic oil used in lieu of DOP for HEPA filter testing.

Polycythemia Too many red blood cells. The condition exists when the hemoglobin, red blood cell (RBC) count, and total RBC volume are all above normal. .

Polygenic disorder Genetic disorder resulting from the combined action of alleles of more than one gene (e.g., heart disease, diabetes, and some cancers). Although such disorders are inherited, they depend on the simultaneous presence of several alleles; thus the hereditary patterns are usually more complex than those of single gene disorders.

Polyhydramnios Polyhydramnios.

Polymer A macromolecule (long chain) consisting of five or more repeating units called monomers. Examples include polyethylene, polystyrene, and PTFE (polytetrafluoroethylene).

Polymerase An enzyme that catalyzes production of nucleic acid molecules.

Polymerase chain reaction (PCR) A method for amplifying a DNA base sequence using a heatstable polymerase and two 20-base primers, one complementary to the (+) strand at one end of the sequence to be amplified and the other complementary to the (-) strand at the other end. Because the newly synthesized DNA strands can subsequently serve as additional templates for the same primer sequences, successive rounds of primer annealing, strand elongation, and dissociation produce rapid and highly specific amplification of the desired sequence. PCR also can be used to detect the existence of the defined sequence in a DNA sample.

Polymorphism Difference in DNA sequence among individuals. Genetic variations occurring in more than 1% of a population would be considered useful polymorphisms for genetic linkage analysis.

Polyolefin The polyolefin polymer is probably one of the most economical and widely used classes of thermoplastics, including such materials as PB, PP, and PE. PB is a semicrystalline polymer based on polybutene, homopolymers, and either polybutene or polyethylene copolymers. The primary use of PB is pipe with hydrostatic pressure rating of 1,000 psi at 73°F. PP is a crystalline polymer that has good resistance to caustics, solvents, acids, and other organic chemicals, but is not resistant to oxidizing-type acids, detergents, alcohols, or chlorinated organic materials. It is suitable for pipe applications. The largest group of polyolefins is linear PE. It includes ULDPE, LLDPE, LDPE, HDPE, HMW-HDPE, and UHMWPE. These density descriptions generally refer to ASTM designations based on unmodified polymers. PE types of higher density have better permeation barrier properties, hardness, abrasion resistance, chemical resistance, and higher surface gloss.

Polyp A spheroidal mass that protrudes upwards or outwards from a normal surface. Polyps may be hyperplastic, inflammatory, or neoplastic.

e.g. pedunculated polyp - a polyp attached by a thin stalk (peduncle).

e.g. sessile polyp - a polyp with a broad base (sessile).

Polypeptide A long chain of amino acids covalently bound by peptide.

Polyphenols Polyphenols are potent and wide ranging in their physiological prperties. They are antioxidants, cancer preventatives, cavity and gingivitis preventatives, prebiotics and even internal deodorizers.

Polypoid Resembling a polyp.

Pons (brainstem) Portion of the central nervous system between the medulla oblongata and the mesencephalon, consisting of the pars dorsalis and pars ventralis. The roof of the pons (the "tegmentum") forms the ventral/ anterior fioor of the fourth ventricle. In a sagittal view, the pons looks like the "pot-belly" of an overweight man.

Popliteal artery A continuation of the femoral artery that branches into the lateral and medial superior genicular, middle genicular, sural, lateral and medial inferior genicular, anterior and posterior tibial, genicular articular, and the patellar rete arteries.

Popliteal bursa The extension of the sheath of the synovial tendon of the popliteus muscle into the popliteal space.

Popliteal vein The vein that parallels the path of the popliteal artery, originating at the junction of the venae comitantes of the anterior and posterior tibial arteries and continuing into the femoral vein at the level of the adductor hiatus.

Population health Organized efforts focused on the health of defined populations in order to promote and maintain or restore health, to reduce the amount of disease, premature death and disease-produced discomfort and disability. Programs, services and institutions here emphasize the prevention of disease and the health needs of the population as a whole. Among a broad scope of disciplines, various knowledge and skills are utilized such as bio-statistics, epidemiology, planning, organization, management, financing and evaluation of health programs, environmental health, application of social and behavioral factors in health and disease, health promotion, health education and nutrition.

Pop-Up Menu In Windows 95 and 98, a pop-up menu is a menu that contains commands for a specific object. You access Pop-Up menus by right clicking an object.

Porcine Of, relating to, or from swine (pigs) such as porcine growth hormone.

Port The portion of a computer through which a peripheral device may communicate; a plug-in/socket on the back of the computer for connecting cables for peripherals.

Portal circulation Refers to the vascular circuit draining the gastro-intestinal tract into the liver via the portal vein.

Portal hypertension High blood pressure in the portal vein that carries blood to the liver.

Portal vein Vein originating from the junction of the superior mesenteric and splenic veins, and divides into smaller branches throughout the liver.

Portfolio A series of professional documents, which will contain- a cover letter, clinical narrative, letters of support, letter of endorsement and a resume.

Portfolio based learning or portfolios A collection of evidence that learning has taken place, usually set within agreed objectives or a negotiated set of learning activities. Some portfolios are developed in order to demonstrate the progression of learning, while others are assessed against specific targets of achievement. In essence, portfolios contain material collected by the learner over a period of time. They are the learner's practical and intellectual property and the learner takes responsibility for the portfolio's creation and maintenance. Because the portfolio is based upon the real experience of the learner, it helps to demonstrate the connection between theory and practice, accommodating evidence of learning from different sources, and enabling assessment within a framework of clear criteria and learning objectives. The use of portfolios encourages autonomous and reflective learning which is an integral part of professional education and development. Candidates are expected to produce evidence and process such evidence with relation to a pre-determined standard. Since the portfolio approach includes both content and a reflective component, one must first determine which components are to be assessed. Portfolios provide a process for both formative and summative assessment, based on either personally derived or externally set learning objectives or a model for lifelong learning and continuing professional development.

Positional cloning A technique used to identify genes, usually those that are associated with diseases, based on their location on a chromosome. This is contrast to the older, "functional cloning" technique that relies on some knowledge of a gene protein product. For most diseases, researchers have no such knowledge.

Positive airway pressure (PAP) Positive airway pressure adjuncts are used to mobilize secretions and treat conditions such as atelectasis, or to keep airways open and unobstructed in patients with sleep apnea. They include continuous positive airway pressure (CPAP), positive expiratory pressure (PEP), expiratory positive airway pressure (EPAP). and bilevel positive airway pressure (BiPAP)

Positive expiratory pressure (PEP) A method of mechanical ventilation in which pressure is maintained to increase the volume of gas remaining in the lung at the end of expiration, thus keeping alveoli open and improving gas exchange.

Sometimes called Positive end expiratory pressure (PEEP)

Positive pressure personnel suit Personnel protection equivalent to that provided by Class III (BSCs). It is a one-piece, ventilated suit worn by the laboratory worker when working with Biosafety Level 3 (BL-3) or Biosafety Level 4 (BL-4) in a "suit area" and using Class I or II Biological Safety Cabinets (BSCs). The personnel suit is maintained under positive pressure with a life-support system to prevent leakage into the suit. In this containment system, the worker is isolated from the work materials. The personnel suit area must be entered through an airlock fitted with airtight doors. A chemical shower is provided as a "dunk tank" to decontaminate the surfaces of the suit as the worker leaves the area. The exhaust air from the suit area is filtered through two HEPA filters installed in series. The entire area must be under negative pressure.

Positive pressure ventilation (PPV) Process of forcing gases down a patient's trachea using either a manual control technique or using an automatic ventilator. PPV can be done using a manual resuscitator or the rebreathing bag on the anesthesia machine; for long term use an automatic ventilator is usually prescribed.

Positive relative accommodation (PRA) A measure of the maximum ability to stimulate accommodation while maintaining clear, single binocular vision.

Post mature baby Pregnancy of 42+ weeks gestation

Post nasal discharge (PND) The sensation of mucus accumulation in the throat or a feeling that mucus is dripping downward from the back of the nose into the throat. Also called Postnasal Drip

Post neonatal mortality rate Number of deaths after 28 days up to, but not including, one year of age during a given time period per 1,000 live births during the same period.

Post-Acute Care Care for residents (patients) who are admitted to a facility following an acute care hospitalization. Care may involve high-intensity rehabilitation or clinically complex care. Most post-acute stays are for less than 30 days. Some post-acute stays lead to long term admissions for chronic care.

Posterior clinoid Two tubercles located on the superior sides of the dorsum sellae of the sphenoid bone, that are part of the attachment for the tentorium of the cerebellum.

Posterior or dorsal Back (example, the shoulder blades are located on the posterior side of the body).

Posterior rib Portion of the rib located on the dorsal side of the body.

Posterior tibial artery Artery originating from the popliteal artery and branching into the fibular circumflex branch, peroneal, medial plantar, and lateral plantar arteries.

Postpartum blues Mild depression after delivery.

Postpartum depression Postpartum depression-Depression after delivery.

Postpartum hemorrhage Bleeding greater than 15 ounces (450ml) at time of delivery. Pre-eclampsia-Combination of symptoms significant to pregnancy, including high blood pressure, edema, swelling and changes in reflexes.

Post-Prandial After meals.

Post-Survey Revisit An on-site provider visit intended to verify correction of deficiencies and/or violations cited during a survey.

Post-void residual (PVR) volume A diagnostic test which measures how much urine remains in the bladder after urination. Specific measurement of PVR volume can be accomplished by catheterization, pelvic ultrasound, radiography, or radioisotope studies.

Potable Suitable for drinking.

Potassium Mineral that helps maintain cellular integrity and water balance, nerve transmission and energy metabolism; necessary for muscle contraction. Potassium helps to lower blood pressure, lower risk of stroke, maintain muscle balance and prevent muscle cramping. Potassium helps to reduce the amount of sodium in the body.

Potent A substance that is "active" in relatively low doses or concentrations.

Pouch A specialized collection bag worn over an ostomy to collect stool.

Power of Attorney Authorization for one person to act in the place of another, which may be triggered by loss of competency of the elderly person, or may be valid even if the other person is still competent. Used to make decisions or sign documents related to property or financial affairs.

PP (polypropylene) A crystalline polymer with a melting point of 330°F (165°C), and heat deflection temperature ranging from 195°F (91°C) to 240°F (116°C) which is higher than other common plastics. Its key properties are high heat resistance (for piping an upper limit of 212°F (100°C)), a specific gravity of 0.91 if unmodified (the lightest of the most common thermoplastics), stiffness, and chemical resistance with respect to handling caustics, solvents, acids, and other organic chemicals. It is not recommended for use with oxidizing type acids, detergents, low boiling hydrocarbons, alcohols, and some chlorinated organic materials. Polypropylene is a relatively inert material and contributes little in the way of contamination to pharmaceutical water.

PPB (parts per billion) Parts per billion (abbreviated ppb only in the U.S.), or micrograms per liter. One part per billion is like seeing a bottle cap on the earth's equator from an orbiting satellite.

PPF A blood plasma fraction. Identical to NHSA but containing no more than 15% w/w A and ß globulins. Dispensed as a 5% solution.

PPLO Pleuropneumonia like organism.

PPM (parts per million) Abbreviation for parts per million, used to describe concentration in liquids or gases, e.g., 10,000 ppm is approximately equivalent to 10 g/liter or a 1% W/V solution.

PQ (performance qualification) Documented evidence that a process or system consistently and reproducibly performs as intended and does what it purports to do. This accomplished through extended time studies or process runs with simulated products or conditions.

Practicability of assessment procedures As there are always restrictions on the resources available to conduct assessments, expertise and creativity are required to develop the best compromise between ideal and practical procedures and tools for assessment. Time and resources are required to develop a proper examination possessing minimally acceptable standards of validity and reliability. This applies particularly to the assessment of clinical skills where much longer or more frequent observations of student performance are required than are usually undertaken. The planning of exams should take into account the number of students to be assessed. An assessment procedure appropriate for 20 students may not be practical where 100-200 have to be evaluated. Important factors are the number of staff available, their status and specialties, number of available patients, available space or accommodation and the end-use of the assessment; for instance, if results are used to determine "pass or fail" status or to probe for areas of competence in which students are deficient.

Prana The yogic concept of a cosmic energy or life force, similar to the Chinese idea of chi, that enters the body with the breath. Prana is thought to flow through the body, bringing health and vitality. It is considered the vital link between the spiritual self and the material self.

Pranayama A term from yoga and Ayurveda meaning breath control.

Pre term Less than 37 completed weeks (less than 259 days) of gestation. Pre-term births are also referred to as premature births.

Preadmission Screening/Annual Resident Review Reports (PASARR) Screening of all nursing home residents, prior to admission, to determine if the individual residents are mentally ill or mentally retarded.

Precipitate An insoluble reaction product. When a solution reaches saturation, solute will begin to come out of solution, as when water precipitates from the air as rain, or calcium carbonate precipitates out of water to form scale, the chalky white substance deposited on the inside of tea kettles.

Precommission Preparing the plant for commissioning (start-up). This includes briefly starting (bumping) all pieces of equipment, verifying their shaft rotation is correct, verifying that valves, gauges, and other inline devices are installed in the correct orientation, and performing functionality runs on all equipment and material. This also includes leak tests.

Predicate rules A previously published set of rules (such as GLPs, GCP, or cGMPs) that mandate what records must be maintained, the required contents of those records, whether signatures are necessary, and how long the record must be maintained.

Pre-epiglottic recess The space between the posterior border of the tongue (at its root) and the anterior margin of the epiglottis.

Prefilter A filter to trap gross particulates located upstream before a HEPA filter. The efficiency of initial prefilters is usually in the 20% to 30% range by the ASHRAE Atmospheric Dust Spot Efficiency, while intermediate prefilters usually have a collection efficiency of 80% to 90% by the same test.

Pregnancy diabetes Pregnancy diabetes.

Pregnenolone The "mother" steroid hormone from which most other steroid (sex) hormones are made, including DHEA. Has beneficial neurotransmitter effects.

Premature delivery Premature delivery—Delivery before 38 weeks gestation.

Premature Rupture Of Membranes ABBR: PROM. In pregnancy, rupture of the amniotic membrane prior to the time labor was expected. This occurs in about 10% of patients. PROM is the single most common diagnosis leading to admission of the newborn to intensive care nursing. PROM is more common in women of poor socioeconomic groups, teenagers, single women, smokers, and women who have a sexually transmitted organism cultured from the cervix or vagina in the first half of pregnancy. PROM increases the risk of intrauterine infection. preterm premature rupture of membranes ABBR: PPROM. Rupture of the fetal membranes before completion of week 37 of pregnancy.

Prenatal Tests Tests performed on the fetus to identify fetal abnormalities. The most common prenatal method for detecting prenatal disorders is fetal karyotyping, a time-consuming process that requires amniocentesis or CVS, and cell culturing for the purpose of chromosome analysis.

Presacral space The retro- and extra- peritoneal soft-tissues that are anterior to the sacrum.

Presbyopia Sometimes called the fourth refractive error, is not truly a refractive error. It is the natural process of the eye losing the ability to accommodate or change the shape of the natural crystalline lens inside the eye to see comfortably at near. This vision defect occurs with the advancement of age; the onset usually occurs between the ages of 40 to 45. Unlike the rest of the body, which stops growing by the age of twenty, the lens of the eye continues to grow throughout life. As the lens ages and grows, it becomes harder in consistency, loses its elasticity, and therefore is resistant to changes in shape. The result is a gradual reduction in accommodation (near eye focus), and a more dependence on reading glasses. A plus lens or multi-focal lens (such as a bifocal lens) is prescribed in the form of glasses or contact lenses.

Presentation Presentation-Describes which part of the baby comes into the birth canal first.

Preservative A bacteriostatic or bacteriocidal agent added to some multiple dose parenterals and most cosmetics. Examples are benzalkonium chloride (BAC), formaldehyde, and thimerosol (merthiolate).

Pressure rating Pressure at which a system is designed to operate, allowing for applicable safety factors.

Pressure Sore/Ulcer An inflamed lesion of the skin or internal mucous tissue caused by pressure or friction. Pressure sores are classified (Stages from 1-4) for increasing severity.

Pressure vessel A closed vessel designed to operate at pressures above 15 psig (103.4 kPa).

Preterm Premature Rupture Of Membranes ABBR: PPROM. Rupture of the fetal membranes before completion of week 37 of pregnancy.

Pretreatment Initial water treatment steps performed prior to final processing to prolong the life of cartridges and filters and to protect downstream elements from premature failure.

Prevalence Prevalence differs from incidence in that it does not convey information about risk. Prevalence is defined as the number of individuals with a certain disease in a population at a specified time divided by the number of individuals in the population at that time.

Prevalence rate The proportion of the population that has the health problem or disease under study. The prevalence rate is expressed as the number of existing cases of the disease at a specified point in time in the total population. The ratio is expressed per 100, 1,000, 10,000 or 100,000.

Prevention The goals of medicine are to promote health, to preserve health, to restore health when it is impaired, and to minimize suffering and distress. These goals are embodied in the word prevention, which is easiest to define in the context of levels, customarily called primary, secondary and tertiary prevention:

Primary prevention refers to the protection of health by personal and community wide effects, such as preserving good nutritional status, physical fitness, and emotional well-being, immunizing against infectious diseases, and making the environment safe.

Secondary prevention can be defined as the measures available to individuals and populations for the early detection and prompt and effective intervention to correct departures from good health.

Tertiary prevention consists of the measures available to reduce or eliminate long-term impairments and disabilities, minimize suffering caused by existing departures from good health, and to promote the patient's adjustment to irremediable conditions. This extends the concept of prevention into the field of rehabilitation. There are no precise boundaries between these levels.

Preventive medicine A specialized field of medical practice composed of distinct disciplines that focus on the health of defined populations in order to promote and maintain health and well-being and prevent disease, disability and premature death. It aims at the application of preventive measures within all areas of clinical medicine. In addition to the knowledge of basic and clinical sciences and the skills common to all physicians, practitioners of preventive medicine possess knowledge of and competence in other disciplines. Among a broad scope of such disciplines are: biostatistics, epidemiology, planning, organization, management, financing, and evaluation of health programs, environmental health, application of social and behavioral factors in health and disease, health promotion, health education and nutrition.

Primary air Air circulating through HEPA filters used to produce unidirectional flow in critical zones.

Primary ciliary dyskinesia (PCD) Condition where cilia in the body fail to beat effectively causing mucus to become trapped in various parts of the respiratory system.

Primary containment The first level of containment, consisting of the inside portion of that container which comes into immediate contact on its inner surface with the material being contained.

Primary health care The World Health Organization defines primary health care as the principal vehicle for the delivery of health care at the most local level of a country's health system. It is essential health care made accessible at a cost the country and community can afford with methods that are practical, scientifically sound and socially acceptable. Everyone in the community should have access to it, and everyone should be involved in it. Beside an appropriate treatment of common diseases and injuries, provision of essential drugs, maternal and child health, and prevention and control locally endemic diseases and immunization, it should also include at least education of the community on prevalent health problems and methods of preventing them, promotion of proper nutrition, safe water and sanitation.

Primary health care provider A practitioner who is directly accessible to clients without referral from a member of another health profession and who is authorized to provide health services within his/her scope of practice without being supervised by a member of another health profession.

Primary immunodeficiency (PIDS) Primary immune deficiency diseases are inherited disorders in which part of the body's immune system is missing or fails to function properly. Often presenting as 'common' infections or conditions (such as asthma or sinusitus), PIDs can go undetected for many years resulting in permanent damage to organs, and even the patient's death.

Primary medical care Primary medical care begins when a patient with a new health problem encounters the first-level provider of care. The provider initiates care, may screen for referral to a specialist, and secures overall responsibility for continuity of care provided by all medical personnel in both outpatient and in-patient settings.

Primary Midwife A midwife who assumes primary responsibility for providing all aspects of midwifery care, including antepartum, intrapartum and postpartum care and care of the newborn. Only one midwife is considered the primary midwife for the intrapartum period for a given client, with the exception of supervised midwifery care where both the supervised midwife and the supervisor are considered to be the primary midwife.

Primer Short preexisting polynucleotide chain to which DNA polymerase can add new deoxyribonucleotides.

Principle of nonrepudiation The ability to say with confident assurance that only one user entered specific data or performed specific actions on a computer system and that the particular user is identifiable. If more than one user can get into the system in such a way that the audit trail cannot specify who performed what action, the principle of nonrepudiation has been violated.

Prions Virus-like proteinaceous infectious agents. Prions differ from viruses in that they are not known to contain either DNA or RNA.

Prior Assessment The assessment that occurs in the most recent four months (46-165 days) preceding the target assessment.

Prism A wedge-shaped lens which is thicker on one edge than the other. This plastic or glass lens bends light (opposite direction from its thicker end). Prisms can be used to measure an eye misalignment and/or treat a binocular dysfunction (eye teaming problem). A prism is sometimes added to glasses to help improve eyesight due to an eye misalignment or visual field loss.

Prismatic effect by lens When light goes through a wedge shaped lens which is called a prism, it bends. Light is also bent when it does not go through the center of a lens. This is an undesirable effect that can occur in glasses. It commonly occurs when the pupillary distance (PD) is not measured or made correctly.

Private Pay Residents or patients responsible for payment of their own care, as opposed to residents whose care will be paid for by a third party, such as Medicare

Proanthocyanadins Potent antioxidant phytonutrient found in some pine needles (pycnogenol) and grape seeds and skins (grape seed extract), it is especially synergistic with vitamin C making them more powerful antioxidants together than by themselves.

Probe Single stranded DNA or RNA molecules of specific base sequence, labeled either radioactively or immunologically, that are used to detect the complementary base sequence by hybridization.

Probiotics Substances such as acidophilus and bifidus that restore the beneficial bacteria normally present in the intestines. Stress, poor diet, antibiotics, and oral contraceptives can throw off the normal balance of bacteria and fungi. This imbalance may be manifested as a yeast infection, or in symptoms such as diarrhea or gastrointestinal disturbances.

Problem based learning (PBL) In this approach, students learn in small groups supported by a tutor. They initially explore a predetermined problem. The problem contains triggers designed to evoke objectives or concepts which are used to set the agenda for individual or group investigation and learning after the initial session. Subsequent group meetings permit students to monitor their achievements and to set further learning goals as required. The tutor's role is to offer support for learning and to help reach the expected outcomes. PBL enables students to develop the ability to translate knowledge into practice at an early stage, encourages individual participation in learning and also allows the development of teamwork skills. Students in PBL courses have been found to place more emphasis on "meaning" (understanding) than "reproduction" (memorization). Students must engage in a significant amount of self-directed learning; lectures are kept to a minimum. PBL originated at McMaster University in Canada, and then at Maastricht University, and is now widely adopted in medical schools in many countries. Each school makes its own adjustments to the basic model. It does require a heavy investment in resources (library books, IT, tutorial rooms) as well as requiring education and training for tutors.

Procedures A documented description of the operations to be carried out, the precautions to be taken and measures to be applied directly or indirectly related to the manufacture of an intermediate or API.

Process aids Materials, excluding solvents, used as an aid in the manufacture of an intermediate or API (Active Pharmaceutical Ingredient) which themselves do not participate in a chemical or biological reaction (e.g. filter aid, activated carbon, etc.).

Process limits Environmental limits that, if exceeded, may affect product quality adversely.

Process suitability The established capacity of the manufacturing process to produce effective and reproducible results consistently.

Process support systems Systems that do not contact product and are generally engineering systems.

Process systems Systems that may contact the drug substance or could otherwise directly impact product quality.

Process validation Establishing, through documented evidence, a high degree of assurance that a specific process will consistently produce a product that meets its predetermined specifications and quality characteristics.

Process validation protocol Documented plan for testing a pharmaceutical product and process to confirm that the production process used to manufacture the product performs as intended. This includes a review of process variables and operational limitations as well as providing the sampling plan under actual use conditions.

Proctitis Benign inflammation of the rectum from various causes.

Proctosigmoidoscopy An examination of the rectum and last portion of the colon using a tubular speculum and a light source.

Product campaign The production of more than one product in a facility, with strict adherence to accepted cleaning procedures between these products. The products may be run in the same equipment, but not at the same time.

Product contact surface A surface that contacts raw materials, process materials, and/or product.

Product mix The types and number of different products produced in a facility.

Product water The water produced as a result of a treatment process.

Production All operations involved in the preparation of an API (Active Pharmaceutical Ingredient), from receipt of materials, through processing and packaging, to its completion as a finished API.

Productive cough A cough in which mucus or phlegm is dislodged, enabling a person to clear the lungs.

Professional Accountability Professional accountability means being responsible for one's actions and decisions, and accepting the consequences. Nurses demonstrate accountability through their decision-making, competency and integrity. This is reflected through nurses' actions and through accurate documentation.

Professional Misconduct Defined in the Regulated Health Professions Act as a violation of the ethical standards set out for the profession, a failure to meet or a breach of the standards of practice, or crossing the boundaries of the therapeutic relationship.

Professionalism Adherence to a set of values comprising both a formally agreed-upon code of conduct and the informal expectations of colleagues, clients and society. The key values include acting in a patient's interest, responsiveness to the health needs of society, maintaining the highest standards of excellence in the practice of medicine and in the generation and dissemination of knowledge. In addition to medical knowledge and skills, medical professionals should present psychosocial and humanistic qualities such as caring, empathy, humility and compassion, as well as social responsibility and sensitivity to people's culture and beliefs. All these qualities are expected of members of highly trained professions.

The American Board of Internal Medicine's Project Professionalism indicates the most important elements of professionalism to be: altruism, accountability, duty, excellence, honor and integrity, and respect for others.

Professional Altruism: constitutes the essence of professionalism and is based on the rule that the best interest of patients and not self-interest is the professional obligation.

Professional Accountability is an important element of professionalism which is required of physicians at several levels: to their patients for fulfilling the implied contract governing the patient/physician relationship, to society for addressing the health needs of the public, and to their profession for adhering to medicine's time-honored ethical precepts.

Professional Duty can be expressed by the free acceptance of a commitment to service, availability and responsiveness when "on call," accepting inconvenience to meet the needs of ones patients, enduring unavoidable risks to oneself when a patient's welfare is at stake, and 0advocating the best possible care regardless of the patient's ability to pay. It is willingness to seek an active role in professional organizations and volunteering ones skills and expertise for the welfare of the community.

Professional Excellence entails a conscientious effort to exceed ordinary expectations. Commitment to excellence is an acknowledged goal for all physicians and includes a commitment to life-long learning.

Professional Honor and Integrity implies being fair, being truthful, keeping one's word, meeting commitments, and being straightforward. It also requires recognition of the possibility of conflict of interest and avoiding any situation in which the interest of the physician is placed above that of the patient or allowing personal gain to supersede the best interest of the patient. It constitutes an integral part of professionalism. The importance of professionalism in the patient/physician relationship cannot be overstated.

Professional Respect for Others is reflected in the respect towards the patients and their families, other physicians and professional colleagues such as nurses, medical students, and residents. It is the essence of humanism, and humanism is both central to professionalism and fundamental to enhancing collegiality among physicians.

Profunda femoris artery Atery which origintes from the femoral artery, and branches into the medial and later circumflex arteries of the thigh and perforating arteries.

Progesterone Progesterone is a hormone produced in in every menstrual cycle after ovulation. This hormone plays a very important role in pregnancy.

Prognosis A prediction of the outcome of the pathological process or disease.

Programmer Not a person, but a computer-based equipment used to communicate with the pulse generator. It provides information during testing and follow-up exams. The doctor uses the programmer to adjust the pulse generator so that it senses and treats your arrhythmias. The programmer can, for example, help your doctor to determine when the pulse generator needs to be replaced.

Progressive systemic sclerosis One of two types of scleroderma, an autoimmune disease characterized by thickening of the skin and by hardening of the tissue of some internal organs. The other form of scleroderma is called CREST.

Projection fibers One of three basic classifications of nerve fibers within the white matter (centrum ovale) of the cerebral hemispheres. Projection fibers (also known as itinerant fibers) project to widespread areas of the cerebral cortex from subcortical loci and from distant loci to the cortex.

Prokaryote A unicellular organism having a less complex structure than a eukaryote. It is characterized by the absence of a nucleus and by having the genetic material in the form of simple filaments of DNA. The sizes of most prokaryotes vary from 0.5μm to 3μm in equivalent radius. Different species have different shapes such as spherical or Coccus (for example, Staphylococci), cylindrical or bacillus (E. coli), or spiral or spirillum (Rhodospirillum).

Prolapse When part of the body (for instance, a section of intestine) slips from its normal position.

Promoter A site on DNA to which RNA polymerase will bind and initiate transcription.

Prompt A character or message provided by the computer to indicate that it is ready to accept keyboard input. Usually an on-screen question or instruction that tells the user which data to enter or what action to take; for example, "Enter name:".

Prone Having the front or ventral surface downward; lying facedown.

Prophylactic surgery Surgery to remove tissue that is in danger of becoming cancerous, before cancer has the chance to develop. Surgery to remove the breasts of women at high risk of developing breast cancer is known as prophylactic mastectomy.

Prophylaxis The prevention of, or protective treatment for disease.

Proportion A fraction where the numerator is a subset of the denominator.

Proprius (fasciculus) An exclusively intrinsic spinal pathway that consists of short acsending and descending fibers interconnecting various spinal cord levels. This fasciculi proprii or spinospinal fasciculi system is located adjacent to the gray matter of the spinal cord and participates in intersegmental reflex activity.

Propylene glycol A common solvent for antibiotics, particularly the tetracyclines. Miscible (soluble) in water, but often filtered as pure propylene glycol prior to combination with the antibiotic. Its high viscosity controls absorption of the dissolved drug.

Propylthiouracil Propylthiouracil-Medication used to treat thyroid disease.

Prosencephalon The most rostral of the three primary vesicles of the mbryonic brain. The adult derivatives of the forebrain are the cerebral hemispheres, striatum, diencephalon, lateral and third ventricles.

Prospective Payment System Program for reimbursing Skilled Nursing Facilities based on the expected, or prospective, cost of providing care, using an assessment of the resident's condition as scored on the Minimum Data Set. This program is being phased in to replace the Cost-Based Reimbursement System used prior to 1999. Under PPS, each resident gets a per diem rate based on the geographical area in which they are receiving care and their MDS scores. MDS scores are grouped into 44 distinct categories, each of which has its own reimbursement rate.

Prospective Rates Rates paid based an expectation of what costs will be. Sometimes prospective rates are coupled with "settlements," where actual costs are compared to the prospective reimbursement, and the difference is due to/from the program.

Provider Tax Taxes imposed by the state on health care providers, generally based on the number of licensed beds or on gross revenues.

Prospective validation Establishing documented evidence that a system does what it purports to do based on a preplanned protocol.

Prostaglandin Any of various oxygenated unsaturated cyclic fatty acids of animals that have a variety of hormonelike actions (as in controlling blood pressure or smooth muscle contraction).

Prostate Gland surrounding the neck of the bladder and urethra in males. Prostatic secretions are combined with spermatocytes to form semen, and provide nourishment for the spermatozoa.

Prostatectomy Surgical removal of the prostate.

Suprapubic / Retropubic Prostatectomy This involves the removal of obstructing prostatic tissue through a supra-pubic incision (a cut below the belly button). The Prostate is not wholly removed.

Suprapubic Prostatectomy requires incising the bladder to remove the obstructing tissue while a

Retropubic approach involves incising the Prostatic capsule to remove the obstructing tissue. Both approaches utilize an abdominal incision.

Radical Retropubic Prostatectomy Removal of prostate through an abdominal incision. The prostate is completely removed. The advantage is that the lymph nodes can be sampled at the time of the operation and the nerve-sparing procedure is easier to do via this operation.

Perineal Prostatectomy A Perineal incision is utilized. The advantages are: less blood loss, easier visualization of the bladder / urethral anastomosis and decreased recovery time because the incision does not involve muscle or any other vital tissue.

Prostatic stent Inserted through a cystoscope, it is a wire device that expands after placement thus pushing prostate tissue away from passageway allowing for easier urination.

Prostatic urethra Portion of the urethra that passes through the prostate.

Prostatitis Inflammation of the prostate.

Prostatron Also called TUMT or Transurethral Microwave Thermotherapy. A catheter is placed within the bladder and positioned within the prostate, then the antenna emits microwaves. This procedure increases the passageway allowing for easier urination.

Prosthetic groups Organic and/or inorganic components other than amino acids, contained in proteins.

Protease A proteolytic enzyme; a protein that can cleave other proteins into smaller fragments.

Protein One of a group of substances constituting the greater part of the nitrogen-containing components of animal and vegetable tissues. They are of very complex constitution, all containing carbon, hydrogen, nitrogen, and oxygen and some containing in addition iron, phosphorous, or sulfur; chemically they are regarded as peptides (polypeptides) or combinations of amino acids and their derivatives. They are colorless, odorless, generally tasteless, and of varying degrees of solubility; they are putrefiable and readily undergo chemical change, hydrolysis, under the influence of ferments and on boiling with dilute acids or alkalis.

Protein (Egg) Source of protein with high Protein Efficiency Ratio, usually in egg white form (albumin) when used in protein powder to avoid cholesterol in egg yolk. Egg protein is the standard by which all other proteins are measured because of its very high ration of indispensable amino acids (also called essential amino acids because they must be supplied to the body from food or supplements) to dispensable amino acids.

Protein (Soy) Soy protein does not offer much benefits to a bodybuilder. Soy protein does not form a good curd in the stomach, thus making it a fast protein. The amino acid pattern in soy is inferior to that of milk proteins, and not as favorable toward promoting growth. However, it is a unique vegetarian protein that contains all of the Essential Amino Acids you need.

Protein (Whey Hydrolyzed) When you hydrolyze whey protein, you permanently modify the native protein structure, meaning that the protein has been denatured. A denatured whey protein has little or no biological activity. The hydrolysis process breaks apart peptide bonds, which destroys the protein structure and the bital whey protein biological activity. However, you still get the amino acids of whey proteins from the hydrolyzed whey protein. Half the reason bodybuilders eat protein is to obtain these healthful smaller protein chains.

Protein (Whey Ion-Exchange) This special process revolved around the positive and negative charges or ion properties of whey protein. It featured the use of a resin to isolate the protein material from the whey. This is followed by ultrafiltration methods to furthur concentrate the protein. This contains 90% protein, and less than 1% lactose. True ion exchange whey protein is clear in a solution.

Protein (Whey Microfiltration) Microfiltration Whey Protein features filtering membranes with microscopic holes. This is also sometimes called Cross-Flow filtration, or Nanofiltration, depending on the size of the holes of the filtering membranes.

Protein (Whey Protein Concentrate) This type of protein contains 80% protein. The remaining 20% include moisture, lactose, fat and minerals. They have more 'fractions' and biologically active proteins than whey protein isolates. There is no difference between whey protein isolates and concentrates in the ability to spport muscle growth and recovery.

Protein (Whey Protein Isolate) This type of protein contains 90% protein, and about 10% moisture. There is almost no lactose and fat in this type of protein. They normally taste better, are easier to digest, and is much more expensive than Whey Protein Concentrate. There is no difference between whey protein isolates and concentrates in the ability to spport muscle growth and recovery.

Protein (Whey) Dairy source of protein (other than cassein), known for high levels of BCAA's and high nitrogen retention. Made from milk curd, whey protein is the Rolls Royce of proteins because it has a superior amino acid composition (including high levels of leucine, arguably the most important branched chain amino acid), superior biological value (meaning that more of what you eat gets digested and into your system), is very low in lactose (a milk sugar that most adults have difficulty digesting).

Protein sequencer An instrument that will determine the sequence of amino acids, which make up a particular protein.

Proteinuria Proteinuria is a term used when protein is found in the urine. Protein in the urine can be symptomatic of some prental complications and is probably tested for at your prenatal visits.

Proteolysis Protein hydrolysis, the decomposition of protein.

Proteolytic enzyme (protease) Any enzyme that takes part in the breaking down of proteins. A system of several such enzymes is necessary to break down proteins to their constituent amino acids.

Proteomics A concept more than a defined technology, it refers to any protein-based approach that has the capacity to provide new information about proteins on a genomewide scale. 75% of the predicted proteins in multicellular organisms have no known cellular function.

Protocol A prospective plan, that when executed as intended, produces documented evidence that a Process or System has been properly qualified.

Proton pump inhibitors Medicines that affect how acid is produced by the stomach's "proton pump" system, thereby decreasing stomach acid.

Protoplasm A semifluid, viscous, translucent mixture of water, proteins, lipids, carbohydrates, and inorganic salts found in all plant and animal cells.

Protozoa Nucleated microorganisms, some of which are large enough to be detected with the naked eye. They consist of a single cell and or an aggregation of nondifferentiated cells loosely held together and not forming tissues. The protozoa are divided into four classes: Sarcodina, Mastigophora, Sporozoa, and Infusoria (Ciliata).

Provera Provera is a synthetic progesterone often given to women to bring on a period after a seven or more week delay, when she is not pregnant.

Provider Initiative Project (PIP) A quality indicator information system for long term care developed by the Center for Health Systems Research and Analysis (CHSRA) at the University of Wisconsin-Madison that utilizes MDS assessment data.

Proximal Toward or nearest the trunk or the point of origin of a part (example, the proximal end of the femur joins with the pelvic bone).

Proximal vergence A convergence response attributed to the awareness of, or the impression of nearness of an object of regard.

Pruritis gravidarum Itching during pregnancy.

Psaltarium A thin sheet of commissural fibers which bridges across the crura of the fornix beneath the splenium of the corpus callosum. It interconnects the hippocampal formations. It is also known as the hippocampal commissure.

Pseudomyopia The condition Accommodative Excess/Spasm causes an individual to experience blurry distance vision after prolonged near work such as reading or using a computer. The individual may appear to be nearsighted (myopia). Treatment options may include prescription lenses and/or vision therapy.

Pseudonomas diminuta The bacterium used for validation of sterilizing filters. Recognized as the challenge organism for 0.2µm filters, its size is 0.3 x 0.8µm approximately. According to the HIMA (Health Industries Manufacturers Association) standard, filters must be successfully challenged to a titre of 107 per cm^2 to be validated as sterilizing grade 0.2µm rated.

Psoas muscle Originates at the lumbar vertebrae and fascia and inserts into the lesser trochanter of femur. It contributes to the flexion of the trunk and the flexion and medial rotation of the thigh. Note: Pork tenderloin and filet mignon are psoas muscles.

Psoriatic Arthritis Psoriatic arthritis is a condition characterized by the concurrent development of both arthritis and psoriasis. It is affects both the joints and the skin.

Psychotropic Medications Psychoactive medications used to change, modify, or alter an individual's behavior or mood. This general term includes antianxiety, antidepressant, antipsychotic, and hypnotic medications.

Psychrometer A hygrometer that uses the difference in readings between two thermometers, one having a wet bulb ventilated to cause evaporation and the other having a dry bulb, as a measure of atmospheric moisture.

Psychrometry Determination of the properties of gas-vapor mixtures. The air-water vapor system is by far the one most commonly encountered.

Psychrophile An organism that requires temperatures below 20°C (68°F) for growth.

PTFE (polytetrafluoroethylene) Teflon A fluoroplastic that is resistant to practically every known chemical or solvent in combination with the highest useful temperature limit of commercially available plastics. PTFE has a melt point of 620°F (327°C), a useful temperature range from -436°F (-260°C) to 500°F (260°C), high impact strength, and exceptionally low coefficient of friction. Usual processing techniques like injection molding are not possible with PTFE due to a very high molecular weight which results in a melt viscosity about 1 million times higher than is acceptable for conventional thermoplastics. PTFE resin is pressed into shapes under high pressure at room temperature and then heated to 700°F (371°C) to complete the molding (sintering process) and adjust the crystalline content.

Ptosis Droopy upper eyelid, causing the eye to remain partially closed.

PTS computerized perceptual home vision therapy system A home-based computerized perceptual therapy program, which was designed to enhance visual information processing. The therapy procedures address simultaneous processing, sequential processing and/or speed of information processing. This computer program contains 6 activities that are specifically for the following problems: a weakness with visual information processing skills such as figure-ground, form constancy, spatial relations, visual closure, visual discrimination, visual memory, and visualization skills, slow speed of information processing, and acquired brain injury with perceptual-cognitive deficits. This program is available only from a licensed eye care practitioner.

Pubic symphysis Pubic symphysis—Bony prominence in the pelvic bone found in the midline. Landmark from which the doctor often measures during pregnancy to follow growth of the uterus.

Public health Organized efforts of society to protect, promote, and restore people's health. It is the combination of science, skills, and beliefs that is directed to the maintenance and improvement of the health of all the people through collective or social actions. The programs, services and institutions involved emphasize the prevention of disease and the health needs of the population as a whole. Public health activities change with variations in technology and social values but the goals remain the same: to reduce the amount of disease, premature death, and disease-produced discomfort and disability in the population. Public health is thus a social institution, a discipline, and a practice.

Public key certificate (PKC) A data file issued by a certified authority to a person or company that acquires a digital signature service. The certificate includes information identifying the subject, the issuing authority, and the period of validity, and it provides the related public key. The certified authority signs the PKC digitally.

Pubovaginal Sling A surgical procedure in which a man-made or cadaveric piece of material is placed under the bladder neck to support and immobilize. This technique improves sphincter function and decreases bladder neck movement, improving continence.

Pudendal block Local anesthesia during labor.

PUID The Personal User ID (PUID) is an individual logon that is unique to each staff member who uses the ePIP system. New IDs can be requested at any time by contacting the ePIP help desk.

Pulmonary arteries and trunk The large vessel which originates from the conus arteriosus of the right ventricle (pulmonary trunk). It divides into the right and left pulmonary ateries. The pulmonary arteries deliver deoxygenated blood to the lungs for gas exchange.

Pulmonary embolism Blood clot from another part of the body that travels to the lungs. Can cause closed passages in the lungs and decrease oxygen exchange.

Pulmonary veins The four veins (right/left superior and inferior) that return oxygenated blood from the lungs to the left atrium.

Pulmonology Medical Specialty dealing with diseases of the lungs.

Pulse generator The part of the pacemaker or defibrillator system that contains the electronics and the battery. It is implanted under the skin in the abdominal or pectoral area.

Pulvinar The cushion-like nuclear mass in the posterior dorsal thalamus overhanging the geniculate bodies of the midbrain. It has reciprocal connections with areas of parietal, temporal and occipital cortex.

Pupil The opening at the center of the iris of the eye. It contracts (dilates) in the dark and when the eye is focused on a distant object.

Pupillary distance (PD) The distances between the pupils of the eyes, in millimeters – a necessary measurement for proper lens prescription.

Pupillary reflex The automatic contraction or enlargement of the pupil when confronted with the presence or absence of light, accommodation, or emotional change.

Pupillometer A device used to measure the distance between the pupils of the eyes, in millimeters, which is a necessary measurement for proper lens prescription. It also measures the diameter of the pupil.

Pure culture A culture containing only one species of microorganism.

Pure steam Steam that is produced by a steam generator which, when condensed, meets requirements for WFI.

Purification The removal of impurities of concern. The term has one meaning when applied to the preparation of drinking water, another when applied to reagent grade water for the laboratory, and still another when applied to water used to rinse ICs (Integrated Circuit devices).

Purified water,. Water rendered suitable for pharmaceutical purposes by processes such as distillation, ion-exchange treatment (deionization or demineralization), or reverse osmosis. Common uses are: a rinse for equipment, vials, and ampoules, and as make up for cosmetics, bulk chemicals, and oral products. For FDA acceptance, purified water must contain less than 0.5 mg/l of TOC (Total Organic Carbon), and less than 100 CFU (Colony Forming Units).

Purine A nitrogen-containing, double-ring, basic compound that occurs in nucleic acids. The purines in DNA and RNA are adenine and guanine.

Purity The ratio of desirable to undesirable components in a liquid as determined on a weight basis per unit volume of sample.

Purpura A hemorraghic disease characterized by extravasation of blood into the tissues producing spontaneous ecchymoses and petechiae.

Purslane It is a weed that is edible, and sometimes put on salads, mostly in Europe. It is loaded with linolenic acid, and omega-3 fatty acid that may help reduce the risk of heart attack, and improve the health of cell membranes in the eyes and brain. It is also an excellent source of Vitamin E, providing 6 times as much as spinach.

Pursuit dysfunction A condition in which the individual's ability to follow a moving target is inadequate. Vision therapy is an effective treatment option.

Pursuit test Measures the eyes ability to follow a moving target.

Pursuits The eye's ability to smoothly follow a moving target.

Pus A protein-rich liquid inflammation product comprised of leukocytes, a thin fluid and cellular debris.

Putamen The largest component of the lenticular nucleus, situated lateral to the globus pallidus and separated from it by the lateral medullary lamina. The putamen is continuous with the caudate nucleus rostrally.

PVC (polyvinyl chloride) The largest volume of the vinyl family of plastics. Overall it has excellent basic properties, may be easily processed and welded, and is exceptionally economical in cost. Homopolymers grades of PVC comprise over 80% of all PVC used, and contain 56.8% chlorine by weight. When the chlorine content is increased to about 67% its heat deflection temperature at 264 psi increases from 155°F (68°C) to 218°F (103°C). Because PVC is a thermally sensitive thermoplastic compounding ingredients such as heat stabilizers, lubricants, fillers, plasticizers, impact modifiers, pigments, and processing aids must be added to make it processible. PVC is prone to produce extractables during start-up in high purity water.

PVDF (polyvinylidene fluoride) kynar, sygef, solef A thermoplastic fluoropolymer with a melt point of 352°F (178°C), and a wide service range from -40°F (-40°C) to 284°F (140°C). It has a very linear chemical structure, and is similar to PTFE with the exception of not being fully fluorinated, i.e. having 3% hydrogen by weight. Its drawbacks in the area of chemical resistance include unsuitability with strong alkalis, fuming acids, polar solvents, amines, ketones, and esters. It has a high tensile strength as well as a high heat deflection temperature. It is readily weldable, offers high purity qualities, and is resistant to permeation of gases. PVDF is a relatively inert material and contributes little in the way of contamination to pharmaceutical water.

Pycnogenol Source of proanthocyanadins.

Pyelonephritis (nephropyelitis) Inflammation of the kidney and renal pelvis often by ascending bacterial infection.

Pyloric sphincter The muscle between the stomach and the small intestine.

Pyloric stenosis An enlargement of the muscle between the stomach and the small intestine, blocking the passage of food and liquids forward into the intestines.

Pyloric valve Fold of mucous membrane located at the pyloric orifice of the stomach.

Pyloroplasty An operation that enlarges the opening between the stomach and small intestine so food and liquid can move forward and be digested normally.

Pylorus The muscular valve separating the stomach from the duodenum.

Pyo (prefix) Pus.

e.g. pyometra - an accumulation of pus within the uterus.

e.g. pyogranuloma - an infiltration of polymorphonuclear cells into an area of chronic inflammation characterized by mononuclear cells, macrophages, lymphocytes and even plasma cells.

Pyramids (medullary) Two longitudinal eminences located on the ventral surface of the medulla oblongata formed by the corticospinal tract fibers.

Pyridoxine (Vitamin B-6) A vitamin which supports glycogen and nitrogen metabolism; production and transport of amino acids; production and maintenance of red blood cells (hemoglobin) Essential for the body's utilization of protein. Needed for the production of red blood cells, nerve tissues, and antibodies. Women taking oral contraceptives have lower levels of B-6.

Pyriform lobe A pear-shaped lobe that is prominent in macrosmatic animals. It includes the lateral olfactory gyrus, and areas (uncus, periamygdaloid, entorhinal) of the anterior parahippocampal gyrus. This corresponds to the primary and secondary olfactory areas of cortex.

Pyrimidine A nitrogen-containing, single ring, basic compound that occurs in nucleic acids. The pyrimidines in DNA are cytosine and thymine, in RNA, cytosine, and uracil.

Pyrogen A foreign substance that produces a fever response in humans and animals, hence the name pyrogen (heat producing). Chemically, the lipopolysaccharide outer layer of gram-negative bacteria. Bacterial pyrogens were at one time believed to be toxic substances released when bacterial cells disintegrate and are therefore still referred to as endotoxins. Parenteral drugs must be essentially pyrogen free. Pyrophoric A chemical that will spontaneously ignite in air at or below a temperature of 130°F (54.5°C).

Pyruvate A key energy metabolite for the breakdown of fuel (glucose, fatty acids, amino acids, etc.) to energy in our bodies, pyruvate can give us increased energy, assist in burning fat as fuel, and have anticatabolic effects (such as producing alanine). Pyruvate acid is alpha - ketopropionic acid. Studies have shown that pyruvate can help decrease fatigue, and increase vigor with only six grams per day.

The human body breaks down carbohydrates for energy though a process called glycolysis. As these sugars and starches are metabolized, pyruvate (pyruvic acid) is produced, which readily enters the mitochondria of cells to create energy fueling the muscles and other parts of the body.

Pyuria The presence of pus in the urine; usually an indication of kidney or urinary tract infection.

Q

QA (quality assurance) The sum total of the organized arrangements made to ensure that all APIs (Active Pharmaceutical Ingredients) are of the quality required for their intended use and that quality systems are maintained.

QC (quality control) Checking or testing, that specifications are met, or the regulatory process through which the industry measures actual quality performance, compares it with standards, and acts on the difference.

QI Domain For the CHSRA QIs, the broad areas of care that represent the common conditions and important aspects of care and life to nursing home residents. Each domain is represented by one or more QIs.

Quadriceps Collective name of the rectus femoris, vastus intermedius, vastus lateralis, and vastus medialis muscles, which all insert into the tuberosity of the tibia via a common tendon. They contribute to the extension of the leg upon the thigh.

Quadrigeminal plate and cistern The posterior part of the brainstem, at the mesencephalon (midbrain), has four knobby bit: two superior colliculi and two slightly smaller inferior collicul. The enlarged subarachnoid space posterior is called the Quadrigeminal Plate Cistern (QP or Kewpee Cister), and is contiguous with the ambient (circum-mesencephalic) cistern. The QP cistern looks like a smile. During brain herniation, the smile become crooked or disappears entirely, as the brainstem shifts and the subarachnoid space is obliterated.

Qualification Action of providing that equipment or ancillary systems are properly installed, work correctly, and actually lead to the expected results. Qualification is part of validation, but the individual qualification steps alone do not constitute process validation.

Qualified Mental Retardation Professional (QMRP) A person who has at least one year of experience working directly with persons with mental retardation or other developmental disabilities and is one of the following: a doctor of medicine or osteopathy, a registered nurse, or an individual who holds at least a bachelor's degree in a professional program service area. The professional program staff must be licensed, certified, or registered, as applicable, to provide professional services by the State in which he or she practices. Those program staff that does not fall under the jurisdiction of State licensure, certification, or registration requirements, must meet specific eligibility qualifications set forth by the CMS. A person who is responsible for ensuring quality care for a group of persons with mental disabilities.

Quality assurance A system of procedures, checks, audits, and corrective actions to ensure that all research, testing, monitoring, sampling, analysis, and other technical and reporting activities are of the highest achievable quality. Quality assurance serves to benefit the quality of care.

Quality assurance (QA) group The group who interprets the GMP regulations and guidelines.

Quality Assurance (QA) Program The Regulated Health Professions Act requires that each regulatory college develop, establish and maintain programs to promote continuing competence among the members of the profession.

Quality control (QC) group The group who enforces the GMP regulations.

Quality function The entire collection of activities from which the industry achieves fitness for use, no matter where these activities are performed.

Quality Improvement Organizations (QIOs) State organizations funded by the CMS "to ensure the quality, effectiveness, efficiency and economy of health care services provided to Medicare beneficiaries," formerly referred to as Peer Review Organizations, or PROs. The 53 QIOs have been designated to provide educational materials and programs to nursing homes in their State to assist them in understanding and using the publicly reported quality measures (QMs).

Quality Indicators (QIs) CHSRA's indicators of provider level and resident (patient) level status derived from MDS (OASIS) information. The QIs are pointers or signposts of potential resident (patient) and/ or provider care problems. QIs are used by surveyors to help structure the survey process and can be used by providers to help monitor and improve their own performance.

Quality Measures (QMs) Publicly reported information made available by CMS to help consumers assess the quality of nursing home care. There are two categories of quality measures: 1. Conditions relevant primarily to long-term residents (patients) (chronic care), including decline in late loss ADLs, pressure sores, residents with pain, physical restraints, and prevalence of infections; and

2. Short-stay (temporary) residents (patients) (post-acute care), specifically prevalence of delirium, residents with pain, and improvement in walking. Many of the QMs are based on, and virtually identical to, QIs.

Quality of care A level of performance or accomplishment that characterizes health care. Ultimately, measures of the quality of care always depend upon clinical outcomes or value judgments, but there are ingredients and determinants of quality that can be measured objectively, such as structure, process or procedures, and outcomes.

Quality of life The degree to which individuals perceive themselves as able to function physically, emotionally and socially. In a general sense, it is that which makes life worth living. In a more "quantitative" sense it refers to a person's time remaining alive, free of impairment, disability, or handicap.

Quality unit(s) An organizational unit independent of production that fulfills both Quality Assurance and Quality Control responsibilities. This may be in the form of separate QA and QC units, a single individual (or group), depending upon the size and structure of the organization.

Quarantine The status of materials isolated physically or by other effective means pending a decision on their subsequent approval or rejection.

Quercetin This bioflavonoid occurs in many plant foods. Quercitin has a synergistic effect with ephedrine and caffeine, increasing and prolonging their properties.

Queue Documents lined up and waiting to be printed, or commands lined up and waiting to be serviced. Use the Printer window to view the print queue for a printer.

QWERTY Refers to the standard English language keyboard configuration. The name QWERTY is formed by combining the first six letters on the top row of keys

Quick stop DNA mutants of E. coli cease replication immediately when the temperature is increased to 42°C.

Quickening Feeling the baby move inside the uterus. Often described as butterflies fluttering, gas, or bubbles.

R

Radiation sterilization Sterilization using gamma radiation emitted from radioactive materials such as cobalt-60, or cesium 137. If proper dosage of nuclear radiation can be documented, sterility testing is not required.

Radio immunoassay (RIA) A highly sensitive method of detecting and measuring the concentration of biological compounds in vivo.

Radioactive material A material or combination of materials that spontaneously emits ionizing radiation.

Radius One of the two bones of the forearm, it has a large articulation with the carpal bones that form the wrist.

Rami (communicantes gray) Nerve bundles that extend from the sympathetic trunk to all 31 pairs of spinal nerves. They consist of unmyelinated postganglionic sympathetic fibers originating from cell bodies within the sympathetic trunk and distributed with the spinal nerves to cutaneous effectors (smooth muscle and glands).

Rami (communicantes white) Twelve pair of nerve bundles that connect the sympathetic trunk to spinal nerves T1 to L2,3. They are composed of myelinated preganglionic sympathetic fibers that originate from cell bodies within the intermediolateral cell column of the thoracolumbar cord and synapse in the sympathetic trunk.

Ramus R. (Anterior Ascending) A branch of the lateral fissure (of Sylvius) extending vertically from its stem into the inferior frontal gyrus and separating the pars triangularis from the pars opercularis.

R. (Anterior Horizontal): A horizontal branch of the lateral fissure (of Sylvius) extending forward from the stem of fissure and separating the pars orbitalis from the pars triangularis of the inferior frontal gyrus. It sometimes has a commo n origin with the anterior ascending ramus.

R. (Posterior)): That branch of the lateral fissure (of Sylvius) distal to the point of origin of the anterior ascending and anterior horizontal rami.

Random Access Memory (RAM) This is the memory used by your computer to perform tasks, like running programs, doing calculations etc and it's analogous to short-term memory in humans. When you run a software program, your computer copies it to the RAM and does all the work there. This allows the computer to run the software faster. RAM needs power (electricity) to work, however, so when your computer's power is turned off, the RAM is erased. The software program is still on your system because your computer copied the working parts of it to RAM but any new information that you created whether text, spreadsheets, graphics and is kept in RAM until you save it. That is why you need to continuously save your information to your hard drive or disk.

Random sampling A method of selecting a sample whereby each element in the population has an equal chance (probability) of being selected for the sample.

Range of Motion (ROM) The extent or magnitude of a 'resident's (patient's) joint movement.

Raphe The midline plane of the midbrain, pons, or medulla oblongata.

Raphe nuclei Cells groups located along the midline of the medulla, pons, and midbrain whose fibers are distributed widely in the neuraxis. They use serotonin as a neurotransmitter although not exclusively.

Rapid exchange (RX) A feature available on balloon catheters, also known as monorail or rail segment, which allows for easy exchange of the balloon catheter without removing the original guidewire.

Rate A measure of the frequency of some event in a defined population at a specified time. In a rate, the numerator is a subset of the denominator. The rate is expressed per 100, 1,000, 10,000 or 100,000.

Ratio A measure of the frequency of one group of events relative to the frequency of a different group of events (e.g., maternal mortality ratio is the number of maternal deaths per 100,000 live births). The ratio is expressed per 100, 1,000, 10,000 or 100,000.

Raw material A general term used to denote starting materials, reagents, intermediates, process aids, and solvents intended for use in the production of intermediates or APIs (Active Pharmaceutical Ingredients).

Raynaud's syndrome (Raynaud's phenomenon) This is a condition characterized by blood vessel spasms in the fingers, toes, ears or nose, usually brought on by exposure to cold. Raynaud's phenomenon can occur in people with autoimmune disorders such as rheumatoid arthritis, lupus and scleroderma.

RDNA (recombinant DNA) The hybrid DNA produced by joining pieces of DNA from different sources.

Read Only Memory A solid-state microchip programmed at the time of its manufacture, that cannot be reprogrammed by a user. Any type of storage media that is manufactured with data in storage that cannot be reprogrammed.

Reading Requires the use of good visual skills, which are distance and near acuity, accommodation skills, binocularity skills (convergence), oculomotor skills (saccadic), peripheral vision, figure-ground, form constancy, spatial relations, visual closure, visual discrimination, visual memory, and visualization.

Reagent A substance used (as in detecting or measuring a component, in preparing a product, or in developing photographs) because of its chemical or biological activity.

Reagent grade water Water suitable for use in making up reagents or for use in sensitive analytical procedures. There are several grades of reagent grade water as defined by various professional organizations, such as ASTM, CAP, NCCLS, and ACS:

1. Type I: Used for procedures requiring maximum accuracy and precision, such as atomic spectrometry, flame photometry, enzymology, blood gas, pH and specific ion determinations; reference buffer solutions; and reconstitution of lyophilized materials used as standards. ASTM to produce Type I water specifies distillation pretreatment of feedwater.

2. Type II: Recommended for most analytical or general laboratory testing such as hematological, seralogical, and microbiological procedures as well as chemical

methods not specifically stated or proven to require Type I quality. ASTM specifies preparation of Type II by distillation and recommends it whenever freedom from organic impurities is important.

3. Type III: Satisfactory for some general laboratory tests; for most qualitative analyses such as urinalysis, parasitology, and histological procedures; for rinsing of analytical samples; preparation of stock solutions; and for washing or rinsing of glassware (final glassware rinsing should be performed with the water type specified for the procedure performed). Distillation, mixed-bed deionization, and reverse osmosis (with high quality feedwater) can be used to generate Type III.

Reasonable and Customary Charge Long term care insurance terminology. This provision limits reimbursement based on what the insurer determines is a reasonable charge for care in the policyholder's geographic area. This limit may or may not be published or available to the policyholder.

Rebirthing Also known as conscious-connected breathing or vivation. A technique in which the therapist guides clients through breathing exercises to help them re-experience past memories - including birth - and let go of emotional tensions stored in the body.

Recalcification A technique producing serum from anticoagulated plasma. Citrate and oxalate act as anticoagulants because they are Ca++ (Calcium Ion) chelating agents; Ca++ as calcium chloride is added in excess (1/40 Molar). Ca++ is a coagulation co-factor (catalyst) and promotes clot formation.

Recessive allele A gene that is expressed only when its counterpart allele on the matching chromosome is also recessive (not dominant). Autosomal recessive disorders develop in persons who receive two copies of the mutant gene, one from each parent who is a carrier.

Recirculation Continuous recirculation may be necessary to maintain uniformly high purity in larger water systems. Water is continuously recirculated and reprocessed to prevent stagnation and to rinse out residual impurities in the system. Bacteria flourish in stagnant water, especially if temperature is conducive to growth.

Recognition Acknowledgement that a clinician has achieved and consistently demonstrates the identified level of practice for a minimum of the previous six months.

Recombinant Pertaining to the recombining of generic material from one species into alternate sequences. Plasmids may then be used to incorporate the genetic material into other organisms such as E. coli bacteria.

Recombinant clone Clone containing recombinant DNA molecules.

Recombinant DNA (rDNA) The hybrid DNA produced by joining pieces of DNA from different sources.

Recombinant DNA molecules In the context of the NIH Guidelines, recombinant DNA molecules are those constructed outside living cells by joining natural or synthetic DNA segments to DNA molecules that can replicate in a living cell, or molecules that result from the replication of those described above.

Recombinant DNA techniques Procedures that transfer genetic material between organisms or species.

Recombinant DNA technology Procedure used to join together DNA segments in a cell-free system (an environment outside a cell or organism). Under appropriate conditions, a recombinant DNA molecule can enter a cell and replicate there, either autonomously or after it has become integrated into a cellular chromosome.

Recombination The process by which progeny derive a combination of genes different from that of either parent. In higher organisms, this can occur by crossing over.

Recovery Any treatment of materials by a process intended to make them suitable for further use.

Recovery time The time after an upset in a room's HVAC environmental parameters for the room to return to "normal" conditions, such as a return to acceptable humidity levels after a room wash down. This occurs within a certain number of air changes after the upset source is removed, minimally six to ten, depending on the severity of the upset, the quality of the air supply, and the degree of mixing of room air.

Recreational Therapist (RT) A person certified, by a recognized certifying organization, to perform as a recreational therapist.

Rectal manometry A test that measures the movements and strength of the rectal and anal sphincter muscles.

Rectocele A herniation of rectum into vagina.

Rectum The distal portion of the large intestine, between the sigmoid colon and the anal canal. Functions as a storage cavity to collect fecal material prior to defecation.

Rectus abdominus muscle Muscle which contributes to flexion of the lumbar vertebrae and provides abdominal support. It originates at the pubis and inserts into the xiphoid process and the cartilage of the fifth, sixth, and seventh ribs.

Rectus femoris muscle Muscle which contributes to the extension of the leg and flexion of the thigh. It originates at the anterior inferior iliac spine and the rim of the acetabellum, and inserts into the patella and tubercle of tibia.

Recycle Bin A special folder in Window 95 and 98 where deleted files are sent when the user gives the command to delete them. They reside in the recycle bin until the user gives the command to permanently erase them ('Empty Recycle Bin'), giving the user the chance to recover any information accidentally deleted.

Reference standard, primary A substance that has been shown by an extensive set of analytical tests, to be authentic material of high purity. This standard may be obtained from a recognized source or may be prepared by independent synthesis or by further purification of existing production material.

Reference standard, secondary A substance of established quality and purity, as shown by comparison to a primary reference standard, used as a reference standard for routine laboratory analysis.

Referential integrity Relationship between records that ensures data integrity by maintaining unbreakable links between related electronic records. It ensures confidence that a specific record (such as a calculated chromatographic result) is unmodified, unmanipulated, and otherwise uncorrupted after its creation and that still carries the references to the other electronic records that were used to generate it.

Reflective learning process An important model of learning that is based on the principle of gaining from the learner's own

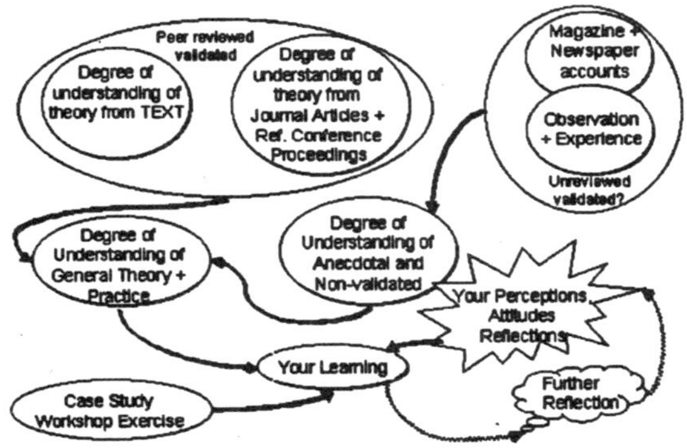

Fig. Reflective learning process

experience; this is significantly different from the traditional model of undergraduate medical education. It has very clear links with the model of self-directed learning based on a portfolio which gives evidence of activity, reflection and the outcomes of learning. Students use their knowledge, skills and attitudes to solve problems in the workplace. However, many problems are ambiguous and create surprises. Recognition of these surprises causes the student to review problems and create alternative hypotheses, which is termed "reflection in action". This leads to a search for more information, seeking help from colleagues or experts, reading texts or searching on-line to solve the problem. In order to turn the new information into new learning, a further step is required, which takes place after the problem has been solved: Reflecting on action' involves looking back critically over the initial 'surprise' and the resolution of the problem. The process of reviewing and evaluating information leads to learning and this in turn adds to expertise. The process of learning itself tends to generate new questions and motivates the professional to undertake further inquiry, which results in the learning process being determined more by the learner than by the person who designed the activity. This process of reflection provides a stimulus for learning and helps learners to derive maximum benefit from their own experiences.

Reflective Practice A component of the Quality Assurance Program. This five-step process helps nurses maintain their competence in today's rapidly changing health care environment. Every year, all nurses practicing are required to complete the Reflective Practice program and declare their participation in the program.

Reflexology Based on the idea that specific points on the feet and hands correspond with organs and tissues throughout the body. With fingers and thumbs, the practitioner applies pressure to these points to treat a wide range of stress-related illnesses and ailments.

Reflux Digestive juices, food, and liquids moving backward from the stomach into the esophagus, and possibly into the mouth.

Reflux esophagitis Irritation of the lining of the esophagus due to movement of digestive juices backward from the stomach into the esophagus.

Refraction test Determines the eye's refractive error and the best corrective lenses to be prescribed. There are several methods of performing refraction: Retinoscopy, Automated Refractor, and Subjective Refraction.

Refractive error Defects in vision caused by the eye's inability to bend, or refract light and focus it clearly on the retina. Astigmatism, hyperopia, and myopia are common conditions of refractive error, also called ametropia.

Refractive media The parts of the eye that light travels through before being focused on the retina includes the cornea, crystalline lens, aqueous, and vitreous.

Refractive power A lens' ability to bend parallel light rays into focus, as measured by power diopters. In general, the greater the curvature of a lens and the greater the difference between center thickness and edge thickness, the higher the index of refraction and the greater its refractive power. Refractive power can also refer the strength of a person's contact lenses or glasses.

Refrigerants Fluids used for heat transfer in a refrigerating system; the refrigerant absorbs heat and transfers it at a higher temperature and higher pressure, usually with a change of state. Refrigerants can be: 1. Primary refrigerants. Liquids with low boiling points that change from a liquid to a gas after absorbing heat.

2. Secondary refrigerants. Substances that act only as heat carriers, such as brine, air, and water.

Regenerate Restore ion exchange of resins by reversing the process. An acid rinse is used to restore cation resin capacity and a sodium hydroxide rinse is used to restore anion resin capacity.

Regional Office (RO) CMS Offices that serve ten distinct CMS regions. (Office Locations: Region 1 Boston; Region 2 New York City; Region 3 Philadelphia; Region 4 Atlanta; Region 5 Chicago; Region 6 Dallas; Region 7 Kansas City; Region 8 Denver; Region 9 San Francisco; Region 10 Seattle.)

Registered Dietitian (RD) A person registered as a dietitian by State statute or the American Dietetics Association.

Registered Nurses Registered nurses (RNs) work to promote health, prevent disease, and help patients cope with illness. RNs are educated in baccalaureate, associate degree and diploma programs which require about 3-4 years to complete. They are advocates and health educators for patients, families, and communities. When providing direct patient care, they observe, assess, and record symptoms, reactions, and progress; assist physicians during treatments and examinations; administer medications; and assist in convalescence and rehabilitation. RNs also develop and manage nursing care plans; instruct patients and their families in proper care; and help individuals and groups take steps to improve or maintain their health. While State laws govern the tasks that RNs may perform, it is usually the work setting that determines their daily job duties.

Registered Pharmacist (RPh) A person registered as a pharmacist by State statute.

Registered Practical Nurse An individual who has been recognized and registered as a Registered Practical Nurse.

Registry A database of configuration information central to Window 95 and 98 operations. This file contains program settings, associations between file types and the applications that created them, as well as information about the types of OLE objects a program can create plus hardware detail information.

Regression Psychological defense mechanism, viewed as a return to an earlier mode of behavior, thought, or feeling. The unconscious process that helps the mind resolve conflicts or lessen anxiety by returning to forms of gratification previously abandoned.

Regulatory affairs Drug companies must show that their products consistently meet standards set by government agencies. Regulatory affairs departments document those activities, submit proposals, and follow those proposals through completion or approval.

Regulatory region or sequence A DNA base sequence that controls gene expression.

Reiki practitioners of this ancient Tibetan healing system use light hand placements to transmit healing energies to the recipient. While the practitioners may vary widely in technique and philosophy, Reiki is commonly used to treat emotional and mental distress as well as chronic and acute physical problems, as well as to assist the recipient in achieving spiritual focus and clarity.

Reject stream In reverse osmosis and ultrafiltration, those impurities not able to permeate the membrane are said to be rejected (removed). They are flushed away in the reject (waste) stream.

Relational database management system (RDBMS) A type of database system that stores data in related tables. A relational database is powerful because it does not assume how data are related or how they will be extracted from the database. As a result, the same database can be viewed in many different ways.

Relative amblyopia Functional amblyopia can co-exit with a pathology abnormality. Treatment is possible.

Relative humidity (% RH) The ratio (measured in percent) of actual water vapor pressure in air to the pressure of saturated water vapor in air at the same temperature and pressure.

Relative risk A measure of the incidence of a condition in those exposed to a particular factor in relation to the incidence of that condition in those not so exposed.

Release The discharge of a microbiological agent or eukaryotic cell from a containment system.

Reliability Trust in the accuracy or provision of one's results; in the case of tests, it is an expression of the precision, consistency and reproducibility of measurements. Ideally, measurements should be the same when repeated by the same person or made by different assessors. In tests, contributing factors to reliability are the consistency of marking, the quality of test and test items, and the type and size of the sample. Satisfactory reliability of objective tests can be achieved by having large numbers of well-constructed test items marked by computer. Reliability is characterized by the stability, equivalence, and homogeneity of test.

Stability or test-retest reliability is the degree to which the same test produces the same results when repeated under the same conditions;

Equivalence or alternate-form reliability is the degree to which alternate forms of the same measurement instrument produce the same result

Homogeneity is the extent to which various items legitimately team together to measure a single characteristic, such as a desired attitude.

In a clinical examination, obtaining reliability depends on three variables: the students, the examiners and the patients. Such complexity makes it difficult to reproduce a comparable situation for tests of clinical skill and clinical problem-solving. In a reliable assessment procedure, the variability due to the patient and the examiner should be removed. Wherever possible, a subjective approach to marking should be replaced by a more objective one and students should be tested by a number of examiners. It is important to note that students are usually examined using different patients, which may enhance the performance of some students and harm the performance of others. Therefore, tests which aim to assess clinical skills and clinical problem-solving have to contain many samples of student performance if they are to achieve adequate levels of reliability. The development of the multi-station objective structured clinical examination (OSCE) represents an effort to do so.

Remibursemet Model A type of Long Term Care Insurance which reimburses costs of covered services for eligible individuals up to a maximum daily amount. In this model, insurance benefits are directly related to the incurred long-term care costs.

Renal artery Artery which originates from the abdominal aorta and provided branches for the ureters and the inferior adrenal (suprarenal) artery.

Renal cortex The outer portion of the kidney, containing most of the glomeruli.

Renal hilus The inner medullary portion of the kidney, containing the urine collecting tubules.

Renaturation The restoration of biological activity to a denatured protein or nucleic acid. The strands of a DNA duplex, for example, are denatured at high temperatures but can be correctly reformed by a slow cooling.

Reniform Shaped like a kidney.

Report Set Report Sets are a new feature of ePIP that allows you to create a collection of reports using parameters you define. They can be saved and run whenever they are needed. It is completely up to you to choose which reports and parameters you want to include in your Report Sets and you can also include multiple copies of the same report with different parameters if that is what you need. For example, if you would like a list of residents with weight loss QI or a decubitus ulcer for your nutritionist every month, define a new report set with the proper Individual QI Series reports selected, and save it. Each month a simple click or two will generate a new, up-to-date list for you.

Representative sample A sample that consists of a number of units that are drawn based on rational criteria such as random sampling and intended to assure that the sample accurately portraits the material being sampled.

Reprocessing A system of reworking batches that do not conform to standards or specifications, including "the steps taken to ensure that the reprocessed batches will conform to all established standards, specifications, and characteristics".

Reproducibility of assessment Consistency in producing the same results if a test is repeated is a vital attribute of any test. It is important to know that if the same examinees were given the same test after some time and learned nothing in the interim, the same scores would result. Reproducibility is especially important in making licensure and certification decisions.

Reproductive Endocrinologist A reproductive endocrinologist is a specialist in handling high risk pregnancies and in diagnosing causes of miscarriage. This type of doctor receives specialized training beyond the standard ob/gyn.

Reproductive toxicology Studies of whether exposure affects male or female fertility.

Research Scientific inquiry or an organized quest for new knowledge and better understanding, such as of the natural world or determinants of health and disease. Research can take several forms: empiric (observational), analytic, experimental, theoretical and applied.

Residency The period of training in a specific medical specialty. It occurs after graduation from medical school and its length varies from three to seven years, depending upon the specialty.

Resident The preferred terminology for a person living in a long term care facility, as opposed to a patient.

Resident Assessment Instrument (RAI) A tool to help facilities identify residents' needs and strengths and develop an appropriate care plan.

Resident Assessment Protocols (RAPs) Eighteen problem-oriented guides for care planning with "trigger" conditions to signal the need for additional assessment and review (e.g., Activities RAP, Mood State RAP, Pressure Ulcer RAP, etc.)

Resident or resident physician An individual at any level in a Graduate Medical Education program, including subspecialty programs. Other terms used to refer to these individuals include interns, house officers, house staff, trainees, or fellows. The term "intern" is often used to denote physicians in their first year of training. The term "fellow" is frequently used to denote physicians in subspecialty programs (versus residents in specialty programs) or in Graduate Medical Education programs that are beyond the eligibility requirements for first board certification in the discipline.

Residential Care Residential care is provided to frail older people and people with a disability who cannot live independently at home and who have been assessed by an Aged Care Assessment Team (ACAT) as needing this care.

Residential Care Facility Terminology used by some states for facilities which provide long term care to residents who cannot live independently, but who need a minimal level of supervision and direction. In some states, this terminology is being changed, and any facility formerly licensed as a RCF will become an Assisted Living Facility.

Resilient Having the ability to return to an original shape after having been compressed or deformed.

Resin ion exchange resins are usually bead-like spherical materials with an affinity for particular ions. Cation exchange resins made of styrene and divinylbenzene containing sulfonic acid groups will exchange hydrogen ions for any cations they encounter. Similarly, anion exchange resins made of styrene and divinylbenzene containing quaternary ammonium groups will exchange a hydroxyl ion for any anions.

Resistance (filter) The pressure drop across a filter at a stated flow and under given conditions; generally expressed in millimeters water gauge or PSI, or in SI units as N/m^2 or Pascals.

Resistivity The reciprocal of conductivity (R=1/C). A measure of specific resistance to the flow of electricity. In water, provides an easy mean of continuously measuring the purity of very low Total Dissolved Solids (TDS), or ionic concentration. The fewer the dissolved ions in water, the higher its resistivity. Resistivity is normally expressed in Megohm-cm and is equivalent to one million ohms of resistance measured between two electrodes one centimeter apart. The theoretical maximum ionic purity of water is 18.3 Megohm-cm at 25°C.

Resolution A term used to describe the amount of information a computer screen can display. The resolution is expressed in pixels. A common resolution is 640x480 pixel which means the screen in 640 pixels wide by 480 pixels tall. The higher the resolution, the better the graphic image since pixels will be smaller and closer together.

Resource Utilization Groups (RUGS) A collection of nursing facility resident classification systems used in a variety of case mix indexed reimbursement systems. Using assessment tools like the MDS 2.0, these systems group residents by expected level of resource utilization, usually based upon staff time measurements per resident per day. Relative resource utilization is reflected in a case mix index (CMI) value assigned to each RUG cell.

Respite Care Many Carers don't know what is meant by the term respite. Basically, it means "time out". Taking a break from your care-giving role, to allow you time to attend to other matters or have a well-earned rest. There are many different types of respite. These are determined by what best suits your needs and the needs of the person being cared for. Sometimes Respite can feel like more trouble than its worth. At first, taking a break can be difficult but if you persevere the benefits will usually outweigh the effort. Family Carers frequently claim that respite is the support they need most, but often reject respite when it is offered because of the initial disruption and strain it has on their routine.

Restorative Care Restorative care goes beyond rehabilitation and into services designed to restore or improve a person's functional independence. Examples of restorative care include physical or occupation therapy, speech therapy, range-of-motion exercises, bowel and bladder training, assisted walking. It can be provided by home health agencies, rehabilitation units of hospitals, free standing inpatient rehabilitation facilities (IRF), rehabilitation clinics, adult daycare centers, assisted living and skilled nursing facilities.

Restore To return data on a disk to its previous state, typically by using a backup copy of the files. You can restore files that have been damaged or corrupted back to the state they were in when you backed them up.

Restore Button In Windows environments, a button usually in the upper right corner of a Window that, when clicked, returns the window to its previous size. When the window is at its previous size, the restore button switches to the maximize button, which resizes the window to its maximum size

Restriction enzyme cutting site A specific nucleotide sequence of DNA at which a particular restriction enzyme cuts the DNA. Some sites occur frequently in DNA (e.g., every several hundred base pairs), others much less frequently (rarecutter; e.g., every 10,000 base pairs).

Restriction enzyme, endonuclease A protein that recognizes specific, short nucleotide sequences and cuts DNA at those sites. Bacteria contain over 400 such enzymes that recognize and cut over 100 different DNA sequences.

Restriction fragment length polymorphism (RFLP) Variation between individuals in DNA fragments sizes cut by specific restriction enzymes; polymorphic sequences that result in RFLPs are used as markers on both physical maps and genetic linkage maps. RFLPs are usually caused by mutation at a cutting site.

Retest date The date when samples of the API (Active Pharmaceutical Ingredient)a material should be re-examined to ensure that material is still suitable for use.

Retina The innermost layer of the eye, a neurological tissue, which receives light rays focused on it by the lens. This tissue contains receptor cells (rods and cones) that send electrical impulses to the brain via the optic nerve when the light rays are present.

Retinoblastoma An eye cancer caused by the loss of a pair of tumor-suppressor genes; the inherited form typically appears in childhood, since one gene is missing from the time of birth.

Retinol (Vitamin A) A vitamin with antioxidant properties, important for eye protection and bone growth; protein and hormone synthesis (including GH and testosterone); supports tissue maintenance. Helps reduce susceptibility to infection. Essential for healthy skin, good blood, strong bones and teeth, kidneys, bladder, lungs and membranes.

Retinoscopy This technique determines the eye's refractive error and the best corrective lenses to be prescribed. An instrument called a retinoscope which consists of a light, lens, mirror, and handle, is used to shine light into a patient's eye. There are two types of retinoscope: streak and spot retinoscope. When light is shone into patient's eye, the light is reflected back ("reflex"). If the reflection is in the same direction ("with movement") of the retinoscope then the refractive error is hyperopia (farsightedness) and a plus lens is prescribed. If the reflection is in the opposite direction ("against movement") of the retinoscope then the refractive error is myopia (nearsightedness) and a minus lens is prescribed. The strength of the prescription is determined when the pupil is suddenly filled with light ("neutralized") with the appropriate lens powers (strength). There are other types of retinoscopy such as Static retinoscopy or Dynamic retinoscopy.

Retrogastric area The area behind the stomach.

Retrospective validation Establishing documented evidence that a system does what it purports to do based on review and analysis of historic information.

Retrovirus An oncogenic, RNA-containing virus, which replicates through a double-stranded DNA intermediate necessitating the presence of an RNA-dependent DNA polymerase.

Revalidation Extent of validation necessary to assure that changes made to qualified or validated equipment, utilities, systems and process do not adversely affect the finished product. Implemented changes should be tracked and evaluated through a thorough, dynamic, change control program.

Reverse Mortgage A loan program to provide one-time or monthly cash payments for the equity in an older person's home without selling the home. Reverse mortgages provide a stream of income for an older person who has most of their equity tied up in a house and who needs cash for day-to-day expenses. A financial institution will provide a series of monthly payments, based on the value of the house, in exchange for all or part of the ultimate proceeds from the sale of the house.

Reverse osmosis (RO) The reversal of osmosis to purify water. In osmosis, water diffuses through a semipermeable membrane from a region of higher concentration (such as pure fresh water) into one of lower concentration (such as a solution of water and salt). The flow of water can be reversed with an opposing pressure that exceeds osmotic pressure. With RO, water is forced out of the lower concentrated solution (such as the salt solution), leaving the solute (impurities) behind.

Reworking Subjecting an intermediate or API (Active Pharmaceutical Ingredient) that does not conform to standards or specifications, to one or more processing steps that are different from the established manufacturing process so that its quality may be made acceptable (e.g., recrystallizing with a different solvent).

A molecule consisting of a number of ribonucleotides attached together to form a long strand one nucleotide thick. Each nucleotide contains the sugar, ribose, and one of four different bases: cytosine, adenine and guanine (as in DNA) and uracil (as opposed to thymine in DNA). The major portion of cellular RNA occurs as ribosomal RNA (rRNA), to a lesser extent as transfer RNA (tRNA) and less still as messenger RNA (mRNA), all three forms being concerned with transformation of the DNA sequence into the complementary protein sequence. It also occurs in some viruses where it acts as the hereditary material.

Rh Factor Rh Factor Rh factor is a protein that attaches to red blood cells in most people. People who have Rh factor (composing most of the general population) are said to be Rh positive; those who do not have it are Rh negative. The presence of Rh factor in a person's blood can be easily determined through a laboratory test.

rH incompatibility A situation where the mother's blood type is rH negative, and the father is rH positive. This is not a concern during a first pregnancy, but if the mother is sensitized to rH-positive blood during pregnancy, subsequent pregnancies may be attacked by her immune system. A shot is given to the rH negative mother at the end of any pregnancy, regardless of length or outcome, to prevent the production of harmful antibodies.

Rh Incompatibility Rh Incompatibility Rh incompatibility occurs when a mother is Rh negative and her fetus is Rh positive. If the fetus's blood travels through to the placenta, it interacts with the mother's blood. When this happens, the mother's body perceives the Rh factor in the fetus's blood as a harmful substance, and produces antibodies to fight it. The production of these antibodies is termed sensitization. These antibodies will fight the Rh factor back to its source: the fetus.

If sensitization occurs early in the pregnancy, the antibodies may begin to attack the current fetus during the third trimester. Fetal damage from Rh incompatibility can include anemia, illness, brain damage, and even death. Worse, once a mother is sensitized, any future Rh positive fetus she bears will run an increased risk of sustaining damage due to the antibodies.

Rhage, rrhage, rrhagia (suffix) Discharge.

e.g. hemorrhage - discharge of blood.

Rheumatoid Arthritis Rheumatoid Arthritis (RA) is an autoimmune disease, caused by improper immune reactions that occur when the one's immune system attacks one's own body, mistaking it for a foreign invader. RA causes inflammation in the lining of the joints and, sometimes, of other internal organs.

Rheumatoid Factor A blood test used to help diagnose rheumatoid arthritis (RA). The test may also be used to help diagnose the arthritis-related condition called Sjögren's syndrome.

Rheumatology A field of internal medicine devoted to the diagnosis and treatment of rheumatic diseases, which involve pathologies of the muscles, tendons and joints. Rheumatic symptoms may have underlying causes not related to rheu-matology.

Rhinencephalon Parts of the brain concerned with olfactory function (reception and integration). In the narrow sense it refers to those parts directly involved with reception of olfactory stimuli only (olfactor y bulbs, tract, striae, anterior olfactory nucleus, part of the amygdala and the pyriform cortex).

Rh-negative Absence of rhesus antibody in the blood.

RHogam Rhogam RhoGAM is the common name for Rho (D) immune globulin. This product is used during and after pregnancies to resolve an incompatibility in Rh factor between mother and unborn child.

RhoGAM Medication given during pregnancy and following delivery to pre- vent isoimmunization.

Rhombencephalon The hindbrain; most caudal of the three primary vesicles of the embryonic brain. The adult derivatives of which are the cerebellum and pons (metencephalon) and the medulla oblongata (myelencephal on).

Rhomboid fossa The diamond-shaped fourth ventricle.

Riboflavin (Vitamin B-2) A vitamin which helps with energy production and amino acid production. Helps body obtain energy from protein, carbohydrates, and fats. Helps maintain good vision and healthy skin.

Ribose Ribose is a simple sugar that is extremely important in many processes in the body. Ribose is found in all living cells. It is the backbone of genetic material, and it is the starting point for production of ATP. Ribose effectively increases ATP and TAN (Total Adenine Nucleotide) recovery, while impriving performance in heart and muscle cells. Ribose also fortifies muscle ATP but through a different pathway than creatine. Ribose also bolsters muscle recovery after your train. Ribose promotes more effcient salvage pathway, thus allowing better ATP recycling and consequent increased muscular recovery after training. If the body does not use the salvage pathway, when ribose is insufficient, it must make ATP from scratch.

Ribosomal RNA (rRNA) A class of RNA found in the ribosomes of cells.

Ribosomes Small cellular components composed of specialized ribosomal RNA and protein; site of protein synthesis.

RIBS There are 12 pairs of thin curving bones, like struts, that extend around from the spine to support the chest cavity.

Rib Fx.

Rickettsias Gram-negative microorganisms that are often carried by arthropod vectors and may infect humans and other mammals. Generally smaller than other bacteria, they require living cells for growth.

Ridesharing A program in which a coordinating agency or dispatcher is responsible for matching potential riders with cars or vanpools.

Right atrium Chamber on the right side of the heart that recieves blood from the superior and inferior vena cavi, directing it to the right ventricle.

Right colic artery Artery which originates from the superior mesenteric artery and supplies the ascending colon.

Right gastroepiploic artery Artery originating from the gastroduodenal artery and branching into the gastric and omental (epiploic) arteries.

Right mainstem bronchi Derived from the trachea, the right main bronchus that enters the right lung.

Right marginal artery Artery which originates from the right coronary artery, passing along the inferior of the heart and apex, suppling the right ventricle.

Right ventricle Chamber of the heart that directs the blood to the pulmonary trunk and into the lungs.

Right click (On a mouse that has more than one button) To quickly depress and release the right mouse button.

Rinse The operation that follows regeneration, a flushing out of excess regenerant solution.

Risk Adjustment A method of statistically controlling for resident (patient) level differences that can affect the measurement of a QI or QM. Risk adjustment is used to "level the playing field," so that fair comparisons can be make between providers who serve residents (patients) with different risk of experiencing a QI or QM. There are several different methods of risk adjustment. The QIs use a stratification approach; the QMs use a regression-based approach.

Risk factor An aspect of personal behavior or lifestyle, environmental exposure, or inborn or inherited characteristic, which on the basis of epidemiological evidence is known to be associated with an unfavorable health-related condition and considered important to prevent, if possible. It is used as an indication of increased probability of a specified health outcome such as the occurrence of a disease but is not necessarily a causal factor. The term risk factor is further used to mean a determinant that can be modified by intervention, thereby reducing the probability of occurrence of disease or other specified outcomes.

Risk Groups An assessment of a 'resident's (patient's) likelihood for development of a condition incorporated into a QI itself. QIs flag for either those persons identified at HIGH risk or those who are not at risk LOW risk. This concept has implications for assessing how providers intervene with residents (patients) who are vulnerable to certain conditions because their diagnosis or physical/mental status, and also how facilities intervene with residents (patients) who are not as vulnerable. LOW risk groups should get special attention because residents (patients) in this group have developed the QI condition in the absence of factors related to their diagnoses or physical/mental condition. High and low risk QIs should be considered as separate QIs.

Rod A receptor cell which is sensitive to light and is located in the retina of the eye. It is responsible for night vision (non-color vision in low level light).

Rolfing Uses deep manipulation of the fascia to restore the body's natural alignment, which may have become rigid through injury, emotional trauma, and inefficient movement habits. The process, developed by biochemist Ida P. Rolf, involves ten sessions, each focusing on a different part of the body.

Roller bottles Small cylindrical bottles often used as bioreactors in the production of products by cell culture. The bottles are kept on a device that rotates them slowly to help assure proper growth. Automated systems may also be used for large arrays of roller bottles introducing sterile media and harvesting finished product automatically.

ROM BIOS Read Only Memory Basic Input Output System. A special chip used to send instructions to the computer when it is turned on and before the operating system is loaded.

Roof of acetabulum The superior portion of the acetabulum.

Roof of orbit The superior wall formed by the "orbital process" of the frontal bone and lesser wing of the sphenoid bone.

Root of penis The proximal, attached, portion of the penis.

Rostrum (of corpus callosum) The most rostral part of the corpus callosum located below the septum pellucidum and extending from the genu to the lamina terminalis.

Rotator cuff (shoulder) The muscles and tendons of the upper arm and shoulder joint that form a 'cuff' about the glenohumeral joint.

Rotavirus A virus that causes diarrhea. It is the most common cause of infectious diarrhea in the United States, especially in children under 2 years old.

Rouge Form of surface corrosion that occurs in some stainless steel piping systems.

Roughness Consists of the finer irregularities of the surface texture, usually including those irregularities that result from the manufacturing process. These are considered to include traverse feed marks and other irregularities within the limits of the roughness sampling length.

Round ligament pain Pain caused by stretching ligament on the sides of the uterus during pregnancy.

Rrhea (suffix) Abnormal or excessive flow.

e.g. steatorrhea - excessive lipid in the feces.

Rubenfeld synergy method gentle touch, movement, verbal exchange, and imagination used to access memories and emotions locked in the body. Integrates elements of the Alexander Technique, Feldenkrais Method, Gestalt and Hypno-therapy. Combines bodywork and psycho-therapy. May be used for physical or emotional problems or for personal growth.

Rule State requirements promulgated to "flesh out" the State Statutes .

Rupture of membranes Loss of fluid from the amniotic sac. Also called breaking of waters.

S

Saccades The eye's ability to direct and coordinate movement as it quickly and voluntarily shift from one target to another.

Saccades dysfunction A condition in which the individual's ability to scan along a printed page and move his eyes from point to point is inadequate. Symptoms include frequent loss of place while reading, skip or transpose words, and have difficulty comprehending because of an inaccurate eye movement. Vision therapy is an effective treatment option.

Saccadic test Measures the eyes ability to move quickly and precisely from point to point.

Saccharin An artificial sweetener. It is nearly 700 times sweeter than sugar, yet leaves an aftertaste. It is not metabolized by the human body. It is useful in diabetic diets in which the patient must lower sugar intake. The FDA has listed saccharin as an 'anticipated' human carcinogen. This means that in certain individuals, the sweetener may increase the risk of cancer.

Saccharomyces cerevisiae Better known as beer yeast, ordinary yeast. Yeast used in rDNA research.

Sacral ala The superior surface of the lateral portion of the sacrum.

Sacroiliac joint The joint made between the articular surfaces of the sacrum and ilium. Partly fibrous and partly synovial.

Sacrum The triangular bone made up of five fused vertebrae that is situated below the lumbar vertebrae and between the hip bones.

Safe Mode A special mode for starting Windows 95 or 98 that uses simple, default settings so that you can at least get into Windows and fix a problem that makes it impossible to work with Windows otherwise. The default settings use a generic VGA monitor driver, no network settings, the standard Microsoft mouse driver, and the minimum device drivers necessary to start Windows.

Safe/Competent Nursing Practice Competence is the ability of a nurse to integrate the professional attributes required to perform in a given role, situation or practice setting. These attributes include knowledge, skill, judgment, attitudes, values and beliefs. Incompetence occurs when a member's professional care of a client displays a lack of knowledge, skill or judgment, or a disregard for the welfare of a client to an extent that demonstrates that the member is unfit to continue to practise, or should have their practice restricted.

Safranin A base, obtained from aniline; aniline pink; used as a stain in histology.

Sagittal Plane (Lateral Plane) A verticle plane running from front to back; divides the body or any of its parts into right and left sides.

Sagittal view An anteroposterior (AP) vertical plane, parallel to the median plane of the body. The perspective is similar to a Lateral view.

Salatrim This is a reduced calorie fat that has only five calories per gram, as opposed to nine normally.

Salience The condition where certain aspects stand out as more or less important in a situation. Salience is a perceptual stance or embodied knowledge whereby a person does not deliberately have to calculate which aspects of the situation are more or less important; they just appear as more or less important.

Salinity The concentration of soluble minerals (mainly salts of the alkali metals or of magnesium) in water.

Saliva A fluid made by glands in the mouth that helps moisten and soften foods we chew, and begins the digestive process.

Salmonella A large genus of the tribe Salmonellae, family Enterobacteriaceae, containing motile, gram-negative, rod-shaped organisms that ferment dextrose, forming acid and usually gas. Several species occur as intestinal pathogens in acute inflammations in humans and domestic animals. Salmonella typhimurium causes food poisoning in humans.

Salt A compound formed by the interaction of an acid and a base, the hydrogen atoms of the acid being replaced by another positive ion derived from the base.

Salt rejection In reverse osmosis, the ratio of salts removed (rejected) to the original salt concentration.

Salvage plasma Plasma obtained by centrifugation of outdated (older than 21 days) whole blood. This type of plasma is difficult to convert to serum because most coagulation factors have lost their activity.

SAM-e (S-Adenosyl-L-Methionine) SAM-e is a naturally occurring molecule in virtually all body tissues and fluids. It is fundamentally important in a number of biochemical reactions involving enzymatic transmethylation, contributing to the synthesis, activation and metabolism of such compounds as hormones, neurotransmitters, nucleic acids, proteins, phospholipids and certain drugs.

Sanitization That part of decontamination that reduces viable microorganisms to a defined acceptance level, normally achieved by using a chemical agent or heat.

Saphenous vein (Magna) The vein that extends from the dorsum of the foot to just below the inguinal ligament, making it the longest vein in the body. Used to supply vascular grafting material for cardiac (coronary artery) bypass surgery.

Saponification The hydrolysis of a fat by alkali with the formation of a soap and glycerol.

Sarcoma A type of cancer that starts in bone or muscle.

Sartorius muscle Muscle which originates at the naterior superior iliac spine and inserts into the medial side of proximal end of tibia. It contributes to flexion of the thigh and leg. The "tailor's" muscle.

Saturated air When there is a state of mutual equilibrium between the moist air and the liquid or solid phases of water. Saturated air holds as much water vapor as it can for a given temperature and pressure.

Saturated fatty acids Fatty acids containing fully saturated alkyl chains.

Saturation humidity The air is saturated when the partial pressure of water vapor in the air at a given temperature equals the vapor pressure of water at the same temperature.

Saturation index The relation of calcium carbonate to the pH, alkalinity, and hardness of water to determine its scale-forming tendency.

Saw Palmetto Herb shown to have protective properties for the liver. It is also shown that Saw Palmetto reduces the size of epithelial tissue in the prostate, especially in the transitional zone.

Scale The mineral deposit that can coat the insides of boilers or the surfaces of RO membranes. It consists mainly of calcium carbonate that precipitates out of solution under certain conditions of pH, alkalinity, and hardness.

Scale up To take a biopharmaceutical manufacturing process from the laboratory scale to a scale at which it is commercially feasible.

Scanner An optical input device that creates a photographic copy of text, drawings, and images for storage and manipulation by graphic and wordprocessor programs in the computer.

Scaphoid A "boat shaped" bone of the hand and foot. Also called the navicular. Note: In the hand, this bone is prone to develop aseptic necrosis after a fracture.

FX Scaphoid (Carpal Navicular)

FX Scaphoid (Carpal Navicular)

FX Tarsal Navicular.

Scapula A complex flat bone that forms the shoulder girdle (joint). Also called the 'shoulder blade'.

Science A branch of knowledge that produces theoretical explanations of natural phenomena based on experimentation and observation.

Sclera The white protective covering of the eye.

Sclero (prefix) Hard.

e.g. scleroma - a hardened patch of skin or mucous membrane.

Scleroderma Scleroderma is an autoimmune disorder marked by hardening of the body's connective tissue, but can also involve internal organs such as the heart, lungs, kidneys and the gastrointestinal tract. There are two types of scleroderma: CREST, which is limited to the skin, and progressive systemic sclerosis, which affects internal organs.

Sclerose To scar.

Sclerotherapy Treatment by injection of an agent which causes a destructive reaction.

Scope The extent or magnitude of deficient facility practice on resident (patient) outcome.

Scratch An elongated mar in the metal's surface not associated with the predominant surface texture pattern, which is visible to the unaided eye.

Screen Saver A varying pattern or graphic that appears on the screen when the mouse and keyboard have been idle for a user-definable period of time. Originally used to prevent a static background from being "burned into" the screen phosphors, this is rarely a problem with modern monitors.

Scroll Arrow Located at either end of a scroll bar, it can be clicked to scroll up or down (vertical scroll bar) or left or right (horizontal scroll bar). Clicking the scroll arrow will move your window in that direction.

Scroll Box A small box located in the scroll bar that shows where the visible window is located in relation to the entire document, menu, or list. You can click and drag the scroll box to make other portions of the document, menu, or list visible.

SCSI Small Computer Systems Interface. SCSI is a standard for connecting peripherals and other computers to a computer. SCSI, used extensively in Macintosh computers, and growing in use among PCs, is very fast and can support several devices on a single card. (Contrast with IDE)

Scutum Latin for spur. The Tympanic scutum forms the bony division between the upper portion of the tympanic cavity and the mastoid cells.

Second Attendant A skilled person whose role is to provide assistance to the midwife during birth and immediate postpartum. The second attendant is trained to deal with obstetrical and neonatal emergencies. The presence of a second attendant does not preclude the attendance of other support persons, e.g. doula, labour companion. In Manitoba, a midwife and a second attendant trained and currently certified in cardio-pulmonary resuscitation and neonatal resuscitation are required to attend each birth.

Secondary containment Level of containment that is external to and separate from primary containment.

Secure retention The ability to generate accurate and complete copies of records in both human-readable and electronic form suitable for inspection, review, and copying by FDA. Records must be protected to enable their accurate and ready retrieval through the records retention period.

Sedimentation A primary step in municipal water treatment. Water is allowed to stand long enough for solids to settle by gravity. Also called settling.

Sedimenters For sedimentation, batch and continuous centrifuges are available. There are three types of centrifuges for continuous sedimentation.

a. Disc - constructed on the vertical axis, disc centrifuges are solid-bowl units. All are capable of separating liquids from solids, solids from two immiscible liquids and two immiscible liquids. Disc-stack centrifuges differ in their ability to handle different volumes of solids in the feed stream, and in the way that the separated solids are removed from the separation vessel: solids-retaining, solids-ejecting, and nozzle-bowl separators.

b. Decanters - consists of a cylindrical settling section with a tapered end. Inside the bowl is a scroll conveyor that is driven usually at a slightly faster rate than the bowl and can be controlled by a differential speed device or back drive.

c. Tubular - a vertical solid-wall cylinder provided with caps on both ends; a tubular centrifuge generally has a bottom feed inlet. When two liquids of different specific gravities are fed, the heavier phase is concentrated against the wall, while the lighter phase "floats" on the heavier phase.

Seed lot system A seed lot system is a system according to which successive batches of a product are derived from the same master seed lot at a given passage level. For routine production, a working seed lot is prepared from the master seed lot. The final product is derived from the working seed lot and has not undergone more passages from the master seed lot than the vaccine shown in clinical studies to be satisfactory with respect to safety and efficacy. The origin and the passage history of the master seed lot and the working seed lot are recorded.

Master Seed Lot - A culture of a microorganism distributed from a single bulk into containers in a single operation in such a manner as to ensure uniformity, to prevent contamination and to ensure stability. A master seed lot in liquid form is usually stored at or below -70°C. A freeze-dried master seed lot is stored at a temperature known to ensure stability.

Working Seed Lot - A culture of microorganism derived from the master seed lot and intended for use in production. Working seed lots are distributed into containers and stored as described above for master seed lots.

Seed stock The initial inoculum, or the cells placed in growth medium from which other cells will grow.

Seed Tank Industrial fermentations are generally started in tanks smaller than a

1,000 to 50,000 gallon main fermenter. This small "seed" tank may be up to 100 gallons and propagate enough organisms to "kick-off" the main fermentation. Often, a seed tank may be large enough to require its own seed tank.

Segregated Storage in the same room or inside area, but physically separated by distance from incompatible materials.

Seizure Sudden onset of a convulsion.

Select To specify a section of text or graphics for initiating an action. To select also can be to choose an option in a dialog box.

Selenium Trace mineral with potent antioxidant effects; component in sulfur bearing amino acid production and fetal development during pregnancy; recent clinical evidence of cancer preventive properties. You can get it from rice, wheats and meats. Selenium helps prevent the formation of free radicals, and can possobly help prevent forms of cancer.

Self actualization Fully realizing one's individual human potential.

Self assessment The process of evaluating ones own deficiencies, achievements, behavior or professional performance and competencies. Self-assessment is an important part of self-directed and lifelong learning because it creates a need for improvement while it justifies confidence in ones competence.

Self assessment questionnaire (SAQ) Assessment completed by the learner about him- or herself to provide indirect, inexpensive measures of skill attainment and real-life performance. SAQ's serve as an evaluation of ones own deficiencies and achievements, professional behavior, performance and competence. Though important as a tool in motivation for improvement of competence, it has the weakness of being subject to rating biases.

Self awareness Self-conscious state of focusing attention on oneself.

Self directed learning A form of education that involves the individual learner's initiative to identify and act on his or her learning needs (with or without assistance), taking increased responsibility for his or her own learning.

Self draining Capable of elimination of all fluid from the system due to the force of gravity alone.

Self empowerment An event or process whereby an individual or group gains control over decisions and actions affecting their health.

Self referral Ordering of laboratory tests, diagnostic procedures or treatment for a patient by a physician from businesses in which the physician has a financial interest. Many physicians who have such financial interests contend that their participation improves access or quality of care, but results of a number of studies suggest that physician-owned enterprises are detrimental, promoting excessive use of diagnostic tests and treatments and potentially increasing total costs of health care as well as harming the physical and financial well-being of the individual patient.

Self-reflection Process by which a clinician reviews each theme and the behaviors noted in the levels of practice and identifies examples of their own practice that fit with the behaviors at that level. Through this thoughtful process the clinician determines at what practice they live at.

Self-regulation Self-regulation means that the profession governs itself, individually in the sense that each member is responsible for practising according to the standards of the profession and for keeping current and competent throughout their nursing careers.

Sella turcica Refers to the configuration of the hypophysial fossa relative to the clinoid processes of the body of the sphenoid bone. The term is used interchangeably for the depression or fossa itself in the body of the sphenoid bone which lodges the pituitary gland.

SEM (scanning electron microscopy) Utilizes an electron beam to produce images over a very broad magnification range of 10X to 105X. The technique is somewhat limited by the conductivity of the material but works very well to inspect 316L stainless steel. Typical magnification levels for surface defect evaluation are from 100 to 4,000.

Semiautomatic arc welding Arc welding with equipment that controls only the filler metal feed. The advance of the welding is manually controlled.

Semicircular canals Three looped bone canals within the petrous pyramid, forming part of the bony labryrinth of the ear, that produce five openings into the vestibule.

Seminal vesicles Paired pouches attached to the posterior portion of the bladder. The seminal ducts join with the ipsilateral ductus deferens to form the ejaculatory duct.

Semipermeable Membranes that do not have measurable pores but through which smaller molecules can pass.

Sensible heat (SH) Heat that causes a change of temperature without causing a change of state.

Sensible heat ratio The ratio of room sensible heat to room total heat as expressed in the formula: Sensible Heat ratio (SHR) = Room Sensible Heat (SH)/Room Total Heat (TH).

Sensitizer A chemical that causes a substantial proportion of exposed people or animals to develop an allergic reaction in normal tissue after repeated exposure to the chemical.

Sensor The part of a pacemaker system that senses the body's need for blood flow. The pacemaker uses sensor information to monitor body activity and provide the proper heart rate.

Sentinel Health Events Significant conditions or events that exist for only a single case or a few cases. For the CHSRA QI, they may represent a significant problem that needs to be investigated (e.g., Fecal Impaction, Dehydration, Pressure Ulcers Low Risk).

Sepsis The presence of various pus-forming and other pathogenic organisms or their toxins in the blood or tissues; septicemia.

Septal area Paraterminal (subcallosal) gyrus and the medial and lateral septal nuclei located rostral to the anterior commissure and lamina terminalis.

Septate Uterus A uterus with a band of tissue coming down the middle. The septum may be very minor and paper thin, causing no problem to a pregnancy, or may be very thick and unmovable, adding to your risk of miscarriage and premature labor. An HSG test is used to diagnose this condition, which is usually treated with surgery if necessary.

Septum pellucidum A thin lamerllar partition that extends between the corpus callosum and the fornix forming the medial wall of the anterior horn and body of the lateral cerebral ventricle.

Sequence tagged site (STS) Short (200 to 500 base pairs) DNA sequence that has a single occurrence in the human genome and whose location and base sequence are known. Detectable by polymerase chain reaction, STSs are useful for localizing and orienting the mapping and sequence data reported from many different laboratories and serve as landmarks on the developing physical map of the human genome. Expressed sequence tags (ESTs) are STSs derived from cDNAs.

Sequencing (of DNA or RNA) Determination of the order of nucleotides (base sequences) in a DNA or RNA molecule or the order of amino acids in a protein.

Sera One of the plural forms of serum.

Serial Port A port through which only one unit of data can pass at a time on a single wire. Contrast with Parallel Port.

Serosa Any serous membrane.

Serous membrane The membrane lining the walls of the body cavities and enclosing the contained organs. It is a mesothelium lying upon a connective tissue layer and secretes a watery serous fluid.

Serpiginous Having a wavy border.

Serrated Having a saw-like edge.

Serratia marcescens They are minute, rod-shaped or coccoid, aerobic, gram-negative organisms, found on various foodstuffs as a pink or reddish growth, nonpathogenic. Used to validate 0.45μm removal rated filters.

Serum The liquid portion remaining after clotting whole blood or plasma.

Service life The life expectancy or number of cycles for which a processing unit will maintain its performance.

Sesamoid bone A bone within a tendon.

Sessile Attached by a broad base.

Sestamibi Technitium 99 Sestamibi is a radioactive isotope used in nuclear medicine for cardiac function studies and for localizing parathyroid adenomas.

Setup Most common in Windows, the practice of copying a program's files to a computer's disk drive and setting the operating system to run it.

Severity The effect or seriousness of deficient facility practice on resident (patient) outcome.

Sex chromosomes Those whose content is different in the two sexes - usually labeled X and Y (or W and Z), female sex has XX (or WW), male is XY (or WZ).

Sexually Transmitted Disease (STD) Infections that are most commonly spread through sexual intercourse or genital contact.

Shaman Among tribal peoples, a magician, medium, or healer who owes his powers to mystical communion with the spirit world. Characteristically, a shaman goes into auto-hypnotic trances, during which he contacts spirits. Shamans are found among the Siberians, Eskimos, Native American tribes, in S.E. Asia, and in Oceania. There is also now a development of shamanic healers and practitioners in North America.

Shared Housing Programs that help older people find other people to live with them and share a home. Sometimes a younger, healthier person will live with an older person and provide housekeeping or other light assistance and general supervision in exchange for free food and board.

Shared Primary Care Occurs when both a midwife and another regulated primary health care provider take responsibility for the care of a woman/baby during normal childbearing care. When there is an insufficient number of midwives in an area to provide on-call coverage for clients, a shared primary care arrangement may be approved by the CMM if there is a solo practice or a small practice serving a large geographic area.

Shareware Refers to a method of software distribution. Shareware are programs that are written and distributed for free for users to install and try out. If a user likes the program and decides to use it, they are expected to "register" the program with its creator for a small fee. If the user decides not to register, they are expected to remove it from their system, and pass it on to another user—thus the "share" in shareware.

Shark cartilage A supplement touted as a cancer treatment. Sharks, whose frames are composed of cartilage not bone, get cancer infrequently. Proponents of this treatment claim sharks get cancer infrequently because something in their cartilage inhibits the ability of tumors to create the blood supply needed to continue growing. Shark cartilage is also promoted as an immune system stimulant and remedy for joint pain, swelling, and stiffness.

Shiatsu A form of acupressure, used in Japan for over 1,000 years to treat pain and illness and for general health maintenance. Practitioners apply finger pressure at specific points on the body in order to stimulate chi, or vital energy. Used to treat stress, circulatory problems, depression, asthma, headaches, diarrhea, bronchitis.

Shielded metal-arc welding (SMAW) An arc welding process that produces coalescence of metals by heating them with an arc between a covered metal electrode and the work. Shielding is obtained from decomposition of the electrode covering. Pressure is not used and filler metal is obtained from the electrode.

Short Term Stay Admission and discharge of a nursing home resident (patient) that occurs in less than 14 days.

Shortcut Another name for a Hotkey Combination (also called a keyboard shortcut). I n Windows95 or 98, a file used to "point" to a file or object in another location. When you open the shortcut, you are, in effect, opening the file the shortcut points to the Target.

Shotgun method Sequencing method that involves randomly sequencing tiny cloned pieces of the genome, with no foreknowledge of where on a chromosome the piece originally came from. This can be contrasted with "directed" strategies, in which pieces of DNA from adjacent stretches of a chromosome are sequenced. Direct strategies eliminate the need for complex reassembly techniques. Because there are advantages to both strategies, researchers expect to use both random (or shotgun) and directed strategies in combination to sequence the human genome.

Shoulder This is a ball and socket joint, without "weight bearing", formed by the distal clavicle, the scapula, and the proximal humerus.

Shoulder Anatomy

Shoulder Position

Shoulder Dislocation.

Siamese twins Siamese twins are twins connected at the body; they may share vital organs. Also called Siamese twins.

Sickle crisis Painful episode caused by sickle-cell disease.

Sickle-cell anemia An inherited, potentially lethal disease in which a defect in hemoglobin, the oxygen-carrying pigment in the blood, causes distortion (sickling) and loss of red blood cells, producing damage to organs throughout the body.

Sickle-cell trait Presence of the trait for sickle-cell anemia. Not sickle-cell disease itself.

Side Effect Undesirable effect of a medication that causes minimal discomfort in some people.

Sigmoid colon The lower part of the large intestine that empties into the rectum.

Sigmoid sinus An S-shaped dural venous sinus which extends along the the mastoid process of the temporal bone to the jugular foramen connecting the transverse sinus to the internal jugular vein.

Sigmoidoscopy A test that uses a thin, flexible tube with a camera lens at the end to look at the inside of the rectum and lower large intestine for abnormalities.

Signed (signature) (ICH API definition) The record of who performed a particular action or review. This record may be initials, full handwritten signature, personal seal, or authenticated and secure electronic signature.

Significant Change in Condition A substantial modification in a resident's (patient's) ' physical, mental, emotional, cognitive, or functional status that requires a new assessment using the MDS instrument, and also generally requires notification of the resident's (patient's) attending physician, family, or guardian.

Significant Medication Error Medication error that causes a resident (patient) discomfort and/or jeopardizes his/her health and safety.

Silica silicon Dioxide ($SiO2$) and its hydrated forms are classified as reactive and nonreactive. Generally, reactive Silica is removed by the anion exchange resin. Reactive Silica is only slightly ionized and is held lightly by the anion resin. It is for this reason that Silica is the first thing to break through when the resin nears exhaustion. Nonreactive Silica is generally considered to be particulate (colloidal) in nature.

SIMM Single Inline Memory Module. A SIMM is a piece of computer hardware that holds pre-assembled RAM chips. The SIMM is plugged into your computer's motherboard to give you more RAM.

Simulated patient (SP) Simulated patients are healthy persons who have been trained to reliably reproduce the history and/or physical findings of typical clinical cases. Sometimes actors are used to accomplish this goal but more often, health care providers are used. Use of an SP is designed to assess students' clinical skills while making the examination as objective as possible. Note that teaching an SP to simulate a new clinical problem takes eight to ten hours.

Simulations and models Tools for assessment of clinical performance in an environment closely resembling reality and imitating real clinical problems to rate the examinees' performance on clinical problems that are difficult or even impossible to evaluate effectively without harming a real patient. They permit examinees to make life-threatening errors and provide instant feedback so examinees can correct a mistaken action.

Models are mannequins constructed to respond realistically to actions, allowing examinees to reason through a clinical problem without risk to a real patient.

Simulation formats have been developed as paper-pencil patient management problems (PMP), computerized versions of PMP called clinical case simulations (CCX), role-playing situations, e.g., standardized patients (SP), clinical team simulations, anatomical models or mannequins, and combinations of all of the above formats.

Virtual reality simulations (VR) use computers sometimes combined with anatomical models to mimic realistic organ and surface images and the touch sensations a physician would expect examining a real patient. Written and computerized simulations have been used to assess clinical reasoning, diagnostic plans and treatment for a variety of clinical disciplines. They are expensive to create.

Single gene disorder Hereditary disorder caused by a mutant allele of a single gene (e.g., Duchenne muscular dystrophy, retinoblastoma, sickle cell disease).

Sino atrial (SA) node The small area in the upper right chamber of the heart that signals an electrical impulse to run through the heart to cause the heart to beat. It is often called the "pacemaker" of the heart.

Sinus rhythm The normal, regular rhythm of the heart, as seen on an ECG.

SIP (steam in place) The introduction of steam to sanitize or sterilize a piece of equipment without relocating the equipment.

Sjogren's syndrome Sjogren's syndrome is a disorder in which immune cells attack and destroy the glands that produce tears and saliva, resulting in dry eyes and mouth. Sjogren's syndrome is also associated with other autoimmune disorders such as rheumatoid arthritis. The hallmark symptoms of the disorder are dry mouth and dry eyes. In its more severe forms, Sjogren's syndrome may cause skin, nose, and vaginal dryness and also affect other organs including the kidneys, blood vessels, lungs, liver, pancreas, and brain.

Skill The ability to perform a task well, usually gained by training or experience; a systematic and coordinated pattern of mental and/or physical activity.

Skilled Care A level of care which requires the training and skills and 24 hour-a-day supervision of a Registered Nurse, is prescribed by a doctor, and which may not be provided by less skilled or less intensive care. Skilled Care may be defined differently by Medicare than by insurance companies. Medicare will generally pay for Skilled Care only for limited periods of time, when such care is expected to improve the medical condition of the patient, and when it is delivered in a Participating Skilled Nursing Facility. Medicare will not pay for such care when no medical improvement is expected, as is the case in many Chronic Conditions.

Skilled health personnel or skilled attendant Doctors (specialist or nonspecialist), and/or persons with midwifery skills who can diagnose and manage obstetrical complications as well as normal deliveries. (Traditional birth attendants, trained or untrained, are not included.)

Skilled Nursing Care Skilled Nursing Care is medical care provided by a licensed nurse, usually under the supervision of a physician. Examples of skilled nursing care include monitoring a patient's condition, intravenous therapy, phlebotomy, tube care, oncology care, rehabilitation and other. Skilled nursing care is provided by home-health agencies and skilled nursing facilities. This skilled nursing care is noted by service, not by location.

Skilled Nursing Facility (SNF) The term used by most States to define the type of nursing home that is licensed to provide the highest level of care.

Skilled Nursing Unit A section of a hospital which is licensed to provide skilled nursing services for longer periods of time than the usual hospital stay. SNUs are generally Medicare-certified. They are sometimes called Step-Down Units, to reflect the fact that patients are moved there subsequent to the original hospital stay, once hospital level care is no longer required.

Skin tag Flap or extra buildup of skin sometimes caused by pregnancy, generally, in places of high friction.

SLE Systemic lupus erythermatosus (SLE)-Connective-tissue disorder common in women in the reproductive ages. Antibodies made by the person act against his or her own tissues.

Sleep Apnea A condition in which, during sleep the soft tissues of the larynx relax and close the airway, thus stopping breathing. A person so afflicted is aroused from sleep continuously through the night.

Sling Procedures Surgical methods for treating urinary incontinence involving the placement of a sling, made either of tissue obtained from the person undergoing the sling procedure or a synthetic material. The sling is anchored to retropubic and/or abdominal structures.

Slit lamp (biomicroscope) This instrument can examine ocular tissue from the front of the cornea to the back of the lens. A narrow "slit" beam of very bright light produced by a lamp. This beam is focused on to the eye which is then viewed under magnification with a microscope. A joystick control is employed to enable instrument to be moved left-right and up-down. A chin rest, head rest and fixation target is also required. Some slit lamps have a tilting mechanism to enable the lamp to be directed from different angles.

Slope An incline or deviation from the horizontal. A tube or pipe installed in the horizontal plane is said to slope if one end is positioned higher than the other.

Small group teaching A very popular form of instruction since it permits the working through of learning material, not just in terms of knowledge but also in terms of attitudes. Within a small group, participants are more likely to éxchange opinions and feelings. Usually such sessions are structured with the help of specific exercises such as patient interviews or discussion topics.

Small intestine The section of the digestive tract between the stomach and the large intestine. Most of digestion occurs here as nutrients are absorbed from food.

Smoke control The use of physical barriers and mechanical ventilation to control the spread of smoke from a fire.

Smoke purge The use of mechanical ventilation to remove smoke resulting from fire.

Smoke test Visualization of airflow streams in a clean space using artificially generated smoke, such as Titanium smoke, CO2, or glycol fog.

Social Security A program of the United States, established in 1935, which includes a retirement income program, as well as disability and survivors benefits.

Sodium Also known as Salt. Regulates body fluid volume, transports amino acids to cells and plays a role in muscle contraction and nerve transmission. Sodium is an important mineral found in our bones, in the fluids surrounding our cells and in the cardiovascular system. Sodium, with potassium, assists nerve stimulation and regulated water balance. It is also involved in carbohydrate absorption.

The average person requires a minimum of one tenth of a teaspoon of salt a day. Any athlete who sweats needs more. A teaspoon a day of salt does not cause problems, nor does eating fresh foods high in natural salt such as fish, carrots, beets and poultry. Easting processed and junk foods, can lead to high, potentially dangerous levels of sodium intake.

Soft palate The posterior fleshy portion of the horizontal partition separating the nasal from the oral cavity.

Softener Water treatment equipment that uses a sodium-based ion-exchange resin, principally to remove cations.

Softening A pretreatment process which uses cation exchange resin to remove hardness elements (calcium and magnesium) from water. The cation resin is regenerated with Sodium Chloride (NaCl) and during the exchange process, the calcium and magnesium are removed from the water and replaced with sodium ions (Na^+). The resulting sodium salts are much more soluble and do not precipitate, which provides better feed water to the RO system.

Software Generic term for any computer program or file. Instructions that make the computer work.

Soldering A metal joining process wherein coalescence is produced by heating to suitable temperatures and by using a nonferrous alloy fusible at temperatures below 427°C (800°F) and having a melting point below that of the base metals being joined. The filler metal is distributed between closely fitted surfaces of the joint by capillary attraction. In general, solders are lead-tin alloys and may contain antimony, bismuth, and other elements.

Solid tumors Cancer cells which grow as a solid mass.

Soluble antigen Generally used in reference to vaccine production. As opposed to a whole live or attenuated virus, a soluble antigen is a fragment of the virus that produces immunity. Also refers to large molecular weight polysaccharides from some bacteria which can act as vaccines.

Solute The substance that dissolves to form ions in solution.

Solvent An inorganic or organic liquid used as a vehicle for the preparation of solutions or suspensions in the manufacture of an intermediate or API (Active Pharmaceutical Ingredient).

Somatic cell Any cell in the body except gametes and their precursors.

Somatotropin Known in the medical community as GH or Growth Hormone. It is a powerful anabolic hormone that affects all systems of the body and plays an important role in muscle growth. It is a peptite hormone, which is composed of many amino acids (191 of them) linked togethers. It is rapidly metabolized by the liver and has a half-life in the blood of approxiamately 17 to 45 minutes. Because of this, detecting GH in a drug screen is very hard.

Somoclonal variation Genetic variation produced from the culture of plant cells from a pure breeding strain; the source of the variation is not known.

SOP (standard operating procedures) The description of necessary activities to respond to normal and abnormal situations in an operating system. The SOP may include a troubleshooting checklist, list of personnel to contact, etc. SOPs should also describe normal operation, maintenance, and cleaning of the system, and normal operating parameters. An SOP may be created for any system but an SOP must be created for each system requiring qualification.

Sound Card A hardware device that makes it possible for the computer to play digitally recorded or created sounds, and CD audio. Creative Labs' Soundblaster sound card is the standard in PC audio, therefore, most manufacturers will label their sound cards as "Soundblaster compatible".

Sounding the body A diagnostic and therapeutic technique used in sound healing. Sound healers read a patient's body by singing a series of tones and listening for imbalances in the natural frequencies of the body or its' energy fields. Imbalances are said to be indicated by changes in the tone of the healer's voice. To correct a problem, the sound healer applies sound to the patient's body by singing certain tones near the affected organ, or by applying tuning forks or electronic vibratory instruments to the body.

Source Code The original copy of a software program as it is written by programmers in a language they understand. The source code is then compiled (converted) into machine language, a language that computers understand. Now the program is able to work on a users computer in a language the user understands.

Southern blotting Transfer by absorption of DNA fragments separated in electrophoretic gels to membrane filters for detection of specific base sequences by radiolabeled complementary probes.

Soy Protein Primary vegetable source of protein found in protein powders; lower in nitrogen retention and BCAA's than whey and egg, but higher in arginine and glutamine and contains isoflavones with antioxidant properties.

Sparger A device used to agitate, oxygenate, aerate, or add a chemical to a liquid by means of compressed air or gas entering through small holes in a pipe below the liquid surface.

Spasm Movement of a muscle that causes cramping and pain.

Spatial relation The ability to judge the relative position of one object to another and the internal awareness of the two sides of the body. These skills allow the individual to develop the concepts of right, left, front, back, up, and down. This ability is needed in reading and math.

Specific conductance The reciprocal of specific resistance usually expressed in micromhos/cm.

Specific humidity Also known as Humidity Ratio, and Absolute Humidity, is the weight of water vapor in each pound of dry air expressed in grains of moisture per pound of dry air, or pounds of moisture per pound of dry air. NOTE: 7,000 grains = 1.0 pound.

Humidity of air mixtures is normally discussed in terms of grains of moisture per pound rather than the more common term of relative humidity because the grains of moisture in an air stream do not change when it is heated or cooled, unless condensation takes place.

Specific ion determinations Electrochemical measurement of trace ion levels in solution.

Specific resistance The resistance of a one-centimeter cube of water to the passage of electricity under standard conditions, expressed in ohms/cm. A measure of the Total Ionized Solids concentration.

Specific volume In Psychrometry, the cubic feet of the mixture per pound of dry air.

Specification A list of testes, references to analytical procedures, and appropriate acceptance criteria that are numerical limits, ranges, or other criteria for the test described. It establishes the set of criteria to which an intermediate or API (Active Pharmaceutical Ingredient) should conform to be considered acceptable for its intended use. "Conformance to Specifications" means that the intermediate or API, when tested according to the listed analytical procedures, will meet the listed acceptance criteria.

Specificity Exerting a definitive and distinctive influence on a particular part of the body and on the course of a particular disease.

Speech Pathologist (SP) A person licensed, certified, or registered by State statute to perform as a speech pathologist.

Speech Therapist (ST) A person licensed, certified, or registered by State statute to perform as a speech therapist.

Spenddown The process whereby a person who is nearly destitute enough to qualify for medicare uses up their remaining assets. In many states, nursing home residents may be put on spenddown, and their assets which exceed the allowable resource limit are applied against the cost of their nursing home care, until the limit is reached.

Spermatic cord The tissues extending from the abdominal inguinal ring to the testis, containing the ductus deferens, testicular artery, pampiniform (venous) plexus, and nerves.

Sphenoid sinus Made up of two cavities, separated by a bony septum, in the anterior portion of the body of the sphenoid bone. The sphenoid sinus communicates with the nasal cavity.

Sphere An ophthalmic lens with no cylindrical power or addition. It has the same power in all parts of the lens.

Sphincter A circular muscle that opens and closes at an entrance to an organ. Examples include the lower esophageal sphincter and the anal sphincter.

Spicer veins Spicer veins-Dilatation or swelling of a small blood vessel. Sometimes called an angioma or Telangiectasias. During pregnancy, another common name is a spider angioma.

Spider Angiomata Varicosities of small superficial cutaneous veins and capillaries.

Spina bifida Malformations that result from the defective development of the spinal cord and/or the encasing vertebrae of varying severity. They most commonly occur in the lower thoracic, lumbar and sacral regions.

Spinal anesthesia Spinal anesthesia-Anesthesia given in the spinal canal.

Spinal cord Portion of the central nervous system within the vertebral canal, running from the foramen magnum to the upper part of the lumbar region, ending as theconus medullaris.

Spine of scapula Plate of bone attached to the back of the scapula, with the tip at the vertebral border and ending laterally as the acromion process.

Spinner flasks Small laboratory bioreactors used for the initial growth of mammalian cells lines.

Spinous process The portion of the vertebrae that projects backward from the arch and is a point of muscular attachment.

Spiritual/shamanic healing Practitioners who regard themselves as conductors of healing energy or sources from the spiritual realm. Both may call upon spiritual helpers such as power animals, angels, inner teachers, the client's Higher Self, or other spiritual forces. Both forms of healing can be used for a range of emotional and physical illnesses.

Spleen Gland-like but ductless organ located on the left side of the upper abdominal cavity, lateral to the cardiac region of the stomach.

Note: No natural "vent" is present.

Splenic artery Originating from the celiac trunk and branching into the pancreatic and splenic branches, left gastro-omental, and short gastric arteries.

Splenic flexure Bend within the large intestine where the transverse colon becomes the descending colon.

Splenic portal vein confluence The point where these two veins merge into one.

Splenic vein The vein originating at the junction of several branches at the hilum of the spleen, and joining the superior mesenteric vein, to form the portal vein, at the neck of the pancreas.

Splenium The enlarged posterior portion of the corpus callosum. Fibers of the splenium contribute to the formation of the roof and lateral wall of the occipital horn of the lateral ventricle and the lateral wall of the temporal horn. Remaining fibers comprise the forceps major which interconnects the occipital lobes.

Spontaneous abortion or miscarriage A fetal death in early pregnancy. At what gestational age (point in pregnancy) a miscarriage becomes a stillbirth for reporting purposes depends on the country's policy.

Spontaneous rupture of membranes (SROM) This is when your bag of waters breaks all by itself during labor without any interference from anyone.

Spore A reproductive cell or seed of algae, fungi, or protozoa.

Spore, bacterial A bacterial spore is a resistant body formed as part of the life cycle of some bacteria. Bacterial spores are able to withstand severe environmental conditions (e.g., heat, drying, chemicals) for many years. When conditions are favorable, spores germinate into vegetative bacterial cells capable of replication.

Sporicide An agent that destroys bacterial and fungal spores.

Spray drying Process by which a material in suspension is converted into droplets that may be coated by a substance, either melted or dissolved in the droplet's media. The action in spray drying is primarily that of evaporation, energy is applied to the droplet forcing evaporation of the media with both energy and mass transfer through the droplet. Examples of this technology include, pharmaceutical tablet granulation, and rapid drying which results in free-flowing powders on a continuous basis. Spray drying process consists of the following steps:

1. Formation of a slurry to be sprayed; this slurry may be a simple concentrated solution or the dispersion of an insoluble material in a solution.

2. Liquid atomization into droplets; this action is critical as the droplet size will dictate the equipment size as well as the final product size. There are four types of atomization devices: air, airless, disk (or rotary) spray, and ultrasonic.

3. Exposure of the droplet to a heated gas flow; this gas (normally air) supplies the energy required to vaporize the solvent. Collection of the dry free-flowing powder or encapsulated liquid or solid.

Spreadsheet A program that uses a grid of rows and columns to perform calculations on numerical data. Spreadsheets are widely used in most businesses to perform both simple and complex financial computations.

Squamo-columnar junction The junction between the normal squamous cell lining of the esophagus and columnar cell lining of the stomach.

Squint To be unable to direct both eyes simultaneously toward a point. Also known as strabismus (turned eye).

St. John's Wort Scientific name: Hypericum Performatum. A plant herb that is used to relieve mild depressive symptoms, sleep disorder, and anxiety, although probably not effective against serious depression. In large doses, it may be unsafe as it can make the skin and eyes extra sensitive to light.

Stability Generally, stability refers to the physico-chemical condition of a parenteral, biological, or shelf life of labile drugs. Certain drugs must pass stability tests. For example, human serum albumin must pass certain limits of nephelometric turbidity. Also manufacturers must have documentation of potency of labile products under labeled storage conditions.

Stability index An empirical modification of the saturation index used to predict scaling or corrosive tendencies in water systems.

Stainless steel There are more than 70 standard types of stainless steel and many special alloys. These steels are produced in the wrought form (AISI types) and as cast alloys (ACI types). Generally, all are iron based, with 12 to 30 percent chromium, 0 to 22 percent nickel, and minor amounts of carbon, columbium, copper, molybdenum, selenium, tantalum, and titanium. There are three groups of wrought stainless steels:

1. Martensitic Alloys: characteristically magnetic and hardenable by heat treatment are oxidation resistant. They are exemplified by Type 410 (UNS S41000). Contain 12 to 20 percent chromium with controlled amount of carbon and other additives. Their corrosion resistance is inferior to austenitic stainless steels, and is generally used in mildly corrosive environments and for cutlery, turbine blades, and high-temperature parts.

2. Ferritic Stainless: characteristically magnetic but not hardenable by heat treatment. Contain 15 to as much as 30 percent Cr with low carbon content (0.1 percent). The higher chromium content improves its corrosive resistance. Type 430 (UNS S43000) widely used in nitric acid plants is a typical example. Corrosion resistance is rated good, although ferritic alloys are not good against reducing acids such as HCl.

3. Austenitic Stainless: widely used in bioprocessing, are characteristically non-magnetic, not hardenable by heat treatment, and are the most corrosion resistant of the three groups. These steels contain 16 to 26 percent chromium, 6 to 22 percent nickel. Carbon is kept low (0.08 percent) to minimize carbide precipitation. To avoid precipitation, special stainless steels stabilized with titanium, columbium, or tantalum, have been developed (types 321, 347, 348). Another approach to the problem is the use of low-carbon steels such as 304L and 316L, with 0.03 percent maximum carbon. Type 302 is the basic alloy of this group. Types 304 (UNS S30400) and 304L are low-carbon versions of 302. Types 316 (UNS S31600), 316L, and 317 (UNS S31700), with 2.5 to 3.5 percent molybdenum, are the most corrosion resistance.

Cast Stainless Alloys: are widely used in pumps, valves, and fittings. All corrosion resistant alloys have the letter C plus a second letter (A to N) denoting increasing nickel content. Numerals indicate maximum carbon. Typical members of this group are CF-8, similar to 304 stainless, CF-8M, similar to 316, and CD-4M Cu, which has improved resistance to nitric, sulfuric, and phosphoric acids.

Standard Refers to a model, example or rule for the measure of quantity, weight, extent, value, or quality, established by authority, custom or general consent. It is also defined as a criterion, gauge or yardstick by which judgments or decisions may be made. A meaningful standard should offer a realistic prospect of determining whether or not one actually meets it.

Standards may be mandatory (required by law), voluntary (established by private and professional organizations and available for use), or de facto (generally accepted by custom or convention, such as standards of dress, manners, or behavior).

Standardized oral examination (SOE) A performance assessment using realistic patient cases with a trained physician examiner questioning an examinee in a standardized manner. These exams assess clinical decision-making and the application or use of medical knowledge with realistic patients. The exam begins with the presentation of a clinical problem in the form of a patient case scenario with a request to the examinee to manage the case. An examinee can be tested on a selection of different clinical cases. The examiners need to be trained in how to provide patient data for each scenario, how to question the examinee, and how to evaluate and score the examinee's responses. To create such an exam, extensive resources and expertise are required.

Standardized patient (SP) Individuals who have been trained to reliably reproduce the history and/or physical findings of typical clinical cases. They can be real patients who have been "standardized" or they can be simulated patients, i.e. persons who are not sick but take on a patient's history and role. Sometimes health care providers or actors are used to accomplish this goal. This tool is designed to make examination and assessment of a student's clinical skills as objective as possible. To teach a standardized patient to simulate a new clinical problem takes eight to ten hours.

Standardized patient examination (SPE) An exam used to assess history-taking and physical examination skills, communication skills, differential diagnosis, laboratory utilization, and treatment. A standardized patient examination consists of multiple standardized patients, each presenting a different condition in a 10-12 minute encounter. The examinee performs a history-taking and physical examination, orders tests, provides diagnosis, develops a treatment plan, and counsels the patient. Using a checklist or rating form, the examiner or the Standardized Patient evaluates the student's performance and behavior. Reproducible scores are readily obtained for history-taking, physical examination, and communication skills. Thorough training of raters, whether they are physicians, patients or other types of observers, is critical to obtaining reliable scores. Development of such an examination is often time consuming.

Standards of Practice These set out the expectations for nurses' conduct and practice. The three major components are professional standards, practice expectations, and legislation and regulations.

Stand-By Assistance When a person occasionally requires the physical assistance of another person to perform one or more Activities of Daily Living (ADLs), and needs someone to be available when they perform those activities. The presence of another person within arm's reach of the individual that is necessary to prevent by physical intervention injury while the individual is performing an ADL. In some cases, this help is needed for a person who is physically capable of performing the ADL who forgets how to do it correctly because of cognitive impairments.

Standpipe system A wet or dry system of piping, valves, outlets, and related equipment designed to provide water at specified pressures and installed exclusively for the fighting of fires.

Start Menu A feature of Windows 95 and 98 located the task bar. Clicking the button marked "Start" opens a popup menu that makes Help, the Run command, settings, find, shutdown, a list of programs (actually, program shortcuts) and a list of recently accessed documents available for you to run with a single click. For some items (such as the Documents item), a submenu opens to the side of the main item to display the list of choices. You can configure the Start menu to specify which programs are available to run from it.

Start Up The initial operation of equipment to prove that it is installed properly and operates as intended. Start-Up is considered complete when the selected equipment will adequately process product as specified.

Startup Folder A folder that contains shortcuts to any programs that you want Windows 95 or 98 to automatically run whenever you start your computer.

Stasis (suffix) Standing still.

e.g. hemostasis - arrest of blood circulation.

Stasis Decreased flow.

State of control A condition in which all operating variables that affect performance remain within such ranges that the system or process performs consistently and as intended.

Statement of Deficiency (SOD) A written summary of noncompliance with regulations found during a provider survey or complaint investigation .

Station Estimation of the descent of the baby. Ranges from -4 to +4. 0 = directly at pelvis.

Statistical process control (SPC) A process control method to demonstrate mathematically that a process or system is operating within the limitations established for the parameter(s) in question.

Stea (prefix) Lipid.

e.g. steatorrhea - excessive lipid in the feces.

Steam In place Sterile Absence of life; usually refers to absence of viable microorganisms.

Steatorrhea Loose, greasy bowel movements caused by an inability of the body to absorb fat.

Stenosis A stricture of any canal.

Stent Tiny mesh tubes that are implanted into an artery, providing the necessary scaffolding to hold the artery open and ensuring blood flow to the heart.

Stereopsis test Measures depth perception that is dependent on the accuracy of eye teaming.

Stereopsis The ability to perceive a three dimensional depth which requires adequate fusion (union) of the images from each eye.

Sterile engineering design (fermentation) The application of techniques to prevent contamination of a fermentation process by undesirable organisms. It includes three basic phases relating to the operation of the plant. First, the fermenter with the ancillary equipment, pipework, and valves must be brought to a sterile state. Secondly, the fermenter feed must be sterilized, and finally, sterile barriers at the interface between the fermenter and the outside environment must be maintained.

Sterile water A form in which water is distributed in sterile packages. Sterile Water for Injection is intended mainly for use as a solvent for parenteral products such as sterile solids that must be distributed dry because of limited stability of their solutions. It must be packaged only in single-dose containers of not larger than 1-liter size.

Sterile water for irrigation, This form of water meets most, but not all, of the requirements for Sterile Water for Injection. The exceptions are with respect of container size (i.e., the container may contain a volume of more than 1 liter), container design (i.e., the container may be designed so as to empty rapidly the contents as a single dose), particulate matter requirements (i.e., need not meet the requirement for Large Volume Injections for single-dose infusions), and labeling requirements (e.g., the designation "For Irrigation Only" and "Not For Injection" appear prominently on the label).

Sterilization The act or process, physical or chemical, that destroys or eliminates all viable microbes including resistant bacterial spores from a fluid or a solid. Despite being stated as an absolute, the action of sterilization is usually stated in terms of probability. Examples of sterilization methods are: steam treatment at 121°C, dry heat at 450°F, flushing with a sterilizing solution such as Hydrogen Peroxide (H2O2) or ozone (O3), irradiation, and filtration.

Sterilizing filter A filter that, when challenged with the microorganisms Brevundimonas diminuta, at a minimum concentration of 107 organisms per square centimeter of filter surface, produces a sterile effluent.

Sternoclavicular articulation The joint formed by the junction of the sternal end of the clavicle, the clavicular notch of the manubrium, and the first costal cartilage.

Sternothyroid muscle Muscle which originates at the manubrium sterni, and inserts into the thyroid cartilage. It is responsible for the depression of the thyroid cartilage.

Sternotomy A lengthwise incision through the breastbone (sternum) that may be made when heart surgery is performed.

Sternum The longitudinal midline plate of bone that articulates with the clavicles and cartilages of the first seven ribs, forming the middle portion of the anterior chest wall of the thorax.

Steroids Classified as lipids, naturally occurring steroids are hormones that are important regulators of animal development and metabolism at very low concentrations. A well known steroid, cholesterol, is present in membranes of animal tissues. Other steroids include testosterone (a male sex hormone), cortisone (an adrenocortical hormone), estrone (a female sex hormone), and progesterone.

Stevia A herb from Brazil and Paraguay that is a good replacement for sugar and artificial sweeteners. You can also bake with it.

Stevioside An artificial sweetener. Extracted from the herb Stevia. It is 300 times sweeter than sugar, but has a strong aftertaste.

Stigma Area on the ovary where the egg has been released at the time of ovulation.

Stillbirth A fetal death in late pregnancy. At what gestational age (point in pregnancy) a miscarriage becomes a stillbirth for reporting purposes depends on the country's policy.

Stoma (prefix) Mouth.

e.g. stomatology - the study of the mouth and its diseases.

Stoma A surgically created opening in an organ, such as the stomach (gastrostomy) or intestine (colostomy).

Stomatitis Inflammation of the mucosa of the mouth.

Stool Waste products that remain after food is digested, including fiber, bacteria, mucus, undigested foods, and cells from the inside of the intestine. Passed through the rectum as a bowel movement.

Strabismus (clinical condition) Turned eye (s), the eyes are misaligned. It is caused by a reduction in visual acuity, reduced visual function, high refractive error, traumatic brain injury, oculomotor nerve lesion, or eye muscle injury. In strabismus, the eyes send conflicting images to the brain, and the brain cannot combine these images as it would in normal vision. The brain compensates by ignoring one image in favor of the other, causing a loss of depth perception. Strabismus in more common in children, and affects four percent of all children (although it may also appear later in life).

It is characterized by using the following categories:

Unilateral strabismus: Strabismus in which only one eye deviates.

Alternating strabismus: Strabismus in which the deviating eye can change.

Intermittent strabismus: Strabismus which is not present at all times.

Constant strabismus: Strabismus which is present at all times.

Periodic strabismus: Strabismus which occurs at one testing distance but not at another.

Strabismus is also known as squint. It may also be referred to as cross-eyes (convergent-turning inward) or wall eyes (divergent-turning outward). Treatment options may include one or more of the following: optical lenses, bi-focal lenses, prisms, surgery, vision therapy, or Botulinum Toxin Type A (Oculinum, Botox) injections.

Straight sinus A large venous dural sinus, at the junction of the falx and the tentorium cerebelli.

Straight Umbilical Cord Straight Umbilical Cord During an ultrasound, your baby umbilical cord might be noted as being "straight". 5% of umbilical cords start out uncoiled, but 30% of those become coiled by the time the baby is born. If you baby's umbilical cord remains severely non-coiled it could indicate that there will be problems with the baby/pregnancy.

Strain A population of cells all descended from a single cell.

Stratum zonale (thalami) Thin plate of myelinated fibers covering the dorsal surface of the thalamus.

Streff syndrome Named after the optometrist who originally described it; Dr. John Streff. This functional vision loss is also known as Non-Malingering Syndrome. Signs include reduced visual acuity in both eyes at distance and near. The visual acuity at near is more reduced than the distance acuity. Frequently patients will have reduced stereopsis, large accommodative lag on dynamic retinoscopy, and a reduced visual field (tubular or spiral field). The syndrome is associated with a visual or emotional stress occurring in the child's life. It is more prominent in girls (ages 7-13) than boys. Treatment includes a low plus lens and/or vision therapy. This condition is sometimes incorrectly diagnosed by doctors as hysterical amblyopia.

Strength The concentration of the drug substance (for example, weight/weight, weight/volume, or unit dose/volume basis), and/or the potency, that is, the therapeutic activity of the drug product as indicated by appropriate laboratory tests or by adequately developed and controlled clinical data (expressed, for example, in terms of units by reference to a standard).

Stress test A diagnostic test using an ECG machine and a stationary bicycle or treadmill to look at areas of the heart that may have a decreased blood supply.

Stress ulcer An ulcer in the esophagus, stomach, or upper small intestine caused by excess acid produced as a result of surgery, major burns, head injury, or other trauma.

Stress Urinary Incontinence Urinary Incontinence: The involuntary loss of urine during period of increased abdominal pressure. Such events include laughing, sneezing, coughing or lifting heavy objects.

Stretch marks Areas of the skin that are stretched. Often found on the abdomen, breasts, buttocks and legs.

Stria Composite bundle of fibers that courses along the dorsomedial thalamus to the habenular nuclear complex. It conveys fibers that arise from the septal nuclei, lateral preoptic hypothalamus, and anterior thalamic nuclei to the habenular nuclei (interface between limbic, motor systems, and rostral midbrain.

Stria terminalis One of the extrinsic subcortical fiber systems of the amygdala that courses along the medial border of the caudate nucleus at its junction with the thalamus. It extends to the anterior hypothalamus, bed nucleus of the stria terminalis, and medial forebrain bundle.

Striate cortex Refers to the primary visual area of cortex (area 17) located in the walls of the calcarine sulcus of the occipital lobe. This is a thin cortical area (1.5-2.5 mm thick) which has striated appearance visible to the naked eye. This is due to presence of a conspicuous band of tangential fibers (outer band of Baillarger) located in cortical layer IV. In this region, this band is known as the band of Gennari which represents the terminal portions of the geniculo-calcarine tract.

Striatum (or corpus striatum) Refers to the neostriatum (caudate nucleus and putamen).

Stricture Abnormal narrowing of a part of an organ.

Structural exam/diagnosis An osteopathic diagnostic technique - involves a visual, hands-on assessment by an osteopathic physician of the skeleton, joints, muscles, ligaments, and tendons.

Styloid process A spike/penlike projection from the inferior portion of the temporal bone, anterior to the stylomastoid foramen, that allows for muscular attachment of the stylo-hyoid/thyroid muscles.

Sub-Acute A care level below acute care, but more intense than long term care, usually needed subsequent to a hospital stay. Many nursing homes and hospitals have developed sub acute care services, which are generally provided for a limited period of time, as a part of rehabilitation or recovery from acute care problems.

Sub-acute Care Sub-acute Care is normally required after an acute episode of illness or injury and usually follows acute care. Sub-acute care may require technically complex procedures and services for patients who are out of the hospital but still need specialized medical services. Sub-acute care can be provided by home-health agencies, long-term care units of hospitals, skilled nursing facilities or sub-acute care facilities. Many sub-acute facilities and services may be located in a skilled nursing facility.

Subacute Type of nursing home care that is generally considered above skilled nursing but below acute hospital care.

Subarachnoid cisternae Enlargements of the cerebrospinal fluid filled space between the pia and arachnoid mater (subarachnoid space). A number of these cisternae are identified at various locations (i.e. lumbar cistern, cisterna magnum etc.)

Subarachnoid space Cerebrospinal fluid filled space between the arachnoidea and the pia mater of the central nervous system.

Sub-Chorionic Hemorrhage An area, usually near the edge of the placenta or in fluid just outside of the gestational sac, that is bleeding. This can either bleed out and show as spotting or bleeding, or can form a bruise that does not bleed. A sub-chorionic hemorrhage is not uncommon, and does not mean the pregnancy will end in miscarriage. It most often happens because during the normal course of the uterus stretching and growing, a bit of the placenta peeled away and bled. It will almost always heal on its own. There is a slightly increased risk of miscarriage if the hemorrhage is large (over 200 ml in volume), as it may mean the placenta implantation is weak. Bed rest is not always given, as many hemorrhages are very minor.

Subclavian artery Artery which originates from the brachiocephalic artery on the right side and directly from the arch of aorta on the left side. They branch into the vertebral, internal thoracic arteries, thyrocervical and costocervical trunks.

Aberrant Right Subclavian Artery.

Subconjunctival hemorrhage A blood spot on the eye. It occurs when a small blood vessel under the conjunctiva (the transparent coating that covers the inner eyelid and the white of the eye) breaks and bleeds. A common condition caused spontaneously from coughing, heavy lifting, or vomiting. In some cases, it may develop following eye surgery or trauma. It tends to be more common among those with diabetes, hypertension, and taking blood thinners (including aspirin). A subconjunctival hemorrhage is essentially harmless. The blood naturally absorbs within one to three weeks and no treatment is required. If a mild irritation is present, artificial tear drops can be used. You can speed up the healing process by applying cool compresses for the first two days and then warm compresses in the following days.

Subcutaneous (SQ) Beneath the skin

Subdural space A potential space located between the innermost layer of the dura mater and the arachnoid mater. This interface is a site of rupture of delicate thin-walled veins following head injuries resulting in subdural hematomas which can have profound neurological consequences.

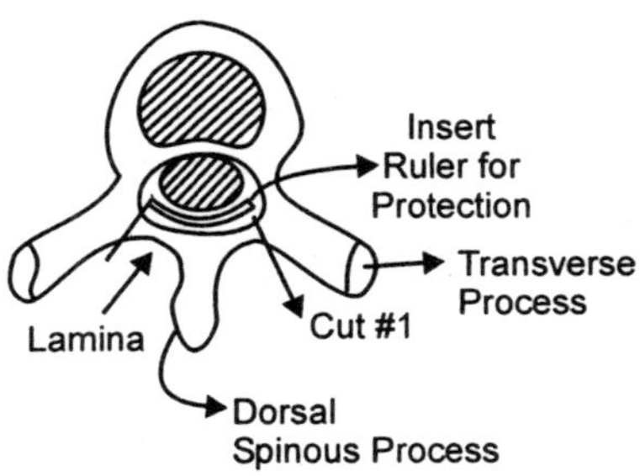

Fig. Subdural space

Subfascial Below the fascia.

Subglottic airway The airway below the "glottis", that is below the true vocal cords.

Subiculum Cortical zone along the medial parahippocampul gyrus. It is along with the presubiculum and prosubiculum transitional from the 6 layered parahi-ppocampul cortex to the 3 layered cortex of the hippocampus and dentate gyri.

Subject based teaching A method of teaching in which each subject area of curriculum is addressed separately. In the past, this model had been very prominent in basic science education. Now, however, it is gradually being replaced with a problem-based learning (PBL) where knowledge and skills unfold as elements in cases that illustrate real life situations.

Subjective refraction The procedure in which the patient is asked to report on which lens combination provides the clearest vision. While this is the method of choice for determining prescription in those able to understand the task and respond to the examiner, it is less reliable in children.

Sublimation The process of vaporizing a solid substance by heat and then condensing it (without its having passed through a liquid state in either direction), a process of purification by separating the nonvaporizable impurities, a process analogous to the distillation of liquids.

Subluxation In chiropractic, a misalignment of bones within joints said to interfere with the flow of nervous impulses and diminish the body's ability to stay healthy.

Submandibular gland Paired salivary gland, located in the middle of the posterior half of the base of the mandible.

Submerged arc welding (SAW) An arc welding process that produces coalescence of metals by heating them with an arc or arcs between a bare metal electrode or electrodes and the work. A blanket of granular, fusible material on the work shields the arc. Pressure is not used and filler metal is obtained from the electrode and sometimes from a supplemental source (welding rod, flux, or metal granules).

Subscapularus muscle Muscle originating at the subscapular (ventral/anterior) fossa of the scapula and inserting at the lesser tubercle of the humerus.

Substandard Care Substandard quality of care is any deficiency in quality of Care that constitutes immediate jeopardy to resident (patient) health or safety; or a pattern of or widespread actual harm that is not immediate jeopardy; or a widespread potential for more than minimal harm that is not immediate jeopardy, with no actual harm.

Substantia gelatinosa (of rolando) A cell column located at the apex of the dorsal horn throughout the length of the spinal cord. It corresponds to lamina II of Rexed and receives pain and temperature input from dorsal root afferents. This input is modified in this location by other sensory input and by excitatory and inhibitory input from the cerebral cortex. Lamina II neurons are entirely interneuronal; ascending or descending several segments in the dorsolateral fasciculus (of Lissauer) before re-entering lamina II.

Substantia nigra A large neuromelanin containing nuclear area ventral to the tegmentum extending throughout the rostrocaudal extent of the midbrain and into the caudal part of the ventral diencephalon. Consists of a ventral pars reticulata and a dorsal part called the pars compacta. Neurons in the pars compacta use dopamine as a neurotransmitter and project primarily to the neostriatum.

Substantial Compliance Minor deficiencies or violations, but a facility generally meets the intent of State regulations.

Substrate Reactive material - the substance on which an enzyme acts.

Subsurface carbon enrichment In metals, a rise in the carbon signal at depths from 15 to 20 angstroms (Å). This indicates that organic material is buried in cracks, crevices, pits, or smeared material. Subsurface carbon is most commonly found in materials having rough morphology generally associated with machining processes.

Subthalamus A subdivision of the diencephalon located ventral to the thalamus, medial to the internal capsule, and lateral and caudal to the hypothalamus. It consists of the subthalamic nucleus, sensory fiber tracts terminating in the thalamus, fibers from the cerebellum, corpus striatum, midbrain motor nuclei proceeding to the thalamus, and forward extensions of the zona incerta, red nucleus, and substantia nigra.

Sub-unit A Sub-unit is a unique group of residents within your facility that has been defined as part of a Classification for use in the ePIP system. Sub-units are mutually exclusive within each classification. Once a Sub-unit has been created, it can be set as a report parameter when requesting reports. Some facilities are using this feature to separate out one floor of a facility from the other floors using the room number field on the MDS. Then, for instance, separate QI Profiles and resident QI summaries can be requested for each floor.

Sucralose An artificial sweetener. Approved by the FDA in 1998. It is 600 times sweeter than table sugar, it is is made from a process that begins with regular sugar. You can bake with it. Sucralose was discovered in 1976. Sucrolose is derived from sugar through a patented, multistep processes that selectively substitutes three choline atoms for three hydrogen oxygen groups on the sugar molecule. The tightly bound chlorine atoms create a molecular structure that is exceptionally stable and is approx 600 times sweeter than sugar. The body does not recognize it as sugar or another carbohydrate. The sucralose molecule passes through the body unchanged, it is not metabolized and is eliminated after consumption. Sucrolose has no calories. The acceptable daily intake for sucralose is 5 mg / kg of body weight per day.

Sudden cardiac death (SCD) A death due to electrical problems in the heart. It is different from a heart attack, which is heart muscle damage from a blockage rather than an electrical problem. Sudden cardiac death usually is caused by ventricular tachycardia or fibrillation. An AICD system, however, greatly reduces the risk of sudden cardiac death.

Sugar Alcohols This group of sweeteners includes Mannitol, Sorbitol and Xylitol. Although found in fruit, they are commercially synthesized and not extracted from natural sources. Sugar alchohols provide a reduced glycemic response (no steep hikes in blood sugar). Sugar alcohols are absorbed slowly, but incompletely. This can cause diarrhea in some people.

Sulcus The valleys or depressions that seperate cortical convolutions.

S. (Hypothalamic): A longitudinal groove that extends along each wall of the neural tube as far cranially as the mesencephalon. It serves to divide the neural tube into a dorsal half called the alar plate and a ventral half called the basal plate.

S. (Limitans): A longitudinal groove that extends along the medial wall of the diencephalon that divides the hypothalamus below from the thalamus above.

Superficial Of, relating to, or located near the surface.

Superficial temporal artery Originating from the external carotid artery and branching into the parotid, auricular, and occipital rami, tranverse facial, zygomàtico-orbital, and middle temporal arteries.

Superficial Thrombophlebitis An infection in a superficial vein caused ro exacerbated by thrombosis within the vein.

Superior gluteal artery Artery originating from the internal iliac artery and branching into the superficial and deep branches of the buttocks.

Superior mesenteric artery Artery which originates from the abdominal aorta and branches into the inferior pancreaticoduodenal, jejunal, ileal, ileocolic, right colic, and middle colic arteries.

Superior mesenteric vein The vein that parallels the superior mesenteric artery and joins the splenic vein to form the portal vein.

Superior or cranial Toward the head end of the body; upper (example, the hand is part of the superior extremity).

Superior pubic ramus Portion of the pubic bone that projects posterosuperolaterally to join the iliopubic eminence, to form part of the acetabulum.

Superior rectus muscle The muscle which originates at the lateral margin of the optic foramen, and inserts into the upper aspect of the sclera. It is responsible for the adduction and upward medial rotation of the eyeball.

Superior sagittal sinus (SSS) Venous sinus within the dura mater of the falx (at it's attachment to the sagittal suture), that extends from the crista galli to the junction with the tentorium and the torcular herophili.

SSS Thrombosis.

Superior thyroid artery Artery which originates from the external carotid artery and branches into the pharyngeal, esophageal, and tracheal rami, inferior laryngeal and ascending cervical arteries.

Superior vena cava The vein created by the joining of the two brachiocephalic veins and empties into the right atrium of the heart. It drains the head, neck, upper extremities and chest.

Superior vesicle artery Artery which stems from the umbilical artery, supplying the bladder urachus, and ureter.

Supernatant The material floating on the surface of a liquid mixture (often the liquid component that has the lowest density).

Supine Lying on the back or with the face upward.

Support group A group of patients and their family members coordinated by medial professionals. The AICD support group provides an opportunity for members to share their experiences with AICD therapy and to discuss any concerns.

Suppression of binocular vision When the brain ignores the image that is seen by one eye. It is the result of weak eye teaming skills (binocularity).

Suppression test Determines if there is any tendency for the visual processing center of the brain to ignore or suppress visual data from one eye.

Suppurative Containing pus.

Suprapatellar bursa A saclike cavity filled with a viscid fluid located between the distal end of the femur and the quadriceps tendon.

Surface iron oxide layer Surface iron oxide layer present when the 316L stainless steel's iron composition signal is higher than its chromium signal at the surface.

Surface residual A foreign substance that adheres to a surface by chemical reaction, adhesion, adsorption, or ionic bonding (for example, corrosion, rouging, and staining).

Surface texture The repetitive or random deviations of the nominal metal surface from the three-dimensional topography of the surface. Surface texture includes roughness, waviness, lay, and flaws.

Surface water Any water where the source is above ground such as rivers, lakes, and reservoirs. Surface waters are usually higher in suspended matter and organic material and lower in dissolved minerals than well water.

Surfactant Surfactant-Phospholipid present in the lungs. Controls surface tension of lungs. Premature babies often lack sufficient amounts of surfactant to breathe without assistance.

Surveillance A dynamic process in which data on the occurrence and distribution of health or disease in a population is collected, organised, analysed and disseminated.

Survey An investigation conducted by an entity that has given a provider a License, Certification, or Accreditation. For instance, states conduct licensure surveys of Nursing Homes where the state surveyors spend several days in the facility observing patients and reviewing records and procedures to determine if the facility is in compliance with licensure requirements.

Suspended solids Undissolved solids that can be removed by filtration. Determined by a filter paper before and after filtration of a water sample.

Suspension A specific category of pharmaceutical product that must be in a colloidal dispersion (suspension) for proper action. For example, Kaolin/Pectin works as an adsorbant because its high surface area in suspension.

Swap File A file that gives Windows the ability to use a portion of hard drive as memory. With the use of a swap file, you can load and run more programs in Windows 95 or 98 than you actually have RAM memory for. A swap file allows Windows 95 or 98 to "swap" chunks of memory containing currently unused information to disk, making room in RAM memory for information you need to run the currently selected program. Using a swap file is slower than holding everything in RAM memory, however.

Sylvian fissure The deep cleft that begins at the anterior perforated substance, continuing between the frontal and temporal lobes, and then posteriorly between the temporal and parietal lobes. It is bound by the overhaning margins ("opercula") of the frontal, temporal, and parietal lobes, as well as deeply by the insular cortex.

Symbiosis The phenomenon of two entities performing a joint function that neither entity can perform alone.

Sympathetic nervous system The thoraco-lumbar component of the autonomic nervous sytem. This system is widely distributed in the body and releases norepinephrine at most terminals. Stimulation of this system has the effect of quickly mobilizing the body for "flight or fight."

Syncope A temporary loss of consciousness due to insufficient cerebral blood flow; fainting.

Syndesmosis (Tibiofibular) A fibrous union between the fibular notch of the tibia and a triangular surface on the fibula.

Synovial fluid A fluid that lubricates the joint and keeps the cartilage smooth and healthy

Synovium A thin membrane inside the joint capsule

Syntax A set of formal rules governing the ways words are put together to make phrases and sentences, and the use of punctuation. On the computer, syntax refers to the rules that must be followed in writing and executing software programs. A syntax error indicates either a programming error or an incorrect response to some software inquiries.

Synthesis Creating products through chemical and enzymatic reactions.

Synthol An oil based solution that swells the muscle region it is injected into giving the muscle a "swollen" appearance without detail or hardness.

System specifications Descriptions of how the system will meet the functional requirements.

Systemic lupus erythermatosus Systemic lupus erythermatosus (SLE)-Connective-tissue disorder common in women in the reproductive ages. Antibodies made by the person act against his or her own tissues.

T

Tachyarrhythmias Abnormally fast heart rhythms.

Tactile Pertaining to the sense of touch.

Tail of pancreas The distal left extremity of the pancreas, next to the medial spleen and the junction between the transverse and descending colon.

Talus The highest tarsal bone which forms the ankle joint by articulating with the tibia and fibula.

Tangential flow filtration A separation method that transfers components of one system (stream) into another. The stream the product is being extracted from crosses the stream that the product is being transferred to, multiple times.

Tanycytes Ependymal cell variants found only within circumscribed regions of the adult mammalian ventricular system. They are distinguished by the presence of a radially directed basal process that extends into the neuropil and terminates on blood vessels, neurons, glia, or the external glial limitans.

Tapetum Fibers of the corpus callosum which course laterally and inferiorly forming the roof and lateral walls of its posterior and inferior horns of thelateral ventricles. The fibers of the tapetum are located between lateral margin of the ventricle and the optic radiations.

Target In Windows 95 or 98, any object pointed to by a shortcut.

Target Assessment The most recent full (AA8a= 01,02,03 or 04) or quarterly assessment (AA8a = 05 or 10) that is available for the time in which the QM score is calculated.

Taskbar An area that runs across the bottom of the Windows 95 or 98 desktop. The Start button is at the left end of the task bar, and the clock can be displayed at the right end of the task bar. Running applications are represented as buttons on the task bar, the current window is shown as a depressed button, all other applications are displayed as raised buttons. Clicking the button for an inactive application activates that application and displays its window as the current window.

Taurine An essential amino acid. Plays a role in cell-membrane stabilization, calcium balance, growth modulation and the regulation of osmotic pressure in the body (water transfer). It is also a key component of bile, which is necessary for fat digestion, absorption of fat-soluable vitamins and control of cholesterol levels. A link has been shown between deficiency in this amino and retinal dysfunction (eye problems).

Taxonomy The development of approaches to organize and summarize our knowledge about the variety or organisms that exist.

Tay-sachs disease An inherited disease of infancy characterized by profound mental retardation and early death; it is caused by a recessive gene mutation.

T-cell (T-lymphocyte) A blood cell, probably originating from bone marrow, but which matures in the thymus. Some T-cells are responsible for cell-mediated immunity and in the production of antibodies.

Teacher centered education An educational system in which the teacher dictates what is being taught and how it is to be learned. The teacher is the central or key figure and activities such as the formal lecture and the formal laboratory are emphasized. Individual students have little control over what they learn, the order in which they learn and the methods they must use. In this approach, learning is rather more passive than active. It is the opposite of the learner-centered approach.

Team biologics A partnership between FDA's Office of Regulatory Affairs (ORA) and CBER to focus on inspectional and compliance issues in biologics. Its goal is to ensure the quality and safety of biologic products and resolve inconsistencies.

Tectum The part of the midbrain situated above the interventricular foramen consisting of the superior and inferior colliculi.

Tegmentum T. Midbrain: The part of the cerebral peduncle of the midbrain located between the basis pedunculi ventrally and the tectum dorsally.

T. Pontine: Small dorsal part of the pons located above the basilar region that forms the floor of the fourth ventricle.

Tela choroidae A thin duplicated layer of pia mater with associated blood vessels that invaginates into the ventricles along with a modified ependymal epithelial lining to form the choroid plexuses.

Telangiectasias Telangiectasias-Dilatation or swelling of a small blood vessel. Sometimes called an angioma. During pregnancy, another common name is a spider angioma or spider veins.

Telecommunications The transfer of information from one place to another over large distances using phone lines, microwaves and/or satellites.

Telemedicine The application of communications technologies for the provision of health care services (diagnosis, treatment, prevention of diseases and injuries) over spatial distance in a situation where remoteness and/or availability of professional expertise is a critical factor.

Telencephalon The rostral subdivision of the forebrain (prosencephalon) which in the adult gives rise to the cerebral cortex, medullary centre, corpus striatum, rhinencephalon, and lateral ventricle.

Telephone Reassurance Friendly calls provided by agencies or volunteers to check up on and offer reassurance, contact, and socialization to elderly people at a predetermined time each day.

Telephony Term used to describe the combined use of a computer and telephone to transmit voice, data, video, or image signals over long distances.

Telomere The end of a chromosome. This specialized structure is involved in the replication and stability of linear DNA molecules.

Temperature A specific degree of heat intensity. There are three temperature designations associated with psychrometrics: 1. Dry Bulb (DB) - The air temperature as measured by a standard thermometer.

2. Wet Bulb (WB) - The air temperature measured by a thermometer with its

reservoir bulb wrapped in a moistened cloth wick and exposed to an air stream moving at a velocity of 1,000 feet per minute.

3. Dewpoint temperature (DP) - Also called Saturation Temperature is the temperature at which condensation of moisture begins (air is holding 100% of the moisture it can) when the air is cooled, measured in °F.

Temporal lobe The lower lateral lobe of the cerebral hemisphere, containing the hippocampal formation and the amygdala.

Temporary Class A short-term registration that enables individuals who have met all the registration requirements, except the national examination requirements, to practise as a registered member.

Temporomandibular joint (TMJ) The joint formed by the condyle (head) of the mandible, the mandibular fossa, and the articular tubercle of the temporal bone.

Tendocalcaneus (achille's tendon) The tendon, located at the back of the heel, which connects the triceps surae muscle to the tuberosity of the calcaneus.

TENS (Transcutaneous electrical nerve stimulation) Delivery of an electric current through the skin to the nerves. Used in physical therapy and to relieve painful conditions such as neuralgia, sciatica, and arthritis. The low voltage electric current blocks the nerves reception of pain signals and possibly stimulates the production of endorphins, the body's pain-killing chemicals.

Tentorium cerebelli A tent-like fold of dura mater that extends horizontally accross the transverse cerebral fissure between the occipital lobes of the cerebrum and the cerebellum forming a roof over the posterior-cranial fossa.

Teratogenic Causes abnormal development.

Teratology Branch of science that deals with teratogens.

Terminal Care Care provided to a dying resident (patient) that may or may not include hospice care . The QIs are not measures of quality, therefore, if your facility flags on a Quality Indicator, it only means that it may be a potential problem and is something that probably should recieve additional review.

Terminal sterilization The process applied to product sealed in its final container that transforms a non-sterile product into a sterile one.

Terminally Ill For an individual, it means that the subject has a life expectancy of six months or less as stated in writing by his or her attending physician and surgeon.

Terminate and Stay Resident Term used to describe a program that loads into memory, then performs functions in the background, without the direct control of the user or operating system.

Test procedure A sequence of activities which when executed successfully provides documentary evidence that part of the system works as specified.

Testosterone Studies says that even minute amounts of it can juice both the male and female sex drives and slightly larger amounts will speed the muscle building process.

Text Box A space in the dialog box where text or numbers can be entered so that a command can be carried out.

Text File A file containing only text characters.

Thalamus The largest of the 4 subdivision of the diencephalon bordering the upper lateral wall of the third ventricle dorsal to the hypothalamic sulcus. It is consists of many nuclei with extensive cortical and subcortical connections. It functions as a motor and sensory relay station, and plays a role in arousal, attention, memory, consciousness, and expression of emotion.

Thalamus Two large egg-shaped gray-matter masses on either side of the third ventricle.

Thalassemia Group of inherited disorders of hemoglobin metabolism, which results in a decrease in the amount of hemoglobin formed. Found most commonly in people of Mediterranean descent.

Theanine A unique amino acid found in green teas. The greater the theanine content in green tea, the higher the price. Theanine increases GABA levels in the brain and counteracts high and even toxic doses of stimulants, such as caffeine. Sleep time is improved, spontaneous physical hyperactivity is decreased and toxicity reactions are markedly reduced. Theanine can help ofset the length and intensity of the stimulatory effects of alpha and beta-agonists and caffeine. It goes beyond helping you relax and sleep well for one night. Be reversing the excitatory state quickly and safely and promoting relaxation and restoration of your brain chemisty, you are in effect priming your body for stimulation once again the following day. That should allow you not only to grow, but to get even beter results from your supplements.

Theoretical yield The quantity that would be produced at any appropriate phase of manufacture, processing, or packing of a particular drug product, based upon the quantity of components to be used, in the absence of any loss or error in actual production.

Therapeutic Diet A diet ordered by a physician as part of treatment for a disease or clinical condition, or to eliminate, decrease, or increase specific nutrients in the diet. (May also be called Medical Nutrition Therapy).

Therapeutic Leave Days when a resident of a nursing facility leaves the facility temporarily for a visit home or a stay in a hospital. Private pay residents are often charged a Bed Hold fee during a leave.

Therapeutic Nurse-Client Relationship Established and maintained by the nurse and the client as the foundation for providing nursing services that contribute to the client's health and well-being. The relationship is based on trust, respect, intimacy and the appropriate use of the nurse's inherent power.

Therapeutic touch Practiced by registered nurses and others to relieve pain & stress. Practitioner assesses where a person's energy field is weak and congested, then uses his or her hands to direct energy into the field to balance it.

Therapy Treatment and care of someone to combat disease, injury, or mental disorder.

Thermogenesis A fancy word meaning heat-producing. To make more heat, your body has to burn more calories. Thermogenesis occurs with training, with food consumption, and with the use of selected herbs.

Thermophile An organism that grows best at greater than 50°C (122°F).

Thermophilic (of a microorganism) With optimum temperature for growth above 45°C, many thermophilic bacteria exist at high temperatures (greater than 80°C) and many of their enzymes which posses high thermal stability, are of great commercial interest.

Thiamin (Vitamin B-1) A vitamin which maintains energy levels, supports brain function (memory). Aids in digestion. Necessary for metabolism of sugar and starch to provide energy. Maintains a healthy nervous system. Alcohol can cause deficiencies of this vitamin and all the B-complex vitamins.

Thoracic cavity The upper ventral, thoracic, or chest cavity contains the heart, lungs, trachea, esophagus, large blood vessels, and nerves. The thoracic cavity is bound laterally by the ribs (covered by costal pleura) and the diaphragm caudally (covered by diaphragmatic pleura).

Thoracic duct The largest lymph channel in the body, which begins in the abdomen at the junction of the intestinal, lumbar, and descending intercostal trunks, and ends at the junction of the left subclavian and internal jugular veins.

Thoracic spine The portion of the vertebral column between the neck and thoracic diaphragm.

Thoracotomy An incision into the chest that may be made when heart or lung surgery is performed.

Threatened abortion Bleeding during the first trimester of pregnancy without cramping or contractions.

Threshold A set point for each CHSRA QI at which the likelihood of a problem is sufficient to warrant further investigation. There may also be a concern below the threshold especially if the percentile rank is close to the threshold. Generally, the threshold point is set at the 90th percentile .

Thrombin (blood coagulation factor II) An enzyme (the activated thrombogen) formed in the blood, after this is shed, that converts fibrinogen into fibrin for clot formation. It is formed from conjunction of prothrombin and calcium salts. It is also a sterile protein substance prepared from prothrombin of bovine origin through interaction with thromboplastin in the presence of calcium. Bovine thrombin is often used to aid production of serum from "salvage" plasma.

Thromboembolism The lesion created by a thromboembolus.

Thromboembolus A clot of material that breaks free from a primary site, is transported in the bloodstream and becomes lodged and adhered at a secondary site.

Thrombosis The use of drugs such as tPA or streptokinase, called thrombolytic agents, to dissolve (lyse) a clot (thrombus).

Throughput volume The amount of solution passed through an exchange bed before the resin is exhausted.

A pyrimidine component of nucleic acid first isolated from the thymus.

Thrush Monilial or yeast infection occurring in the mouth or mucous membranes of a newborn infant.

Thumbnail A miniature rendition of a graphic file. A thumbnail gives a idea of what the full-size graphic looks like, and is usually used as a gateway to view the full-size graphic.

Thymus A bilateral lymphoid organ located in the anterior superior mediastinum.

Thyroid cartilage The largest cartilage of the larynx.

Thyroid disease Abnormality of the thyroid gland and its production of thyroid hormone.

Thyroid hormone Chemical made in the thyroid that affects the entire body.

Thyroid panel Series of blood tests done to evaluate the function of the thyroid gland.

Thyroid stimulating hormone Thyroid stimulating hormone (TSH)-Hormone made in the brain that stimulates the thyroid to produce thyroid hormone.

Tibia The large bone is the Tibia. The thin bone of the lower leg.

Tibial tuberosity Point of attachment for the patellar ligament, located distal to the intercondylar eminence.

Tile To reduce and move windows so that they can all be seen at once.

Time stamp A part of the audit trail that clearly documents the sequence of events in human terms, helping to authenticate an electronic signature and minimizing the chances of signer repudiation. A local time stamp correlates with the whereabouts of the signer. With client-server data systems used by international companies and records accessed from remote sites (such as on business trips), time stamps that reflect the local time of only the user might make the sequence of actions for an individual record appear inconsistent. For example, the approval by a peer reviewer could be signed at 9:00 a.m. on a chromatographic analysis that was performed at 11:00 a.m. in a different time zone. Local time stamps should probably be supplemented consistently with the time stamp of a remote server, with one stamp clearly labeled as local.

Tincture of Iodine A germicidal solution of iodine in aqueous alcohol used primarily as antiseptic on skin and tissue.

Tissue culture Growing mammalian cells in the laboratory in a tissue culture medium (in vitro). For example, this allows researchers to determine the effects of various chemicals on mammalian cells without experimenting directly on live animals or man. Since a molecule of some toxic substances can harm a single mammalian cell, even one part-per-billion of some impurities can affect a tissue culture. Therefore, water used to make up tissue culture media should be extremely pure.

Titer A measured sample - the strength of a solution or the concentration of a substance (as an antibody) in solution as determined by titration.

Title Bar The bar at the top of a program or document window that shows you what its title is. The control menu, maximize, minimize, restore, and task bar buttons can be accessed in the title bar.

Titration Volumetric analysis by means of the addition of definite amounts of a test solution to a solution of a known amount of the substance analyzed.

TNT (tumor necrosis therapy) Therapeutic agents that target dead and dying cells found primarily at the core of the tumor.

Tocolysis Stopping contractions during premature labor.

Tocolytic agents Tocolytic agents-Medications to stop labor.

Toe of weld The junction between the face of a weld and the base material.

Toggle To switch an option to one of two positions (either on or off). The "caps lock", "scroll lock", and "num lock" keys are examples of toggle switches.

Toileting One of the Activities of Daily Living (ADLs). The ability get to and from the toilet, get on and off the toilet, and maintain a reasonable level of personal hygiene for the body. Necessary activities include getting on and off a toilet or commode and emptying a commode, managing clothing and wiping and cleaning the body after toileting, and using and emptying a bed pan or urinal. An inability to do these activities with or without the aid of equipment constitutes a deficit or need in this area.

Tolerance Failure to mount an immune reaction on exposure to what would normally be an antigenic substance.

Tomogram A blurring technique to create a radiograph of a selected plane (layer or cross-section) of the body. Both the location of the plane, and the thickness of tissue in "focus" are controlled by the type of blurring movements used. Largely supplanted by "computerized tomography" - that produces a similar cross-sectional image using a computer.

Ton of refrigeration A unit used to indicate the size of a refrigeration unit. One ton of refrigeration effect is equivalent to removing 12,000 Btu/hr of heat, or melting one ton of ice in a 24-hour period.

Tonic herbal remedy made from herbs taken to maintain health or ward off illness, rather than to treat an illness. Also known as a normalizer.

Tonic vergence Convergence due to the basic tonicity (tension) of the extraocular muscles, which are responsible, in part, for the distance phoria. Deficient tonic vergence would result in exophoria and excessive tonic vergence results in esophoria.

Toning In sound healing, projection of a nonverbal sound to balance the body's energy fields.

Tonometry An instrument that measures the pressure within the eye, which is known as intraocular pressure (IOP).

Tool Bar A collection of buttons that typically make the more common tools for an application easily accessible. Although often grouped in a line under the menus, a toolbar can be located on the left or right side of the working area – or even be relocatable to any area of the screen the user wishes. In some applications (for example, MS Office applications such as Word), the toolbar is user-configurable – the user can display different toolbars, and add or remove tool buttons from the bar.

Topical A medication applied to the skin, an ointment. Usually a medicament suspended in a carrier such as petrolatum or another oil based carrier. Filtration at elevated temperatures is usually possible.

Topical product A pharmaceutical product meant to be applied to the skin or soft tissue in the form of liquid, cream, or ointment, and therefore needs not be aseptic. Sterile ophthalmic products throughout are manufactured aseptically.

Torcular herophili Old term for the confluence of the sinuses located at the internal occipital protuberance first described by Herophilus.

Torus tubarus The bottom lip of the pharyngeal opening of the auditory (Eustachian) tube.

Total bacteria count An estimation of the total number of bacteria in a sample based usually on Standard Methods procedures for collecting, incubating, and counting colony-forming units (cfu).

Total dissolved solids (TDS) The term used to describe inorganic ions in the water. Usually measured by electrical conductance of the water corrected to 25°C, and expressed as ppm (parts per million).

Total fertility rate The number of children who would be born per woman, if the woman was to live to the end of her child-bearing years and bear children at each age in accordance with prevailing age-specific fertility rates.

Total heat (TH) The sum of sensible heat and latent heat.

Total Ionized solids Concentration of dissolved ions in solution expressed in concentration units of Sodium Chloride (NaCl). It determines the operating life of ion exchange resins and is calculated from measurements of Specific Resistance.

Total organic carbon (TOC) A measure of the level of organic impurities in water by their carbon content that determines the operating life of activated carbon beds. This is one of the parameters used to determine the purity of Semiconductor Grade water. Feed water will have TOC measured in ppm (parts per million), and ultrapure water (UPW) will have TOC measured in ppb (parts per billion).

Total solids Total solids in water include both dissolved and suspended solids. Determined by weighing sample before and after evaporation.

Tower Refers to a physical configuration of PC cases. The tower case is taller than it is wide and is usually designed to sit on the floor, rather than on a desk. Towers usually feature more bays for disk drives and slots for peripheral devices than other configurations.

Toxemia Pre-eclampsia.

Toxic Pertaining to a substance that is harmful.

Toxicology A science that deals with poisons, their effects, and the problems involved.

Toxin Any poisonous agent, especially a poisonous substance produced by one living organism that is poisonous to other organisms. Toxins are usually very unstable, notably toxic when introduced into the tissues, and typically capable of inducing antibody formation.

Toxoid An antigenic toxin. Example is tetanus toxoid that is a bacterial vaccine.

Toxoplasmosis Toxoplasmosis-Infection caused by toxoplasma gondii.

TPA (tissue plasminogen activator) A recombinant drug used in the management of heart attacks to prevent clotting. Produced by Genentech and one of the first successful recombinant DNA drugs to be commercialized.

Trace analysis Analyzing constituents present in ppm and ppb concentrations. Trace analysis requires extremely pure reagents, made with ultrapure Type I reagent grade water.

Traceability A prerequisite for trustworthy records, apart from data security. Traceability is the part of the laboratory data system audit trail that holds the evidence of who did what to a record and when.

Tracer A radioactively labeled nucleic acid component included in a reassociation reaction in amounts too small to influence the progress of reaction.

Trachea A cartilaginous and membranous tube beginning at the larynx and extending to the bifurcation, where it branches into the right and left main bronchi.

Tracheoesophageal fistula Caused by improper development of the baby's trachea (windpipe) and esophagus during pregnancy. The esophagus does not connect to the stomach, and there is also an abnormal connection between the esophagus and the trachea. Food cannot pass through to the stomach, and may pass into the trachea and then into the lungs, causing breathing problems.

Trager bodywork Movement-education approach that gently rocks, cradles, and moves the client's body. Meant to promote relaxation, increase mobility and mental clarity. Used by athletes for performance enhancement and by people with musculoskeletal and back problems.

Tranaglyph Red/green targets used with red/green glasses to develop eye teaming skills.

Transcription The process by which the genetic information encoded in the gene, represented as a linear sequence of deoxyribonucleotides (DNA), is copied into an exactly complementary sequence of ribonucleotides known as mRNA (messenger RNA).

Transduction The transfer of genetic material from one cell to another by means of a viral vector (for bacteria, the vector is Bacteriophage).

Transfer panel A panel to which process and utilities are piped, allowing cross connections between different use points. A jumper spool is used to connect the desired process/utility users and mechanically preclude erroneous connections to other lines.

Transfer RNA (tRNA) A class of RNA having structures with triplet nucleotide sequences that are complementary to the triplet nucleotide coding sequences of mRNA. The role of tRNAs in protein synthesis is to bond with amino acids and transfer them to the ribosomes, where proteins are assembled according to the genetic code carried by mRNA.

Transfer systems Equipment allowing the introduction and removal of material, toxic and/or sterile, with continuous protection to both operator and product.

Transferring One of the Activities of Daily Living (ADLs). Moving from one position to another, like moving from a bed to a wheelchair or sofa or coming to a standing position. If a person can move with the help of equipment such as a cane, walker, crutches, grab bars or other support devices, then he or she is considered able to transfer positions.

Transformation A process by which the genetic material carried by an individual cell is altered by incorporation of exogenous DNA into its genome.

Transgenics The alteration of a plant or animal's DNA such that it contains a gene from another organism. There are two types of cells in animal and plants, germ line cells (the sperm and egg in animals, pollen and ovule in plants) and somatic cells (all other cells). Transgenic animals have alterations in their germ line DNA so the alterations are passed on to the offspring. That is done to produce therapeutics, to study disease, and to improve farm animals. Transgenic plants have been created for increased resistance to disease and insects as well as to make biopharmaceuticals.

Transient urinary incontinence Temporary episodes of urinary incontinence that are gone when the cause of the episode is identified and treated.

Translation The process in which the genetic code carried by mRNA directs the synthesis of proteins from amino acids.

Translocation A chromosomal anamoly where two pieces of genetic material are switched in position. A translocation will usually show no symptoms in parents, but may greatly increase their chance of miscarriage, as the chromosomes in the egg and sperm will not align correctly. A karyotype of the parents can uncover this rare problem.

Transportation Services Provide transportation for older adults to services and appointments, using bus, taxi, volunteer drivers, or van services that can accommodate wheelchairs and persons with other special needs.

Transvenous Passed into the heart through a vein.

Transverse Made at right angles to the long axis of the body.

Transverse colon The part of the intestine that lies horizontally in the abdomen, running straight across the abdomen from right to left.

Transverse lie Fetus is turned sideways in uterus.

Transverse process The lateral process of the vertebrae, which stems from the junction between the lamina and the pedicle.

Transversus abdominus muscle Muscle responsible for the compression of the abdominal viscera. It originates at the cartilages of the six lower ribs, thoracolumbar fascia, iliac crest, and inguinal ligament, and inserts into the linea alba and conjoined tendon to pubis.

Trapezium One of the carpal bones of the wrist.

Trapezoid body The name given to secondary auditory fibers in the rostral medulla (specifically the ventral acoustic stria) as they cross the midline through parts of the medial lemniscus.

Trapezoid One of the carpal bones of the wrist.

Trash Can A special folder in the Macintosh operating system where deleted files are sent when the user sends the command to delete them. They reside in the trash can until the user gives the command to permanently erase them, thus giving the user the chance to recover any information accidentally deleted.

Treatment investigational new drug An Investigational New Drug that makes a promising new drug available to desperately ill patients as early in the drug development process as available. FDA permits the drug to be used if there is preliminary evidence of efficacy and it treats a serious or life-threatening disease, or if there is not comparable therapy available.

Triangulation A method of assessment that is required when validity cannot be achieved with the use of a single assessment tool. If multiple testing methods are used to evaluate a single competence, one can be more certain that the competency has been appropriately assessed.

Tribulus Terrestris A herb for sexual deficiency or as a mild aphrodisiac. It may increase libido and serum testosterone.

Trichomonal vaginitis Venereal infection caused by trichomonas.

Trigeminal nerve The 5th and largest cranial nerve having three divisions (ophthalmic, maxillary and mandibular) and an associated sensory ganglion (called the semilunar, gasserian or trigeminal ganglion). The sensory and motor roots of the nerve emerge from the lateral surface of the ventral pons and . The nerve is associated with nuclei located in the pons, midbrain, and medulla. It is the main sensory nerve of the head and innervates the muscles of matication.

Trigone (Lateral ventricle) The triangular area between the temporal and occipital horns at the junction with the body of the lateral ventricle.

Trihalomethanes Compounds present in the feed water that are formed by the reaction of Chlorine and the organic material in the water. Activated carbon and degasification can reduce THMs.

Trimester Method of dividing pregnancy into three equal time periods of about 13 weeks each.

Triple Screen Test Also referred to as a "Multiple Markers Screen". A prenatal diagnostic test for fetal abnormalities performed between the 16th and 18th week of pregnancy. The test measures the levels of three substances circulating in the mother's blood: alpha-fetoprotein (AFP), human chorionic gonadotrophin (hCG) and unconjugated oestriol . Changes in the levels of these three substances are associated with the presence of Down syndrome or other fetal disorders.

Triquetrum One of the carpal bones of the wrist.

Trisomy 13 Caused by an extra copy of chromosome 13, which results in multiple internal and external physical defects and severe mental retardation.

Trisomy 18 A congenital disease caused by an extra copy of chromosome 18. Infants with trisomy 18 rarely survive past six months of age due to multiple internal and external physical defects.

Trisomy 21 The chromosomal disorder (Down syndrome) caused by an error in cell division that results in an extra copy of chromosome 21. Down syndrome is the most frequent genetic cause of mild to moderate mental retardation and associated medical problems.

Trisomy A chromosomal abnormality where three copies of a chromosome exist within a cell nucleus.

Trocar Surgical instrument passed through the body, used to allow easy exchange of endoscopic instruments during endoscopic surgery.

Trophoblast Cell layer important in early development of the embryo and fetus. It provides nourishment from the mother to the fetus and participates in the formation of the placenta.

Trophy (suffix) Nourish.

e.g. dystrophy - defective or faulty nutrition.

True vocal cord The mucous membrane surrounding the vocalis muscle in the larynx, forming the inferior ventricular boundary. Air moving over this fold produces the vibrations of speech.

Tryptophan An essential amino acid, known for its calming and mood enhancing effectcs. It is a naturally occuring ingredient in turkey that mellows you out and makes you want to take a nap after the Thanksgiving feast. Tryptophan can also be called 5-HTP (5-hydrotryptophan) which is make with a slightly different compound that regular tryptophan.

TSH Thyroid stimulating hormone (TSH)-Hormone made in the brain that stimulates the thyroid to produce thyroid hormone.

Tube size Tube is sized by its nominal outside diameter. For bioprocessing equipment, tube does not include pipe.

Tuber cinereum A midline swelling on the ventral surface of the hypothalamus between the optic chiasma and the mammillary bodies. It tapers to form the median eminence from which the infundibular stem or stalk of the neurohypophysis takes oigin. The tuberal and arcuate nuclei are located in this region of the hypothalamus .

Tubercle See clava, cuneate tubercle.

T. (Anterior of Thalamus): Swelling on the dorsal surface of the rostral thalamus produced by the underlying anterior nuclear group. This complex serves as a relay nuclei of the limbic system receiving afferents from the mammillary nuclei (via the mammillothalamic tract) and projecting to the cingulate gyrus, mammillary nuclei and habenula. This complex plays a role in memory, learning, attention, and emotional behavior.

Tubercle of rib A small eminence on the posterior side, where the head and body of a rib join.

Tumor An abnormal growth of cells. Also defined as a circumscribed growth, not inflammatory in character, arising from preexisting tissue, but independent of the normal rate or laws of growth of such tissue, and subserving no physiological function.

Tumor necrosis factor (TNF) A protein produced by white blood cells as means of controlling disease and breaking down developing cancer cells, or neoplasms. As a side effect, this defense mechanism can cause inflammation in the body and may trigger conditions such as rheumatoid arthritis.

Tumor pathogenesis Morphological and physiological changes associated with tumor growth.

Tumor-suppressor genes Genes that normally restrain cell growth but, when missing or inactivated by mutation, allow cells to grow uncontrolled.

Tunnel vision A constriction of the visual field that is commonly caused by chronic glaucoma, retinal degeneration, a tumor, or a brain disorder that interferes with the fibers that connect the optic nerve to the brain. (Please note that a visual stress, emotional stress, or emotional trauma can also cause a constriction of the visual field.)

Turbidity A suspension of fine particles that obscures light rays but requires many days for sedimentation because of small particle size.

Turner Syndrome A congenital condition in females designated by a 45,X genotype. Turner syndrome is a genetic abnormality caused by the complete or partial absence of one of the two X sex chromosomes found.

Turnover Also known as "hand over" in the U.K. It is a formal transfer of custody for a system or unit to another group, department, or operating company.

Turnover package (TOP) A collection of pertinent design, construction, vendor, and operational documentation. This collection of documentation is used for the qualification and process validation activity, as well as reference and single source information for the life of any particular system, process, or piece of equipment.

TWAIN A communication standard used with most scanners.

Two-bed deionizer Separate beds or layers of cation and anion exchange resins. Results in lower purity than mixed-bed deionization, but provides higher capacity in terms of throughput.

Tyrosine A conditionally essential amino acid, tyrosine can elevate mood and is a precursor of the brain neurotransmitters dopamine, norepinephrine and epinephrine.

U

U.S.P. (United States pharmacopeia) A compendium of testing and purity criteria for pharmaceuticals, ancillaries, and raw materials.

Ulcer A sore in the lining of the digestive tract.

Ulcerated Having a local defect or excavation of the epithelium of an organ or tissue through the basement membrane.

Ulcerative colitis A disease that causes irritation and ulcers in the lining of the large intestine and rectum. Also known as Inflammatory Bowel Disease.

Ulna One of the two bones of the forearm, it has a large articulation with the distal humerus and protudes posteriorly as the olecranon process.

Ultra low penetration air filters (ULPA) Extended media dry filters in a rigid frame that have a minimum particle-collection efficiency of 99.999% for particles greater than or equal to 0.12μm in size. Most commonly used in microelectronics, few uses in pharmaceuticals.

Ultracentrifugation The separation of macromolecules on the basis of their density and shape using the gravitational field generated in a high-speed centrifuge. It is used in rDNA work for the separation of RNA and DNA, and for purification of plasmids.

Ultrafiltration Molecular sieves; membranes with pores small enough to remove large molecules. Rated in terms of nominal molecular weight cutoff. A 10,000 Dalton (molecular weight) UF membrane, for example, will remove bacterial pyrogens that are typically in the range of 20,000 Daltons.

Ultrafine particle Particle with an equivalent diameter less than 0,1μm.

Ultrapure water Water with a specific resistance higher than 1 megohm-cm. In the laboratory, it usually refers to Type I reagent grade water. Anything in laboratory water that is not H2O is an impurity. Although chemically pure water is not attainable, ultrapure water systems are now capable of reducing impurities down to the limits of detection.

Ultrasonic scalpel A device using high frequency sound waves fore cutting tissue and controlling bleeding during surgery.

Ultrasonography A non-invasive diagnostic technique, frequently used in the second trimester, where sound waves are used to generate an image of the fetus in order to assess its growth and development, and to identify any physical abnormalities.

Ultrasound A radiologic procedure that produces detailed images using sound waves.

Ultraviolet oxidation Ultraviolet radiation is employed in water purification for the photochemical oxidation of organic impurities resulting in HPLC grade water with organic impurity levels below 0.0005 absorbance units.

Ultraviolet radiation Light in the wavelength region 200-300 nm, used to detect RNA or DNA that has the fluorescent dye, ethidium bromide, bound to it..

Ultraviolet sterilizer Ultraviolet lamps used to kill microorganisms in water.

Ultraviolet TOC reduction An ultraviolet source, which partially oxidizes organic compounds to ionic species that can be removed. It relies on 185 nm (nanometer) radiation from "ozone producing" mercury lamps (along with 254nm germicidal radiation). Generally has a longer contact time than sterilization alone.

Umbilical cord Cord that connects the placenta to the developing baby. It removes waste products and carbon dioxide from the baby and brings oxygenated blood and nutrients from the mother through the placenta to the baby.

Umbilicated Marked by depressed spots resembling the umbilicus.

Umbilicus The scar marking the site of entry of the umbilical cord into the fetus.

Uncinate process Literally a "hook". For the ethmoid bone, a plate of bone down and to the back from the anterior portion of the ethmoid labyrinth.

Uncinate process of pancreas The left and caudal portion of the head of the pancreas that "hooks" around.

Uncoiled Umbilical Cord Uncoiled Umbilical Cord During an ultrasound, your baby umbilical cord might be noted as being "straight". 5% of umbilical cords start out uncoiled, but 30% of those become coiled by the time the baby is born. If you baby's umbilical cord remains severely non-coiled it could indicate that there will be problems with the baby/pregnancy.

Unicellular Composed of only a single cell.

Unidirectional airflow Previously referred as "laminar" airflow, is the "rectified airflow through the entire cross section of a clean zone with a steady velocity and approximately parallel streamlines. This type of airflow results in a directed transport of particles from the clean zone".

Uniform mechanical code A document that provides a complete set of requirements for the design, construction, installation, and maintenance of heating, ventilating, cooling and refrigeration systems; incinerators and other heat-producing appliances.

Uniform zoning code A code dedicated to intelligent community development and to the benefit of the public welfare by providing a means of promoting uniformity in zoning laws and enforcement.

Unilateral Affecting only one side.

Uninstall To completely remove a program from your system. When a program is installed, it's files are copied to the system disk, and changes are made to certain system files and folders to allow the program to work properly. Properly uninstalling a program means deleting all of the files and undoing any changes made to system files fully.

Unit dose Defines an SVP that must be administered in one dose. Unused contents must be discarded.

United states medical licensing examination (USMLE) A 3-step examination procedure that provides a common evaluation system for United States medical licensure applicants. Results of the USMLE are reported to State Medical Boards granting the initial license to practice medicine. Each medical licensing authority requires, as part of its licensing procedure, a successful completion of an examination or other certifications demonstrating qualification for licensure.

Universal Precautions Measures taken to prevent transmission of infection from contact with blood or other body fluids or materials having blood or other body fluids on them.

UNIX UNIX is an operating system that supports multiusers (more than one person can use the computer at the same time) and multitasking (more the one program can be run on the computer at one time). Originally created by programmers to be used by programmers, it is VERY powerful.

Unnecessary Drug Any of the following: drug that is given without a medical reason; drug given in excessive dose; drug given for an excessive amount of time drug without adequate monitoring; drug given with side effects and/or adverse drug reactions indicate the drug should be reduced or discontinued.

Unregulated Care Provider (UCP) A family member, household member or paid individual who is not a member of a regulated health profession and assists with or provides personal care.

Unsafe abortion "A procedure for terminating unwanted pregnancy either by persons lacking the necessary skills or in an environment lacking minimal medical standards or both" (WHO).

Unsaturated fatty acid A fatty acid containing one or more double bonds.

Unstable (reactive) material A material other than an explosive, which in the pure state or as commercially produced will vigorously polymerize, decompose, condense or become self-reactive and undergo other violent chemical changes, including explosion, when exposed to heat, friction or shock, or in the absence of an inhibitor or in the presence of contaminants or in contact with noncompatible materials. Unstable, reactive materials are subdivided as follows:

1. Class 4 - Materials that in themselves are readily capable of detonation or of explosive decomposition or explosive reaction at normal temperatures and pressures. This class includes materials that are sensitive to mechanical or localized thermal shock at normal temperatures and pressures.

2. Class 3 - Materials that in themselves, are capable of detonation or of explosive decomposition or explosive reaction but which require a strong initiating source or which must be heated under confinement before initiation. This class includes materials that are sensitive to thermal or mechanical shock at elevated temperatures and pressures.

3. Class 2 - Materials that in themselves are normally unstable and readily undergo violent chemical change but do not detonate. This class includes materials which can undergo chemical change with rapid release of energy at normal temperatures and pressures and which can undergo violent chemical change at elevated temperatures and pressures.

4. Class 1 - Materials that in themselves are normally stable but which can become unstable at elevated temperatures and pressures.

Update To install the latest version of a program, or to record the latest information in a file or other document.

Upgrade A newer version of a program intended to seamlessly add new features to an existing piece of software without having to purchase and install an entirely new edition. Upgrades typically cost less than buying an all new copy of the software (most are nominal, or even free). Also refers to reconfiguring a computer system to increase its computing power— by installing new hardware components.

Upload To copy or move a file from one computer or drive to another computer or drive.

Upper GI series A test that looks at the organs of the upper part of the digestive system: the esophagus, stomach, and duodenum (upper small intestine). A liquid that shows up well on x-rays called barium is swallowed. X-rays are then taken to evaluate the digestive organs.

Upward compatibility Refers to software that runs not only on the computer for which it was designed, but also on newer and more powerful models. In the context of CFR 21 Part 11, compatibility plays an important role in ensuring that legacy data can be moved (copied) accurately and completely to a new system. Without it, legacy systems would have to be maintained as long as the records contained in them are kept.

Uracil A pyrimidine base important as a component of ribonucleic acid (RNA). Uracil is capable of forming a base pair with adenine.

Urea breath test A test that measures the amount of urease in the breath, which is an enzyme that the bacteria Helicobacter pylori makes. This helps diagnose H. pylori infection, which can help determine the cause for ulcers in the digestive tract.

Ureter A fibromuscular tube that transport urine from the collecting pelvis of the kidney to the base of the bladder, via a "stripping-wave" type of peristalsis.

Urethra A membraneous canal used in the transportion of urine from the bladder to the outside.

Uria (suffix) Urine.

e.g. proteinuria - protein in the urine.

URL Uniform Resource Locator, a string of text used to identify and locate a file on a computer network, like the internet.

Urogram (intra venous urogram or IVU) An imaging study to look at the structure and function of the kidneys, ureters, and bladder. Also called an IVU - intravenous urogram. This test requires the injection of a *contrast agent*.

User A person who operates and uses a computer.

User interface Dials, knobs, operating system commands, graphical display formats, and other devices provided by a computer or a program to allow users to communicate and use the computer or program. A Graphical User Interface (GUI) provides its user with a "picture oriented" way to interact with technology.

User-friendly Programs that have been thoughtfully designed to be intuitive and self-explanatory to the average user, with a minimal chance of mistakes.

Usnic Acid A herbal compound currently being used as an antifungal and antobiotic agent. It elevate body temperature, which can be a potent thermogenic but also dangerous. It works like DNP, which was a popular fat loss drug in the 1930s. Usnic acid shows that it uncouples oxidative phosphorylation.

Uterine atony Lack of tone of uterus.

Uterine cavity The lumen within the uterus that is connected laterally to the uterine (fallopian) tubes and posteriorly/inferiorly with the cervix and vagina.

Uterus A hollow muscular organ in which the fertilized ovum is embedded.

Utility systems Facility wide systems not tailored to a specific process and that do not have contact with the drug substance or potential drug substance.

Uvula A small fleshy mass located on the soft palate above the root of the tongue. (The dangly thing hanging in the back of your throat.) "It'll behoove ya' to take care of your uvula".

V

Vaccine A preparation of microbial antigens that provokes an immune response (i.e. the production of antibodies) on injection, thus conferring immunity on the recipient. There are three types of vaccines:

1. Those containing material from a nonvirulent organism that retains its immunogenicity but does not result in infection.

2. Those containing a modified toxin (a toxoid) that has lost its toxic properties but retain its immunogenicity.

3. Those containing live, attenuated organisms (i.e. genetic variants of a virus or bacterium) that are antigenically similar to the original strain but lack virulence.

Recombinant DNA research has allowed the production of new and more specific vaccines. For example, the gene for the B antigen of hepatitis virus has been cloned in E. coli, the protein expressed and a specific anti-B antiserum produced which can be used as a vaccine.

Vacterl A syndrome involving birth defects affecting several organs. V stands for vertebral defects (spinal cord), A stands for anal deformities, C stands for cardiac problems, TE stands for tracheoesophageal fistula, R stands for renal abnormalities (urinary system and kidneys), and L stands for limb deformities (arms and legs).

Vacuoles Membrane-bound organelles of low density responsible for food digestion, osmotic regulation, and waste product storage. Vacuoles may occupy a large fraction of cell volume (up to 90% in plant cells).

Vacuum degasification The process of removing dissolved and entrained gases from the Reverse Osmosis (RO) product water by creating a vacuum in a tower through which this water flows. The degasifier may be located before the RO system but the majority of the time will be located after. The most prevalent gas present is Carbon Dioxide (CO2), which may have been generated during pH adjustment of the RO feed water. The anion exchange resin can remove CO2 but using the vacuum degasifier can reduce that load. The other gas of concern is Oxygen, which can also be removed by a vacuum degasifier.

Vacuum extractor Device used to provide traction on fetal head during delivery.

Vagina Part of the female genitalia, the canal extending from the vulva to the cervix uteri.

Validation A documented program that provides a high degree of assurance that a specific process, method, or system will consistently produce a result meeting predetermined acceptance criteria.

Validation master plan The documented plan for qualification of a facility or part of a facility that identifies the layout of the operation, the associated utilities and systems, the equipment, and the processes to be validated. The validation master plan also provides preliminary information as to the extent of the qualification and validation (IQ, OQ, PQ), required documentation, SOPs, acceptance criteria and responsibilities. Validation Master Plans should also establish the cross reference of qualification projects by product, system, discipline, etc.

Validation protocol (from ICH API) A written plan stating how validation will be conducted and defining acceptance criteria. For example, the protocol for a manufacturing process identifies processing equipment, critical process parameters/ operating ranges, product characteristics, sampling, and test data to be collected, number of validation runs, and acceptable test results.

Validation protocol A written plan describing the process to be validated, including production equipment and how validation will be conducted. Such a plan would address objective test parameters, product and process characteristics, predetermined specifications, and factors, which will determine acceptable results.

Validity A term that reflects a solid foundation or justification for bringing the intended results. In the case of assessment, validity means the degree to which a measurement instrument truly measures what it is intended to measure. The establishment of validity is the first priority in developing any form of assessment. Without it, all other attributes are of little consequence.

The assessment instrument should accurately represent the skills or characteristics it is designed to measure. Validity may be characterized in these four ways - content, concurrent, predictive or criterion-related validity:

Content validity is the one of greatest concern to teachers as the test must contain a representative sampling of the subject matter the student is expected to have learned. This sampling must be representative and should cross several categories of competence, a range of patient problems and a list of technical skills. Valid clinical examination should assess the components of clinical competence, including the ability to obtain from the patient a detailed and relevant history; carry out a physical examination of the patient; identify the patient's problems from the information obtained and reach a differential diagnosis; identify the appropriate investigations; interpret the results of the investigations; recommend and undertake appropriate management including patient education.

Concurrent validity considers the degree to which a measurement instrument produces the same results as another accepted or proven instrument which measures the same parameters.

Predictive validity examines the degree to which a measure accurately predicts expected outcomes; for instance, a measure of attitudes toward preventive care should correlate significantly with preventive care behaviors.

Criterion-related validity includes concurrent validity as well as predictive validity.

Valine One of the three branched chain amino acids. They are called BCAA's because they structurally branch off another chain of atoms instead of forming a line. Studies have shown that BCAA's help to stimulate protein synthesis and inhibit its breakdown, so BCAA's have powerful anabolic and anticatabolic effects on the body. They may also potentiate the release of some anabolic hormones, such as growth hormone. Regular ingestion of BCAA's help to keep the body in a state of postive nitrogen balance. In this state, your body much more readily builds muscle and burns fat. Studies have shown that athletes taking extra BCAA's have shown a loss of more bodyfat than those not taking BCAA's.

Vallecula A furrow located on the lateral and median glossoepiglottic folds.

Value A term referring to what people believe in, or what they consider important about the way they live. Values influence behavior and culture as persons, groups and communities. Values therefore are an important determinant of individual and community health. They are, however, difficult to measure objectively.

Vanadyl Sulfate Source of mineral vanadium; helps optimize glycogen storage to yield more energy. Vanadyl is supposed to help you attain a little more muscle and inhibit fat storage by controlling insulin release. In theory, Vanadyl works inside the muscle cells by bringing carbohydrates into the muscle without the assistance of insulin. If there is less insulin, there is less chance of carbohydrates being converted to stored bodyfat.

Vapor pressure Dalton's Law for a mixture of perfect gases states that the mixture pressure is equal to the sum of the partial pressures of the constituents. The partial pressure of moisture is called vapor pressure, and is expressed as: Total Pressure (Pt) = Partial Pressure of Air (Pa) + Partial Pressure of Moisture (Pv).

Variable A quantity, attribute, phenomenon or event that may assume any one of a set of values:

Independent variable refers to a characteristic being observed or measured that is thought to influence an event or manifestation (the dependent variable) within the defined area of relationships under study. In medical education, it is a factor that could explain or predict the curriculum's outcomes such as the curriculum itself, previous or concurrent training, environmental factors.

Dependent variable is a manifestation or outcome whose variation we seek to explain or account for the influence of independent variables. It can be a program outcome, such as knowledge or skill attainment, real-life performance, and clinical outcomes.

It is prudent to focus on a few dependent variables that are most relevant to the main evaluation questions and similarly, to focus on the independent variables that are most likely to be related to the curriculum's outcomes.

Variance The granting of an alternate requirement in place of a State regulation.

Varicose veins Blood vessels (veins) that are dilated or enlarged.

Vascular targeting agents (VTAs) Multifunctional agents that are home to the capillaries and vessels of solid tumors.

VEAs (vasopermeation enhancement agents) A new generation of drugs that increase the uptake of therapeutic agents to solid tumors.

Vegetative Form In bacteria, a stage of active growth, as opposed to a resting state or spore formation.

Vectogram A three-dimensional picture that is used to strengthen the binocularity system. Available in fixed and variable styles to provide base-in and/or base-out training. 3D glasses are used to view the picture.

Vector An agent, such as an insect, that can carry a disease-producing organism from one host to another; the agent used to carry new genes into cells. Plasmids currently are the vectors of choice, though viruses and other bacteria may sometimes be used. These molecules become part of the cell protoplasm.

Vehicle Any solvent or carrier fluid in a pharmaceutical product that has no pharmacological role. For example, water is the vehicle for xilocaine and propylene glycol is the vehicle for many antibiotics.

Vein A vessel that carries blood from the body back toward the heart.

Vena cava The large venous channels that return blood to the heart. There is a superior vena cava (SVC above the heart - draining the head and upper extremities) and an inferior vena cava (IVC - below the heart, draining everything else).

Venogram A radiograph or other image of veins, usually obtained by injecting a radiopaque liquid contrast material into a vein. Leg venograms are done to r/o DVT (Deep Vein Thrombosis) that can cause pulmonary embolism.

Venous compression devices External devices attached to the legs to provide intermittent compression and maintain venous blood flow during periods of immobility. Greatly diminishes the likelihood of venous clot formation.

Ventilator A device to mechanically assist a resident (patient) to breathe.

Ventral Being or located near, on, or toward the front or anterior part of the human body.

Ventricle One of the two lower chambers of the heart. The right ventricle sends blood to the lungs, and the left ventricle passes blood carrying oxygen to the rest of the body. The ventricles contract at the same time.

Ventricular fibrillation (VF) A very fast, irregular heartbeat that is caused by abnormal impulses coming from several areas of the heart. These abnormal impulses take over the "pacemaker" function of the sino-atrial node. The heartbeat is so fast that the heart doesn't have time to pump enough blood to the brain and body tissue, which may lead to unconsciousness and heart arrest.

Ventricular tachycardia (VT) A fast heartbeat caused by abnormal impulses coming from a single area of the heart. These abnormal impulses also take over the "pacemaker" function of the sino-atrial node. The rapid heartbeat produces symptoms of fainting, dizziness, weakness, blind spots and, eventually, unconsciousness leading to heart arrest.

Vergence To turn the eyes horizontally (convergence- inward or divergence-outward). Accommodative vergence, fusional vergence, proximal vergence, and tonic vergence are needed to maintain single vision.

Vergence facility A measure of the ease and speed of the eyes to change from a converging to diverging position.

Verification The act of reviewing, inspecting, testing, checking, auditing, or otherwise establishing and documenting whether items, processes, services, or documents conform to specified requirements.

Vernix Fatty substance made up of epithelial cells that covers fetal skin inside the uterus.

Verruca A wart.

Verrucous Rough; wart-like.

Version A specific release of a software product. Version numbers are typically assigned in ascending order, thus the higher the number, the newer the software. Sometimes, to add a small feature or fix a small error, rather than release another version of a program, a manufacturer will release a revision of the software, which is represented in the version number as a decimal (e.g. Paint Shop Pro v 5.1).

Vertebral artery Originating at the subclavian artery, passing vertically through the transverse foramina of the vertebrae, and providing branches for the spinal and muscular rami, anterior spinal artery, and posterior inferior cerebellar artery, before joining with the opposite side to form the basilar artery.

Vertebral body Only the main round, anterior portion of the vertebrae should be called the body. The part from which the other processes extend. However, often incorrectly used as a nickname for the entire vertebra.

Vertex Head first.

Vertigo A disordered state in which the individual is dizzy or feels that the surrounding environment is whirling.

Vestibule (of Ear) The oval cavity within the bony laryrinth that is a confluence for the vestibular endolymphatic channels (semicircular canals). NOTE: There are other vestibules, e.g. for the vagina.

Veterinary Referring to pharmaceuticals or biologicals intended for animal use. Historically veterinary products were made by less than "Good Manufacturing Products". Today, however, the GMP's refer to both human and veterinary products.

VGA Video Graphics Array. The standard analog system used for computer monitors.

Viability Age Usually babies must weigh 500 grams, or 1 pound, to survive, although as technology advances, some babies smaller than this do make it. This point is usually crossed at about the 24th week. Babies can have severe complications however, any time before 32 weeks, and a few complications after that mark. This term also refers to the point in pregnancy when you can no longer seek a legal end to a pregnancy.

Viable living Viable Organism Capable of living and reproducing. Thus, nothing is sterile as long as it contains even a single viable organism.

Vial A final container for a parenteral or diagnostic product. Sealed with a rubber closure and over-seal. Generally required to be class I borosilicate glass.

Viatical Settlement A cash settlement of a life insurance policy prior to death to pay for care needs by selling or transferring the policy to someone else in exchange for a reduced payment.

Vibrational healing / medicine Promotes healing by balancing the body's energy field. Can include acupuncture, homeopathy, flower essences, sound & color healing, crystals, gems, aromatherapy, and energy-based bodywork (Reiki, Therapeutic Touch, Polarity Therapy).

Video assisted thoracic surgery (VATS) Thorascoscopy (aka VATS) is a minimally invasive keyhole surgical procedure which allows the surgeon to directly examine the chest cavity without a big incision.

Videoscopic Generic term referring to performance of a surgical procedure through a scope and viewing the procedure in progress on the video screen.

Villi Projection from a mucous membrane. Most important within the placenta in the exchange of nutrients from maternal blood to the placenta and fetus.

Violation A written summary of noncompliance with regulations found during a State provider survey or complaint investigation . The written document is generally called a Notice of Violation.

Viral antigens Specific proteins on the capsid of a virus that can act as inducers of antibody formation.

Virion A fully formed, mature virus. Infection is initiated in a cell by a virion.

Virucide An agent that destroys or inactivates viruses.

Virulence The disease-producing power of a microorganism.

Virus A simple, noncellular parasite that can reproduce only inside living cells. The simple structure of viruses is their most important characteristic. Most of them consist only of a genetic material - either DNA or RNA - and a protein coating. Some also have membranous envelopes. Viruses are "alive" in that they can reproduce themselves - although only by taking over a cell's synthetic machinery - but they have none of the other characteristics of living organisms. Viruses cause a large variety of significant diseases in plants and animals, including humans.

Visagraph eye movement recording system Records and measures eye movements while an individual reads. The system also measures reading efficiency. Specially created goggles and a computer program are used.

Viscosity The tendency of a fluid to resist flowing because of molecular attraction (cohesion).

Viscous Thick, coagulated; sticky or gummy.

Vision The ability to take in information through our eyes and process the information so that it has meaning.

Vision therapist Optometrist or an optometric vision therapy technician who develops and administers vision therapy programs. (Typically this term is referring to a vision therapy technician rather than an optometrist.)

Please note that there are some individuals that call themselves vision therapists, but they are not optometrists or vision therapy technicians.

Vision therapy technician One who works under the supervision of an optometrist in evaluating clients and in planning and implementing vision therapy programs.

Visiting a Level Occurs when the clinician demonstrates certain behaviors at certain times at one level but does not demonstrate those behaviors consistently at that level.

Visual acuity Sharpness or clearness of eyesight.

Visual analysis Refers to figure-ground, form constancy, spatial relation, visual closure, visual discrimination, visual memory, and visualization.

Visual closure The ability to identify or recognize a symbol or object when the entire object is not visible.

Visual discrimination The ability to discriminate between visible likeness and differences in size, shape, pattern, form, position, and color. Such as the ability to distinguish between similar words like "ran" and "run".

Visual field The total area that can be seen while looking straight ahead. (Note: Perimetry is the method of testing an eye's field of vision.

Visual form dysfunction Difficulty with figure-ground, form constancy, visual closure, and visual discrimination. Symptoms include confusion with similar objects, words, or colors. Vision therapy is a treatment option.

Visual memory dysfunction Difficulty with retention, recall, or recognition of things seen. Symptoms can include poor spelling and poor recall of visual information. Vision therapy is a treatment option.

Visual memory The ability to recall and use visual information from the past.

Visual motor dysfunction The inability to process and reproduce visual images by writing or drawing. Symptoms can include poor pencil grip/writing, poor organization on written page, poor copying/spacing, and excessive erasing. Vision therapy is a treatment option.

Visual motor integration (VMI) After visual data is gathered, it is processed and combined in the brain with information from movement (eye hand coordination).

Visual motor skills The ability of our eyes to guide our hands (eye hand coordination, visual-motor integration).

Visual pathway Route of the nerve impulses from the retina along the optic nerve, and optic nerve radiations to the brain's sensory cortex that is located at the base of the skull.

Visual perceptual disorders Information processing dysfunctions of the visual system. These dysfunctions can be a directionality/laterality disorder, visual form dysfunction, visual memory dysfunction, and visual-motor dysfunction. Vision therapy is a treatment option.

Visual perceptual skills The ability to organize and interpret information that is seen and give it meaning. These information-processing skills include figure-ground, form constancy, spatial relations, visual closure, visual discrimination, visual memory, and visualization.

Visual sensory integration After visual data is gathered, it is processed and combined in the brain with information from hearing (auditory-visual integration), balance (gross-motor/bilateral integration), posture, and movement (visual-motor integration).

Visual sequential memory Ability to recall a sequence of numbers, letters or objects in the order they were originally given.

Visual skills Are accommodation (eye focusing), binocularity (eye teaming), and oculomotor skills (eye movement), which are neuro-muscular abilities that are controlled by muscles inside and outside of the eye and are networked with the brain.

Visualization The ability to crate and manipulate mental pictures of an object or concept on the basis of past visual experience and memory. Essential in reading and playing sports.

Vital capacity (VC) The maximum volume of air that can be exhaled following a complete lung inflation. The difference between Total Lung Capacity (TLC) and Residual Volume (RV).

Vital statistics Data collected from continuous or periodic recording or registration of all "vital events", such as births, deaths, marriages and divorces.

Vitamins Complex organic molecules essential for biochemical transformations necessary for proper metabolism and disease protection. Some popular vitamins are:

A: (Retinol) A vitamin with antioxidant properties, important for eye protection and bone growth; protein and hormone synthesis (including GH and testosterone); supports tissue maintenance. Helps reduce susceptibility to infection. Essential for healthy skin, good blood, strong bones and teeth, kidneys, bladder, lungs and membranes.

B-Complex Vitamins. A group of eleven known vitamins that work together in your body. All play vital roles in the conversion of food into energy. Essential for the normal functioning of the nervous system, and the maintenance of good digestion. Helps promote healthy skin, hair, and eyes. These are water soluble vitamins, which means they cannot be stored by your body and must be replaced every day.

B-1 (Thiamin) Maintains energy levels, supports brain function (memory). Aids in digestion. Necessary for metabolism of sugar and starch to provide energy. Maintains a healthy nervous system. Alcohol can cause deficiencies of this vitamin and all the B-complex vitamins.

B-2 (Riboflavin) Energy production and amino acid production. Helps body obtain energy from protein, carbohydrates, and fats. Helps maintain good vision and healthy skin.

B-3 (Niacin) Important in carbohydrate metabolism, formation of testosterone and other hormones, formation of red blood cells and maintaining the integrity of all cells. Helps body utilize protein, fats, and carbohydrates. Necessary for a healthy nervous system and digestive system. It also lowers elevated blood cholesterol levels when taken in large amounts of more than 1,000 milligrams a day.

B-5 (Pantothenic Acid) Supports carbohydrate, protein and fat metabolism; hemoglobin synthesis. Helps release energy from protein, carbohydrates, and fat. Needed to support a variety of body functions, including the maintenance of a healthy digestive system.

B-6 (Pyridoxine) Supports glycogen and nitrogen metabolism; production and transport of amino acids; production and maintenance of red blood cells (hemoglobin) Essential for the body's utilization of protein. Needed for the production of red blood cells, nerve tissues, and antibodies. Women taking oral contraceptives have lower levels of B-6.

B-12 (Cobalamin) Necessary for carbohydrate, protein and fat metabolism. Important to amino acid and fatty acid synthesis; essential for hemoglobin and nerve cell growth and maintenance. The anti-stress vitamin, sometimes prescribed for stress reduction.

Biotin Energy metabolism, fatty acid and nucleic acid synthesis.

C (Ascorbic acid) Antioxidant, synthesis of hormones, amino acids and collagen (connective tissue); excretion of excess cholesterol. Necessary to produce collagen, the connective material of all body tissues. Important for the health of the teeth and the gums. Strengthens capillaries and other blood vessels. Plays an important role in healing injuries. Aids in the body's absorption of iron. Vitamin C is water soluble, which means it cannot be stored by your body and must be frequently replaced.

D (Calciferol) Supports calcium absorption and deposition into bones. Must be present for your body to use calcium and phosphorus. Essential for growing children to insure that teeth and bones develop properly.

E (d-alpha-tocopherol) Antioxidant, especially protective of polyunsaturated fats and body tissues. Acts as a preservative, preventing many substances, such as Vitamin A, from destructive breakdown by oxidation in the body. Prolongs the life of red blood cells. Necessary for the proper use of oxygen by the muscles.

Folic Acid Necessary for the production of red blood cells. Essential for normal metabolism. A deficiency may cause a form of anemia. Drinking alcohol and taking oral contraceptives can cause lower levels of this vitamin in your body. Especially important during pregnancy to prevent birth defects.

K Supports blood clotting, bone mineralization.

Vitreous body The inner part of the eyeball located between the iris and retina that is made up of a transparent gel (actually a living tissue). Also known as the vitreous humour. The aqueous humour is the watery liquid between the cornea and the iris, in the anterior chamber of the eye.

Vocal cords Above the trachea, there are two pairs of fibromuscular "cords" - superiorly are the false cords, and inferiorly the true vocal cords. Between them is the laryngeal ventricle. Adduction (bringing together) the true cords causes vibration in the air column - speech or phonation. Abduction moves the cords apart.

Volvulus A twisting of the stomach or large intestine that leads to blockage of the digestive tract.

Vomiting The release of stomach contents through the mouth; also known as throwing-up.

VPHP Microbiodecontamination Technology used to decontaminate the exposed, internal surfaces within a sealed isolator and the exposed, external surfaces of materials and components placed within the sealed isolator. It consists of four distinctive phases:
1. Dehumidification - Lowers humidity and increases temperature

2. Conditioning - "Ramp-up" (VPHP) at or below saturation conditions

3. Sterilization - Steady-State (VPHP) at or below saturation conditions

4. Aeration - Reduces the VPHP to Safe Levels.

W

Wallerian degeneration After cerebral infarction, when the cortical neuronal cell bodies have died, there is atrophy of their distal portions (dendrites). This is seen as atrophy in the white matter, especially in the cerebral peduncles.

Wallpaper A graphic used to cover the "desktop" or background of a graphical user interface such as Windows and Netscape. The wallpaper usually serves no purpose other than to improve the appearance of your workspace.

WAN Wide Area Network. A network of computers at many different and distant locations.

Warning letter The most serious FDA postaudit (after inspection) letter notifying a manufacturer of adverse finding and giving it 15 days to reply.

Water hammer A tremendous force produced by rapid interruption of linear flow of a non-compressible fluid. Most commonly occurs when fast acting valves are closed in a high flow liquid system.

Water treatment Water treatment, also referred to as water conditioning, can consist of adding or removing chemicals to change the properties of water. In water softening, for example, sodium ions are substituted for metallic ions that cause "hardness" thus reducing the scale-forming tendencies of water. Water purification on the other hand, always consists of removing undesirable impurities.

Waviness The more widely spaced component of surface texture. Unless otherwise noted, waviness includes all irregularities whose spacing is greater than the roughness sampling length. Waviness may result from such factors as machine or work deflection, vibration, chatter, heat treatment or warping strains. Roughness may be considered as superimposed on a "wavy" surface.

Wegener's Granulomatosis Wegener's granulomatosis is characterized by inflammation of the blood vessels, which in turn interferes with normal blood flow. The condition can cause damage to internal organs in the body, but affects mainly the respiratory tract: the sinuses, nose, trachea and lungs. Wegener's can also affect the kidneys. Wegener's can strike men and women of any age. It is more prevalent in Caucasians than in African Americans.

Western blot A procedure in which a mixture of proteins is separated on a polyacrylamide gel and then transferred to a nylon membrane. The membrane may then be treated with reagents such as specific antibodies to locate a protein of interest.

Wetted surface The surface(s) of any valve or component that will be exposed to a fluid (liquid or gas) when in service.

WFI (water for injection),. WFI is water purified by distillation or by reverse osmosis, it contains no added substance. WFI meets the purity requirements under Purified Water. Although not intended to be sterile, it meets a test for a limit of bacterial endotoxin. It must be produced, stored, and distributed under Sterile Water for Injection.

What's This? A new feature of Windows 95 and 98 help program. In a dialog box, click the small button with a question mark (?) on it. Then, click where you want help. A small description will pop up to explain what the item is and how to use it.

Wheatstone stereoscope An instrument designed to present separate images to each eye. Each eye can see independently. Two plane mirrors are joined at one edge at a 90-degree angle and two target holders, one opposite one mirror and the other, mounted on a screw base which, when turned, synchronously moves the targets toward or away from each other. The Amblyoscope, Troposcope, Synoptophore, and the Bernell Mirror Stereoscope are examples of this design.

Wheezing The sound made by air moving through partially obstructed airways.

Whey protein Dairy source of protein (other than cassein), known for high levels of BCAA's and high nitrogen retention. Made from milk curd, whey protein is the Rolls Royce of proteins because it has a superior amino acid composition (including high levels of leucine, arguably the most important branched chain amino acid), superior biological value (meaning that more of what you eat gets digested and into your system), is very low in lactose (a milk sugar that most adults have difficulty digesting).

White blood cell A blood cell containing no respiratory pigment. In vertebrates it may be a polymorphonuclear leukocyte, a lymphocyte or a monocyte.

White matter The white nervous tissue of the brain and spinal cord consisting of the conducting, myelinated fibers.

Willow Bark White willow bark is a source of salicin, a chemical relative of asparin. The effects of willow bark are milk pain inhibition, and increased blood flow to the skin and greater heat loss.

Win.ini Microsoft Windows' main configuration file. Win.ini is the file that contains all possible options and sets up Windows to your specifications to default to your selections every time you start your computer. Wallpaper, fonts, printers and other devices are all set up by the Win.ini file.

Window A work area in a graphical user interface. Programs run in a window within the operating system. Similarly, documents are often opened in another window inside a program window. Windowing programs makes it easy to switch between different programs and tasks by working in "layers".

Wizard Microsoft's name for a step-by-step set of instructions that guide you through a particular task. For example, there are many wizards included with Windows 95 and 98 for installing new hardware, configuring the Start menu, establishing dial-up networking for modem use, and changing other aspects of the computer environment.

Women of reproductive age (or women of childbearing age) Refers to all women aged 15 to 49 years (WHO).

Word Processing A technique for electronically storing, editing, and manipulating text by using an electronic keyboard, computer, and printer. Word processing differs from typing since a user can type, edit, and reformat text before it is printed, as well as save it on magnetic media so that it can easily be modified.

Word Wrap In word processing, when text that is entered into a paragraph reaches the end of a line, it automatically breaks and continues on the line immediately below.

Works Package Also called integrated software and similar to an Office Suite, a Works package is typically a single program with database, spreadsheet, and word processing functions offered together. Microsoft Works is an example of a works package.

Workstation An open or enclosed work surface, usually with direct air supply.

World federation for medical education (WFME) A non-governmental organization with ties to WHO and UNESCO, the WFME is concerned with global education and training of medical doctors and umbrella organization for six regional associations for medical education. . The WFME's general objective is to strive for the highest scientific and ethical standards in medical education and to take initiatives with respect to new methods, tools and management of medical education. The central office has been located at the University of Copenhagen, Denmark since 1996, in collaboration with Lund University in Sweden.

World Wide Web The most popular feature on the Internet that uses HyperText Markup Language to create and link together graphics, documents and files across the Interriet.

Worst case The highest or lowest value of a given control parameter actually evaluated in a validation exercise.

Wrist The proximal part of the hand, composed of the carpal bones (Latin - 'carpe' to grasp or clutch, as in 'Carpe Diem').

Written interactive test Allows for assessment of clinical reasoning skills, understanding and knowledge of clinical and basic science and application of basic science to clinical problems. test methods such as essays and open-ended interviews are used, providing information about the respondent's perceptions, attitudes, feelings, and experiences. Examples of written objective-type tests are MCQ, PMP, MEQ. Such test should be designed to ensure that they are clinically coherent, containing questions from different disciplines, securing an appropriate discipline balance and ensuring that questions and answers reflect reasonable expectations of students. However, these test methods are often subjective and may contain rater biases. Presently, to enhance their validity and reliability, most of above mentioned methods are computerized with the addition of various audiovisual and holographic inputs (computer-interactive tests).

WYSIWYG Acronym for "what you see is what you get". Referring to a process of designing a document on a computer screen that is a virtual preview of what the printed page will look like.

X

X chromosome A sex chromosome that usually occurs paired in each female cell and single in each male cell in species in which the male typically has two unlike cell chromosomes.

Xantho (prefix) Yellow.

Xenobiotics Industrial chemicals that have a chemical structure not found in natural compounds that may resist degradation by microorganisms.

Xiphoid process The cartilagenous process, with a bony core, connected to the inferior end of the of the sternum. The inferior tip of the sternum. (from the Greek "xiphias" - literally "sword")

XPS(X-ray photoelectron spectroscopy) or ESCA (electron spectroscopy for chemical analysis) A surface-sensitive technique capable of detecting all elements with an atomic number greater than that of helium. ESCA provides data on the outermost several atomic layers of a material, and has a sensitivity in the order of 0.5 atomic percent. A primary advantage of ESCA is that it can both determine and quantify the chemical state of the elements detected (i.e. metallic state or oxide state).

X-ray A diagnostic test which uses invisible electromagnetic energy beams to produce images of internal tissues, bones, and organs onto film.

X-ray absorptiometry (DXA) A test used for measuring bone density.

Y

Y chromosome A sex chromosome that is characteristic of male zygotes in species in which the male typically has two unlike sex chromosomes.

Yeast artificial chromosome A vector used to clone DNA fragments (up to 400 kb); it is constructed from the telomeric, centromeric, and replication origin sequences needed for replication in yeast cells.

Yeasts Unicellular fungi belonging mainly to the Ascomycetes that usually multiply by budding. Their commercial significance lies in their ability to secrete enzymes. For example, in the brewing and baking industries, it is a source of vitamins and proteins. They can also be used as excipients in rDNA technology.

Yield, expected The quantity of material or the percentage of theoretical yield anticipated at any appropriate phase of production based on previous laboratory, pilot scale, or manufacturing data.

Yield, theoretical The quantity that would be produced at any appropriate phase of manufacture, processing, or packing of a particular API (Active Pharmaceutical Ingredient) or intermediate, based upon the quantity of components to be used, in the absence of any loss or error in actual production.

Yoga therapy Emerging field of practices that use yoga to address mental and physical problems while integrating body & mind. Practitioners work one-on-one or in a group setting.

Yohimbe From the bark of an African tree, Yohimbe is a popular herb percieved as a stimulant and aphrodisiac. Yohimbe contains yohimbine, an alkaloid similar to caffeine in it's energizing effects.

Yoked prisms A wedge-shaped lens which is thicker on one edge than the other. The prism bases (thicker end) are in the same direction for both eyes (up, down, left, or right). Yoked prisms are used to train or compensate for a binocular dysfunction (eye teaming problem) or a visual field loss. Sometimes used in optometric vision therapy programs.

Z

Zeolite Naturally occurring or synthetic permutite, a hydrated alkali-aluminum silicate that exhibits limited base exchange. Used as an ion exchange medium for the softening of hard water.

Zero balancing Method for aligning body structure and body energy. Through touch akin to acupressure, practitioner seeks to overcome imbalances in the body's structure/energetic interface, which is said to exist beneath the level of conscious awareness. Zero balancing is often used for stress reduction.

Zeta potential The charge or potential existing at the surface of a particle. It is the positive charge measured at the surface of the membrane across the pH range.

Zinc Mineral important as a cofactor in energy metabolism, amino acid and protein synthesis; Antioxidant effects to protect the immune system. Essential for growth, tissue repair, and sexual development. Plays an important role in healing. Since animal proteins are the best sources, vegetarians are often deficient in zinc.

ZIP files Refers to a the most common file compression format. A zip file is made by compacting the information in a file or set of files to generally make the file smaller. Zip files are easier to store and transport since they require less disk space. A special file-compression and/or decompression utility is typically required, such as WinZip, to work with zip files.

ZMA - Zinc Magnesium Aspartate This compound has been found to increase muscle strength.

Zone therapy Another name for reflexology.

Zoonosis Any disease in humans acquired from one of the lower animals, rabies is an example.

Zygomatic arch The horizontal arch of the cheek bone, formed by the temporal process of the zygomatic bone and the zygomatic process of the temporal bone that attaches the masseter muscle.

Zygote Single cell formed from the conjugation of gametes (egg and sperm cells). The zygote has twice as many chromosomes as do gametes.